EATING DISORDERS IN THE 21ST CENTURY SERIES

ANOREXIA NERVOSA: A MULTI-DISCIPLINARY APPROACH: FROM BIOLOGY TO PHILOSOPHY

EATING DISORDERS IN THE 21ST CENTURY SERIES

Anorexia Nervosa: A Multi-Disciplinary Approach: From Biology to Philosophy
Antonio Mancini, Silvia Daini and Louis Caruana (Editors)
2010. ISBN: 978-1-60876-200-2

EATING DISORDERS IN THE 21ST CENTURY SERIES

ANOREXIA NERVOSA: A MULTI-DISCIPLINARY APPROACH: FROM BIOLOGY TO PHILOSOPHY

ANTONIO MANCINI
SILVIA DAINI
AND
LOUIS CARUANA
EDITORS

Nova Science Publishers, Inc.
New York

LIBRARY OF CONGRESS CATALOGING-IN-PUBLICATION DATA

Anorexia nervosa : a multi-disciplinary approach : from biology to philosophy / editors, Antonio Mancini, Silvia Daini, Louis Caruana.
p. ; cm.
Includes bibliographical references and index.
ISBN 978-1-60876-200-2 (hardcover : alk. paper)
1. Anorexia nervosa. I. Mancini, Antonio. II. Daini, Silvia. III. Caruana, Louis.
[DNLM: 1. Anorexia Nervosa--physiopathology. 2. Anorexia Nervosa--psychology. WM 175 A6149 2009]
RC552.A5A566 2009
616.85'262--dc22

2009037482

Published by Nova Science Publishers, Inc. ✝ New York

CONTENTS

Preface vii

Section I: Biomedical Aspects 1

Chapter 1 Endocrine Alterations in Anorexia Nervosa 3
A. Mancini, V. Di Donna, E. Leone, E. Giacchi

Chapter 2 Anorexia Nervosa and Cytokines 31
A. Mancini, E. Leone, V. Di Donna, R. Festa

Chapter 3 Amenorrhea in Anorexia Nervosa 51
E. Giacchi, E. Leone, V. Di Dònna and A.Mancini

Chapter 4 Anorexia Nervosa: Medical Complications 75
A. Bianchi, F. Veltri, L. Tartaglione, L. Tilaro, L. De Marinis

Chapter 5 Nutrition in Anorexia Nervosa 87
Meniconi Paola, Giraldi Alessandra, Magini Marinella, Meucci Elisabetta and Martorana Giuseppe Ettore

Section II: Psychological Aspects 97

Chapter 6 Infantile Anorexia 99
S. Daini, L. Petrongolo and L. Bernardini

Chapter 7 Anorexia and Parents 115
S. Daini and C. Panetta

Chapter 8 Treating Anorexia in State of Emergency 135
S. Daini, L. Bernardini and L. Petrongolo

Chapter 9 The Logotherapeutic Approach: An Anthropogically founded Method 149
A. Mancini, R. Festa

Section III: Philosophical Aspects **159**

Chapter 10 Anorexia Nervosa: Ethical Issues **161**
Maria Luisa Di Pietro, Andrea Virdis, Dino Moltisanti

Chapter 11 Somatic Semantics: Anorexia and the Nature of Meaning **173**
Louis Caruana

Chapter 12 Anorexia Nervosa: A Case of Self-deception? **187**
Mark Sultana

Chapter 13 Nietzsche's Ascetic Ideal and the Anorexic Condition **203**
Terrance Walsh

Conclusion **225**

About Editors and Contributors **229**

Index **231**

PREFACE

Anorexia nervosa (AN) is a psychosomatic disorder characterized by self-induced and maintained weight loss that, with a vicious circle, leads to progressive malnutrition, with complications in many organ systems and tissues, which can be fatal, even if a clear suicide intention is not present. Many psychological tracts, including disturbance in body image and fear of obesity, are considered key stigmata. It is considered among the enormous field of eating behaviour disorders (even if this definition has the risk to attribute to a symptom, i.e. the alimentary behaviour, the core of the problem; it should be better to speak about "psychogenic alimentary disorders", also including bulimia nervosa and psychogenic obesity).

It is classically considered a disorder with high prevalence in adolescent girls, but it has become a disorder with broader diffusion, both in age (from childhood to adult age, also considering that limits of adolescence itself have been extended), in sex (increasing incidence in males is reported) and geographical distribution (in all continents, due to the diffusion of western models and style of life, not only in alimentary and food availability, but also in values which can overcome traditional view of life of different countries).

To avoid nosographic confusions, specialists must consider the diagnostic criteria of the American Psychiatric Association, which are presented in the table [1]. When comparing the diagnostic criteria which, during the years, have been proposed, it becomes evident that the limit between normal and pathological states is very narrow (for instance the limit of underweight has been reduced from 25 to 15%).

The way of looking to AN has radically changed in the last three centuries [2]. Original descriptions are very ancient: Galeno in his treatise describes fasting performed not for health problems, examples of voracious and insatiable hunger are reported by the Greek philosopher Aristotle and in Hebrew literature. Clear anorexic behaviours are described in the life of Christian saints. An English physician, Sir Richard Morton, reported two cases in adolescent girls, but a systematic description is reported by two other doctors, the English William Gull and the French Charles Lasègue; the term 'anorexia nervosa'. can be attributed to the first, while for the last there is the contribution of an organic peripheral factor (in gastrointestinal tract) with a central, both organic and psychological, factor. To complicate the picture, in 1883 Henri Huchard introduced the term 'mental' anorexia.

From these original description, a great debate developed, with the opposition of "organicistic" and "psychologistic" interpretations. An important benchmark is the article of W.B. Cannon, who underlined the correlation between gastric motility and hunger sensation.

The endocrine interpretation (referring the disorder to altered endocrine milieu) is based on the discover of the pathologist Morris Simmonds, who found an anterior pituitary lobe atrophy in a woman, dead for extreme post-partum cachexia. Only in the fifties Sheehan separated organic causes of weight loss from the nosographic autonomy of AN. Even from the side of psychological research, AN was initially reported to just known psychopathological forms, such as obsessive disorders (Janet), phobic disorders (Sollier), melancholy (Freud), hysteria (Zivieri). Only in the second half of the last century, psychological investigation became more rich and articulated, with the contribution of many different approaches; the most important school are represent by psychoanalytic, cognitive-behavioural, existential analysis, systemic-relational schools. Many sociological and, more recently, ethical approaches have also been tentatively performed. Despite the enormous literature, AN still remains a mystery.

We propose to consider AN among psychosomatic disorders, not in the conventional sense of the somatic appearance of a psychological conflict or in that undefined field intermediate between body and mind, but in that particular view which suggests a need to holistic approach to medicine [3].

Therefore this book attempts to propose itself as a new trigger in the wide world of anorexia nervosa. The originality of its proposal consists in approaching anorexia nervosa, not only by endocrinological and psychological perspectives, but also by anthropological, philosophical and ethical point of view. In this way it's not only an update of specific literature, but also an integration with a new method to study this condition. The purpose of the book is to approach anorexia nervosa from different points of view, to reach a new interpretation which involves notions from biological and human sciences interpreted in an unique model, which could allow a new method to treat the disease. The principal audiences for the book, due to the complete picture of this diffuse disorder which could be delineated by update of more recent advances, are advanced undergraduates, research students, researchers who will profit from an interdisciplinary approach, but also those who are responsible for educational establishments and policy.

The book is divided into 3 sections. The first one consists in endocrine and metabolic advances [4]; starting from a complete nosographic and clinical presentation of the disease, it contains an update of literature data in the following fields:

- *endocrinological aspects*: neurotransmitters control of the hormone secretion (the biochemical language by which central nervous system integrates internal and external stimuli to govern the alimentary habits), low T3 syndrome (the adaptive mechanism of thyroid to food deprivation), growth hormone (the fundamental hormone which controls anabolic function, the 'building' part of our metabolism), the pituitary-adrenal system (which represents the main mechanisms of response to stress);
- *the role of cytokines*, the new frontier of that endocrine mechanism, also called "paracrine", since it refers to biochemical language, mediated not only by blood, but also by cell-to-cell communication; in this section, the new molecules, which are produced by adipose tissue, are also focused, since this tissue is not a fuel deposit, but an active metabolic tissue;

- *mechanisms of amenorrhea*, a symptom included in diagnostic criteria for its importance, which is not simply a consequence of weight loss; to understand this phenomenon, the physiology of pituitary-gonadal axis is reviewed, with underlining of factors which interfere with its function;
- *medical complications*, which cover almost all organ and systems in the body, and are not always reversible with weight recovery;
- *dietetic aspects*.

The second section talks about psychological aspects of this condition, with particular attention on anorexia in the childhood and different pathways of therapy in the emergency, which can happen in this condition. At least, it will describe the experience activated in the Day Hospital of Psychiatry Institute of our University about the management of the disease even from familial point of view [5].

In anorexia, the psychopathologic origin of dietary restriction should be connected, from a psychodynamic point of view, with internalization of persecutory instances regarding ideal Self, that influence perfectionism, lack of self esteem and depression feelings. These internal instances motivate self prescription of dieting in spite of realistic evaluation of body health. The prolonged needs of medical and psychiatric therapies, and their frequent ineffectiveness, suggest the central role of integration of therapies and of the early detection of disordered eating behaviours.

The interdisciplinary integration of carers, and the cooperation of family, implies the search of a delicate equilibrium between group holding of the patient (the group of carers and parents as support of the Self) and acknowledgement of her individual identity.

The third and final section is dedicated to philosophical issues related to anorexia. The most obvious philosophical dimension is the ethical. In this first chapter of the section, a number of ethical questions are raised and addressed. These questions concern both the anthropological aspects of the disorder and the clinical problems involved in its treatment. The authors argue that, to engage in this project, one needs to start with a careful understanding of the cultural and ethical meaning of eating, of body construction and of relationships. Once this understanding is in place, the ethical problems arising from the clinical management of anorexia can be fruitfully addressed. The next chapter in this section concerns the question of meaning. The Author shows how the perceptual-cognitive model used to understand anorexia may benefit from current philosophical studies regarding language, perception and cognition. The central issues discussed here involve two concepts: the concept of introspection and the concept of interpretation. The third chapter in this philosophical section continues on these themes by highlighting the intricate relationship between anorexia and the philosophical problem of self-deception. The Author offers an overview of the current philosophical debates in this area and then highlights essential features of the very meaning of self-deception. He proceeds by investigating whether anorexia qualifies as a case of self-deception, referring especially to the relation between the anorectic's self-image and the self-deceptive beliefs that may be pervasively present in society at large. The final chapter introduces another angle, very seldom considered in the study of anorexia. This concerns the correspondence between the symptoms and etiology of this disorder and Friedrich Nietzsche's theory of the ascetic ideal. Nietzsche's theory deals with the many destructive ways used by humans to seek release from the suffering and aimlessness of existence. This theory illuminates not only the cultural conditions under which anorexia thrives, but also the paradox of a will that seemingly wills to act against its own wellbeing. The Author argues that, in light of Nietzsche's ideas, anorexics can be seen as ascetics without an otherworldly ideal as their goal. The anorexic, who lives in a culture where higher ideals have lost credibility, engages in the self-abnegating practices of the ascetic without the corresponding goal of another, truer world beyond the body.

The first section, which covers biomedical aspects, difficult to be understood for readers who are nor familiar with biological concept, is enriched by schematic figures and summaries, with more important data, to be easily and immediately set by all users.

The method which analyzes different aspects, which is necessary due to the enormous literature in the field, is enriched by a global vision; biological and psychological aspects are separated in heuristic way, but what emerges is the reciprocal influence of the different plans. In such way is particularly provoking for training students and matter of debating for those who are involved in the clinical management of this kind of patients.

The purpose of the book is to approach anorexia nervosa from different points of view, to reach a new interpretation which involves notions from biological and human sciences connected in an unique model, which could allow a new method to treat the disease. The aim is to overcome the traditional approach, based on separate competences organized in watertight compartments.

Therefore, without the presumption to cover all the aspects and overgrowing experimental data, which quickly accumulate in this field, we hope to furnish a useful and provoking tool to think in a new and exciting way to this important disorder of our time.

	DIAGNOSTIC CRITERIA (DSM-IV-TR)
A.	Refusal to maintain body weight at or above a minimally normal weight for age and height
B.	Intense fear of gaining weight or becoming fat, even though underweight
C.	Disturbance in the way in which one's body weight or shape is experienced, undue influence of body weight or shape on self-evaluation, or denial of the seriousness of the current low body weight
D.	In post menarche females, amenorrhea (absence of at least three consecutive menstrual cycles)e
	Specify the subtypes: restricting and binge-eating/purging

REFERENCES

1. *DSM-IV-TR. Diagnostic and statistical manual of mental disorders.* Washington, DC: American Psychiatric Association, 2000.
2. Casper RC. On the emergence of bulimia nervosa as a syndrome: a historical view. *Int J Eat Disord*, 1983, 2, 3-16.
3. Caruana L. *Holism and the understanding of science: integrating the analytical, historical and sociological.* Adershot (UK): Ashgate, 2000.
4. Vigerski RA (Ed). *Anorexia nervosa.* New York, Raven Press, 1977.
5. Daini S. Present subjects of women's psychopathology. *Acta Medica Romana*, XL, 2-3, 2002.

SECTION I: BIOMEDICAL ASPECTS

In: Anorexia Nervosa: A Multi-Disciplinary Approach
Editors: A. Mancini, S. Daini, L. Caruana, pp. 3-30
ISBN: 978-1-60876-200-2

Chapter 1

ENDOCRINE ALTERATIONS IN ANOREXIA NERVOSA

***A. Mancini, V. Di Donna, E. Leone, E. Giacchi*[1]**

Division of Endocrinology,[1] Center for Study and Research on Natural Fertility Regulation, Catholic University of the Sacred Heart, Rome, Italy

ABSTRACT

A complex network of neural, endocrine, and biochemical signals control appetite in humans and the main locus of integration of both external and internal stimuli is the hypothalamus. In turn, it controls the pituitary gland and other glands, that are pituitary-dependent in a cascade manner, closed by a feedback control to maintain stability in the energetic and body composition balance. An alteration of this mechanism is present in eating disorders, even if not a single phenomenon (neurotransmitter, genetic, hormones, and so on...) can alone explain the entire clinical picture. Different hormonal alterations, including hypogonadotropic hypogonadism, hypercortisolemia, growth hormone resistance, and "sick euthyroid syndrome," mediate the clinical manifestations accompanying this condition, which is associated with notable medical complications and increased mortality. Decreases in fat mass result in abnormalities of adipocytokines, produced by adipocytes. Even if most of the endocrine changes that occur in anorexia nervosa represent physiologic and reversible adaptation to starvation, some persist after recovery, leaving an indelible mark in affected persons.

1. INTRODUCTION

Although anorexia nervosa (AN) is increasingly observed among boys and men, the disorder predominantly affects white girls and young women, generally under 25 years old, and is particularly common in adolescence. In women, the complete syndrome of anorexia nervosa has prevalence during life of about 0.5 %, and incidence seems to be augmented in the last decades [1]. The mortality of the disease varies between 5.1% and 13% [2]. This devastating disorder, of unknown etiology, is characterized by anorexia with obstinate refusal of food and behavioral changes, severe loss of weight, and amenorrhoea.

Although most authors agree about the psychiatric origin of this disorder, the effects of starvation are extensive and negatively affect the pituitary gland, thyroid gland, adrenal glands, gonads, and bones. Endocrine abnormalities observed in anorexia nervosa are suggestive of hypothalamic dysfunction, but they are not specific and, for the most part, are similar with those observed in other conditions of extreme loss of weight. These hormonal alterations, including hypogonadotropic hypogonadism, hypercortisolemia, growth hormone resistance, and "sick euthyroid syndrome" (see below), mediate the clinical manifestations accompanying this condition, which is associated with notable medical complications and increased mortality. Alterations in anorexigenic and orexigenic appetite-regulating neuroendocrine pathways have also been described, particularly concerning leptin and ghrelin concentrations. Decreases in fat mass result in adipokine abnormalities. Even if most of the endocrine changes that occur in anorexia nervosa represent physiologic and reversible adaptation to starvation, some persist after recovery, like short stature, osteoporosis, and infertility, and might contribute to susceptibility disorder recurrence.

An interplay between nutritional and hormonal signals, which have a pathological feedback loop of increasing severity, causes a complex physiopathological picture. Single factors have been underlined as the main phenomenon underlying the syndrome, therefore suggesting different theories (neurotrasmitter alterations, genetic transmission, and psychiatric etiology), while they interact in a still mysterious way.

The transfer of information between neurons is mediated, in synapses, by neurotransmitters, molecules interacting with receptors located on postsynaptic membrane. Chemical neurotransmission at synaptic level is influenced by presence of substances different by neurotransmitters, which are not directly involved in impulse transmission, but are able to modulate in various ways the transfer process of nervous informations. These substances, which have peptidic structure, are called neuromodulators and neuropeptides and can act both in presynaptic site, determining variations in quantity or temporal mode of neurotransmitters release, and in postsynaptic one, modulating linking capacity of receptor and determining, in this way, the excitability level of postsynaptic level. The possibility that in the same synapses many modulating neuropeptides exist enhances more the complexity and modulation possibilities of synaptic transmission. Moreover, neurons can be the site of production and metabolism of hormones, therefore called "neurohormones," many of which cover fundamental roles in the control of pituitary gland.

Physiopathology of hypothalamic-pituitary axis is illustrated in Figure 1; strictly related to the hypothalamus, the basal part of Central Nervous System (CNS), the pituitary gland control other glands (thyroid, adrenal, gonads) in a cascade manner, closed by feedback mechanisms devoted to homeostatic maintenance of hormone secretion. After describing the physiological regulation of appetite, we will describe main endocrine alterations, showing that some hormone modifications are adaptive in response to malnutrition (GH, thyroid, glucocorticoids). Other axes are involved as secondary targets (Hypothalamus-Pituitary-Gonadal axis, which will be extensively described in Chapter 3).

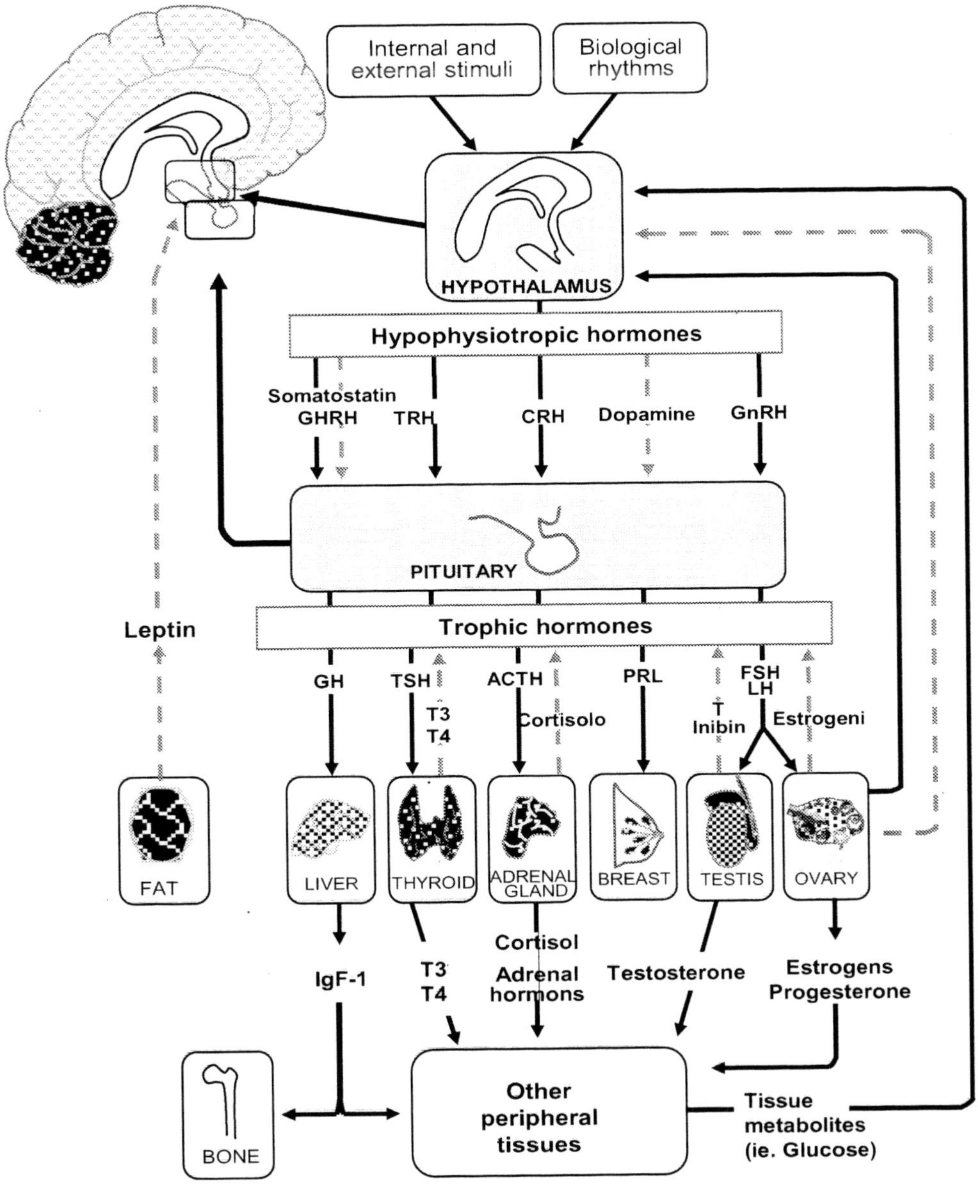

Figure 1. Schematic representation of the hypothamic-pituitary dependent axes. The basal part of the central nervous system (hypothalamus), to which convergence of external and internal stimuli, with a superimposed control by biological clock, produce hormones (hypophysiotropic hormones), which stimulate trophism and secretion by different cell types in the pituitary gland. This, in turn, produces hormones (trophic hormones), which control other glands (thyroid, adrenal, and male or female gonads). The hormones produced by these glands exert a negative feedback (short or long, indicated by dotted lines) to close the circuits. The hypothalamus also exerts a dual control on growth hormone (GH) by a stimulating factor (GHRH) and an inhibitory one (somatostatin); the only hormone with predominant negative control is prolactin (PRL, controlling mammary gland) by the neurotransmitter dopamine (DA). Growth hormone induces the production of proteins (IGF-1) by liver and peripheral tissue to exert its anabolic actions. Finally, adipose tissue produces the hormone leptin that inhibits appetite and has catabolic activities.

2. Hypothalamus and Regulation of Appetite

Appetite and regulation of body weight are modulated by the neuroendocrine system [3,4]. The hypothalamus, in particular, plays an important role in alimentary behaviors, regulation of nutrition, and water intake, but the mechanisms that regulate this control are not entirely known. Areas called "centre of satiety," "centre of hunger," and "centre of thirst" are located in the hypothalamus. For many years, ventromedial nuclei, constituted by cells acting as chemoreceptors sensible to glycaemia and especially to utilization rate of glucose, expressed by artero-venous difference in glucose, have been considered the "centre of satiety," while lateral area of hypothalamus (LH) was the "centre of hunger." This idea, also called the "the dual hypothesis," has not been fully confirmed, for three of reasons. First of all, it has been understood that central nervous system is not organized in distinct structures controlling specifically precise functions, which, instead, are made by neuronal circuits involving different cerebral structures; secondly, other areas in CNS are involved, especially in the attitudes toward food; thirdly, numerous neurotransmitters and neurohormones are implicated in a complex and redundant systems, allowing them to be classified in two categories: orexigenic and anorexigenic principles.

The most important areas, focused upon in the last years, are arcuate nucleus (ARC), in the ventral hypothalamus, near the third ventricle, which can be considered "first-order" neurons; they are the play of secretion of orexigenic Neuropeptide Y (NPY) and Agouti-related peptides (AGRP), on one side, and anorexigenic proopiomelanocortin (POMC) and cocain and amphetamine-regulated transcript (CART), on the other side. These neurons project toward other areas, which can be considered "second-order" neurons, producing again anorexigenic substances (Paraventricular nucleus, PVN, where TRH, CRH and oxytocin are secreted) and orexigenic substances (LH and perifornical areas, with the production of melanin-concentrating hormone and orexins) (Figure 2) [5].

NPY, produced through CNS, stimulates food ingestion and anabolic pathways of metabolism (therefore, it exerts opposite effect to leptin, see below). Two classes of receptors (YY5 and YY1) in rats and humans are assumed to play a major role in NPY-induced food intake [6]. The neuropeptide YY5 receptor gene is expressed in brain regions known to be involved in the central regulation of feeding behavior, including lateral hypothalamus, the paraventricular nucleus, and the arcuate nucleus [7]. Genetic studies on mutation screening within the NPYY5R gene revealed a rare variant (Glu-4-ala) in a single patient with AN. This allele was transmitted from the mother, who had no history of any eating disorder. Also, studies on variations and polymorphism within the NPYY1R and NPYY5R in AN were negative [8].

At variance with NPY, AGRP is indirectly orexigenic, since it inhibits the anorexic action of POMC. In fact, it was discovered as a peripheric antagonist of Melanocyte-Stimulating Hormone (MSH) in the hair (antagonizing the melanocyte stimulating action it induced a yellow appearance of Agouti rats, thus, its name).

On the first-order neurons, a control is exerted by adiposity and nutritional/satiety signals. It is negatively modulated by leptin and insulin (respectively indices of adiposity and nutritional status).

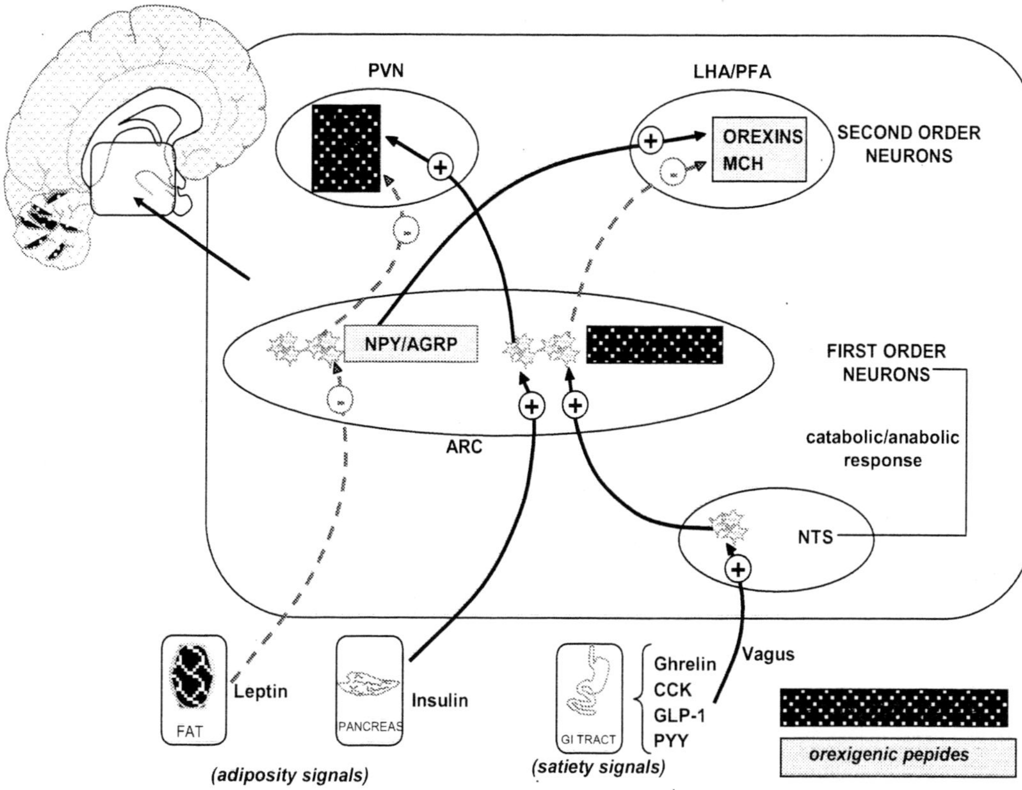

Figure 2. The control of appetite is mainly regulated in the basal part of hypothalamus, the nucleus arcuatus (ARC), where two types of neurons are located: those producing neuropeptide Y (NPY) and agouti-related peptide (AGRP) that stimulate appetite (orexigenic); and those producing proopiomelanocortins (POMC) and CART, that are inhibitory (anorexigenic). These first-order neurons are connected by complex network of both positive and negative signals with other neurons (second-order neurons, producing both orexigenic and anorexigenic factors). A negative control is exerted by adiposity signals (the hormone leptin, produced by adipose tissue) and insulin (produced by pancreas, after ingestion of glucose and aminoacids) and by satiety signals (hormones produced by gastrointestinal tract, GI). The only hormone produced by the stomach that stimulates appetite, is Ghrelin.

Recent studies clarified the importance of adipose tissue and particularly of leptin, a hormone constituted by 167 aminoacids, produced by adipocytes in proportional way to fat stores of the subject (lipostatic hypothesis, see below details on leptin physiology). Leptin acts by a feedback mechanism, augmenting when fat stores increase; in this way, it influences the hypothalamus, inhibiting food intake and energy dissipation. On the contrary, if the fat stores diminish, the serum leptin level also reduces, and this mechanism induces an increased food intake by hypothalamic action.

Satiety signals are generated in gastrointestinal tract during a meal and—via vagal and sympathetic pathways afferent to the nucleus of the solitary tract (NTS) in the caudal brainstem—send a message to ARC to stop food ingestion (they include colecystokinin, GLP-1, PYY, bombesin); the only orexigenic peptides released by gastrointestinal tract is Ghrelin, secreted by oxyntic glands of the stomach and with receptors in NPY neurons. It increases before meals and quickly reduces after food ingestion [5].

Other neuropeptides that stimulate food intake and energy storage are melatonin-concentrating hormone and orexin A and B, which increase in response to fasting and stimulate appetite [9]. The melanocortins (MC) are peptides derived from the precursor POMC and act on specific receptors. The endogenous MC most implicated in food intake and body weight is α-MSH, which has a high affinity for the MC receptors, especially MC3 and MC4 [10]. Mutation screening of the coding region of MC4 receptors in patients with AN and Bulimia nervosa revealed two common polymorphisms in both groups. Allele and genotype frequencies did not differ between these groups and probands of different weight extremes [11].

The paraventricular nucleus is also one of most important efferent nuclei of the hypothalamus. Pancreatic secretion of insulin stimulates food intake, and the vagal efferents direct to pancreas excite the insulin secretion. Projections coming from the paraventricular nucleus and other hypothalamic nuclei modulate these vagal efferents by projections directed to pregangliar neurons of motor dorsal vagal nucleus. Moreover, noradrenalin secretion in medial regions of hypothalamus also stimulates the insulin secretion and let start alimentary behaviours. These projections using noradrenalin have origin principally by locus coeruleus in the brain stem. The presence of insulin receptors in the hypothalamic neurons makes possible that these neurons constantly control insulin-circulating levels.

The main neurotransmitter involved in appetite regulation remains serotonin (5-hydroxytryptamine; 5-HT), which covers a broad range of biological, physiological, and behavioral functions. Since serotoninergic agonists are anorexigenic, the serotoninegic system has been implicated in the development of eating disorders [12], and serotonin antagonists proposed as pharmacological approach [13].

The 5-HT actions are regulated by biosynthetic enzymes (tryptophan hydroxylase), specific receptors, and an inactivation system involving neuronal reuptake (serotonin transporters) [14]. Both 5-HT receptor genes and the tryptophan hydroxylase gene showed polymorphism, and an association a particular allele within the promoter region of the 5-HT2A receptor gene and AN has been reported [15,16]. However, other studies did not confirm this association [17]. An association has been reported between the allele and restrictive AN, but not with the binge/purging subtype [18]. Other authors [19] found that the same allele was associated with lower energy intake and lower alcohol consumption also in obese individuals, reinforcing the hypothesis of such genetic alteration in AN patients. These studies suggest that patients with AN have enhanced 5-HT2A receptor binding and provide further evidence for a serotoninergic dysfunction in eating disorders; but these results need further confirmation [20].

In summary, in last years, we have understood that alimentary behaviour is very complex and requires the interactions of many neurotransmitters, neurohormones, and gastrointestinal hormones, and peptides can play an important role by activation or inhibition of mechanisms of food intake and of maintenance of a correct body weight. A summary of stimulatory and inhibitory substances are presented in Table 1 [4]. Furthermore, neuropeptides, such as beta-endorphin, neuropeptide Y (NPY), galanin and leptin, may affect hormone release; on the other hand, the hormonal status may modulate neuropeptide activity [21]. Glucocorticoids are also implicated. Via their effect on NPY, they act as endogenous antagonists of leptin and insulin [22]. This complex molecular network regulates not only food intake, but also energy expenditure, oxygen consumption, thermogenesis, insulin, and glucocorticoid regulation. Finally, pathologic processes involving areas other than the hypothalamus can cause many disorders in the food assumption, as well as those involving limbic system, strictly connected with the hypothalamus itself [3,4].

A temptative summarizing view is that long-term energy balance is regulated via a system involving hormones secreted in proportion to corporal adiposity, such as leptin and insulin, that act at the level of central nervous systems (CNS). This responds to changes in body fat by activating anabolic or catabolic pathways [23], the first through production of NPY, which stimulates food intake, and the second via the hypothalamic melanocortin system, which reduces food intake and stimulates weight loss [24].

Table 1. The control of appetite

	Stimulating substances	*Inhibitory substance S*
Neurotransmitters	***Noradrenalin (α-receptors)*** ***GABA***	***Serotonin (5-OH-triptamine)*** ***Dopamine*** ***Histamine***
Neuropeptides	***Neuropeptide Y*** ***Agouti-related peptide (AGRP)*** ***GHRH*** ***Opioids*** ***Galanin*** ***Melanocortins (MCH)*** ***Orexines***	***Cocain and amphetamine-regulated transcript (CART)*** ***CRH*** ***MSH*** ***Oxitocin*** ***TRH***
Gastrointestinal hormones	***GHrelin***	***GLP-1*** ***Neurotensin*** ***Bombesin*** ***CCK*** ***CGRP*** ***Peptide YY***
Other hormones	***Insulin (peripheral action)***	***Leptin*** ***Insulin (central action)*** ***Glucagon***

According to some authors [25], anorexia nervosa is the result of a disruption in bioenergy homeostasis induced by lipid dysregulation. This disruption has two major determinants: (1) a biological predisposition to primary multihormonal disharmony linked to post-pubertal growth and development; and (2) an acquired abnormal lipid-induced loop operation precipitated by inappropriate diet. It is so possible to present a step-by-step model describing the cascade of disorders that culminates in anorexia nervosa: defective digestion and absorption of essential fatty acids; diversion of lipids from adipose cells into bloodstream; defective carbohydrate and lipid metabolism, which modifies the blood brain barrier; neuroendocrine membrane alteration causing severe endocrine impairment; changes in the negative feedback mechanism, which escalate the body's use of bioenergy; derangement of the appetite center, which causes a constant sensation of satiety; and replacement of the correct body image with the premorbid one that encourages poor judgement concerning food intake and self-support. The loop-like nature of this mechanism perpetuates the disease.

Characteristic patterns of leptin and ghrelin concentrations have been observed in anorexia nervosa [26]. Fasting plasma levels of the orexigenic peptide ghrelin have been found to be elevated in patients with AN [27]. Studies of the orexigenic peptides neuropeptide Y and the opioid peptides have shown state-related abnormalities in patients with eating disorders [27]. In particular, in patients with anorexia nervosa, plasma leptin and NPY concentrations were low. The disturbances in beta-endorphin release are also observed. The feedback mechanism between leptin and NPY is disturbed in anorexia nervosa, as well as in obesity. An abnormal activity of neuropeptides may lead to disturbed control of appetite and hormonal dysregulation in eating disorders [21].

Moreover, in anorexia nervosa, adrenalin and noradrenalin levels are reduced in blood plasma, urines and cerebrospinal fluid; serotonin and its metabolite 5-HIAA levels are reduced or normal in cerebrospinal fluid; dopamine and its metabolite HVA levels are reduced or normal in cerebrospinal fluid; opioid activity is augmented in cerebrospinal fluid, while β-endorphines are normal or reduced, but only in the extreme thinness [28].

However, despite the large number of studies in this field, an unequivocal pattern that explains all phenomena observed in AN is still lacking, and no single alteration can be considered the unique cause of the disease.

3. GH-IGF-1 Axis

Growth hormone (GH), or somatotropin, with the GH-dependent synthesis of IGF-1 (insulin-like growth factor 1, synthesized in the liver and in peripheral tissue, mediating most GH effects and, therefore, called somatomedin), plays a key role not only in the promotion of linear growth but also in the regulation of intermediary metabolism, body composition, and energy expenditure [29]. On the whole, the hormone appears to direct fuel metabolism towards the preferential oxidation of lipids instead of glucose and proteins, and to convey the energy derived from metabolic processes towards the synthesis of proteins. On the other hand, body energy stores and circulating energetic substrates take an important part in the regulation of somatotropin release. Finally, central and peripheral peptides participating in the control of food intake and energy expenditure (NPY, leptin, and ghrelin) are also involved in the regulation of GH secretion. Altogether, nutritional status has to be regarded as a major determinant in the regulation of the somatotropin-somatomedin axis in animals and humans. In these latter, being overweight is associated with marked impairment of spontaneous and stimulated GH release, while acute dietary restriction and chronic under-nutrition induce an amplification of spontaneous secretion, together with a clear-cut decrease in IGF-I plasma levels. Thus, over- and under-nutrition represent two conditions connoted by GH hypersensitivity and GH resistance, respectively.

A GH resistance, related to malnutrition (as it is observed in malabsorption, diabetes mellitus, liver cirrhosis, and catabolic states), is the main alteration, joint to signs of altered hypothalamic control of GH secretion.

Studies on spontaneous GH secretion show increased frequency of secretory burst superimposed on enhanced tonic GH secretion [30]. Other authors, showing heterogeneity of spontaneous GH secretion at the time of the diagnosis, described mean 24-h GH secretion greater than normal only in 40% of the patients tested, due to modification of amplitude and not frequency of the GH peaks; while in 60% levels below normal range were present; in both cases, the GH abnormalities were reversed by a weight gain of at least 10% of the initial weight [31]. Using a deconvolution method, the half-life of GH was shown to be normal; frequency, duration, and amplitude of the peaks were increased, joint to elevated basal GH levels; these paramethers negatively correlated with BMI [32].

As far as dynamic GH secretion is concerned, an increased GHRH-stimulated GH release was reported [33], and lack of GH suppression after meal was described [34]. We considered such postprandial response as "paradoxical," strangely resembling the response in obese subjects; it was partially inhibited by infusion of an opiate-antagonist (naloxone) [35]. Other abnormalities included: decreased response after hypoglycaemia, clonidine, hexarelin and dexamethasone; and a paradoxical response to TRH or i.v. glucose [36-38] and to LHRH [39]. Our group also tried to correlate alterations of GH dynamic to affective or personality traits in AN: a different cholinergic modulation of GH was observed in different psychological patterns [40].

Ghrelin, a gastrointestinal peptide that stimulates GH secretion in rats and humans [41] presents high plasma levels in AN [42], with a rapid decrease after weight recovery. It indicates a physiological effort to compensate for the lack of nutritional intake and storage energy [43].

Many data concern different steps of GH control and activity: the dual control by GHRH and somatostatin, the GHBP (the circulating from of its receptor), the levels of IGF-1 and its binding proteins (IGFBP, with their 6 isoforms); these data are reviewed by Munoz et al [6].

In fact, these peculiarities in GH secretion depend on an interplay between central and peripheral factors. At central levels, an increase in GHRH and a decrease in somatostatinergic (SS) activity have been hypothesized. Particular resistance to cholinergic manipulation has been demonstrated, suggesting a specific alteration in SS-mediated cholinergic influence on GH secretion. On the other hand, reduced IGF-1 secretion (see below) could have, as a consequence, a reduced feedback, which is normally exerted both at hypothalamic and pituitary levels. A low dose of IGF-1 inhibits, even if not normalizes, spontaneous and stimulated secretion of GH in AN patients. Moreover, hypoestrogenism, due to defective pituitary-gonadal axis, could contribute to increase pulse frequency.

Serum GH-binding protein (GHBP) levels are dramatically reduced and tend to normalize after weight gain. This reduction in GH receptors is most likely one of the principal causes of GH resistance. It has been suggested that in malnutrition, low GHBP levels could be related to hypoinsulinemia, alterations in thyroid function, and hypoestrogenism. Many studies showed a correlation between serum GHBP and BMI, or percentage of body fat, specifically visceral fat. Since it has not been demonstrated that circulating GHBP is uniquely derived from liver GH receptors, it is possible that other tissues, such as adipose tissue, could contribute to GHBP levels; therefore, low levels in AN could be related to the extreme reduction in adipose tissue.

Extremely reduced IGF-1 levels were demonstrated and tended to normalize with weight recovery; the time for this recovery may be prolonged; the lack of IGF-1 correlation with GH suggests the GH-resistance. Contradictory data concern free IGF-1, which were found to be normal or decreased. There are also similar considerations with concern to IGF-II levels.

Another important factor, directly correlated with the nutritional status, is the level of IGF-binding proteins; elevated IGFBP-1 and -2 have been reported and explained by hypoinsulinemia, increased glucagon or glucocorticoids, or decreased intracellular glucose and other substrates. Serum IGFBP-3 are decreased as consequence of GH resistance, as it is GH-dependent; again, a normalization has been reported after weight gain. IGFBP-3 decreases significantly with caloric restriction, but in adults only after protein restriction; no increased proteolysis of IGFBP-3 is present, at variance with other catabolic situation. All the components of the trimolecular complex formed by IGFBP-3, IGF and the acid-labile subunit (ALS), were, as expected, reduced. A dramatic decrease of IGFBP-4 and -5, without normalization with weight gain, was reported; it must be remembered that they are very important in the process of bone formation. The decrease in IGFBP-3, which impedes the retention of IGF in vascular space, could, therefore, be synergic with an increase in IGFBP-1 and -2, which can cross the vascular barrier, allowing movement to tissue with augmentation of IGF activity at tissue level.

Some thyroid dysfunction (low T_3 syndrome), observed in AN as in subjects with deficiency of GH action, can be due to insufficient GH-mediated conversion of T_4 to T_3 (see below section of hypothalamic-pituitary-thyroid axis). Based on these considerations, it is possible to suppose that insufficient GH action plays a role in the progression of this syndrome. It has been hypothesized that the amount of endogenous GH is not enough to increase IGF-I.

Important observations have been made after exogenous administration of rhGH [44]: it induced an increase of plasma IGF-1 levels, accompanied by a decrease in GH levels (suggesting that not only GH action but also normal GH-IGF-1 axis was restored by administration of rhGH). Serum level of triiodothyronine, but not thyroxine and TBG, increased during treatment with rhGH; increase in serum level of T_3 accompanied a decrease in serum TSH concentration, suggesting that thyroid hormone action is improved by recovering GH-dependent conversion of T_4 to T_3.

Various metabolic alterations of AN were corrected by rhGH. Hypoglicemia (one of the indicators for the presence of insufficient energy utilization) was corrected, with restoration of glucose metabolism. Hypercholesterolemia was similarly corrected, possibly due to the normalization of thyroid hormone-accelerated utilization of LDL-cholesterol. On the other hand, the high level of HDL-cholesterol is known to be one of the AN-specific features; its level was normalized by rhGH, indicating that this AN-specific metabolism of HDL-cholesterol is partly related to the insufficient action of GH in this syndrome.

Depressed body temperature increased during rhGH, revealing that thermogenesis is restored by increasing energy utilization. Improvement of thyroid hormone-mediated energy generation may partly contribute to this recovery. Also, BMI increased during treatment with rhGH. In addition to these increments, an increase in caloric intake was observed during rhGH. These results suggest that administration of rhGH is essentially important in maintaining overall energy metabolism.

Administration of rhGH positively influenced other systems, such as the hematopoietic system, (correction of trombocitopenia), and cardiac system (improvement of cardiac output). Finally, an increase in food intake was observed during administration of rhGH, even if it is not normalized, indicating that the habit of food intake may directly be influenced by GH action.

In summary, increased GH secretion, together with reduced GH sensitivity, is observed; it is mostly reversed by weight recovery, suggesting that they are adaptive to malnutrition.

4. Hypothalamic-Pituitary-Thyroid-Axis (HPT)

The changes in thyroid function in AN are still controversially discussed, due to contrasting studies [45-47]. It is unclear whether the changes in TSH and peripheral thyroid hormones are a cause or a consequence of being underweight. The main concept is that most AN patients exhibit a low-T_3 syndrome, with low T_3, normal or low T_4 and normal TSH [45], due to altered peripheral deiodination that preferentially transforms T_4 into the inactive metabolites reverse T_3. This condition is also called "euthyroid sick syndrome." These alterations normalize with weight recuperation [48].

For readers who are not confident with endocrine disorders, we remember that the thyroid gland, under the stimulation of TRH-TSH axis, preferentially synthesizes the pro-hormone thyroxine (T_4), which is converted to active hormone T_3 (or alternative inactive reverse—T_3, so called for the different position of iodine atoms in the molecule) in peripheral tissue. Different kinds of enzymes (deiodinases) are responsible for this metabolism. The way of dieting profoundly influences freeT_3 concentrations: over-nutrition leads to high T_3 serum levels, while hypocaloric diet leads to an increase in the production of rT_3.

These different levels of the axis have been separately investigated in AN.

First of all, ultrasonographic studies showed reduced thyroid gland volume in AN compared to sex- and age-matched controls and to the expected thyroid volume predicted from body weight and age, indicating thyroid atrophy [49]. TSH normally plays a major role in thyroid growth. However, since TSH levels were not different from the control group and since , in very aged hospitalized euthyroid geriatric patients, thyroid volume has been reported to be decreased, it has been suggested that thyroid atrophy could be a common feature of chronic illness. Low circulating levels of IGF-1 can be responsible, as there is evidence that thyroid size is significantly influenced by IGF-1 [50], and, in vitro, TSH had little effect on thyroid growth in the absence of IGF-1 [51]; the low IGF-1 level may contribute to the thyroid atrophy in AN patients.

As far as TSH secretion is concerned, generally TSH levels are normal or slightly decreased; the response to TSH to exogenous TRH is normal or reduced; often, it is delayed as it can be observed in hypothalamic disease.

The T4 concentration is generally normal and sometimes subnormal because of a modest decrease in iodothyronine-binding proteins; the T_3 one is often reduced with, not always [45], an increase of reverse T_3 (biologically inactive), not because of a major increase in the production but because of a decrease in its clearance. Since thyroid hormones regulate both the resting energy expenditure (REE) and thermogenesis, this hormonal pattern, by the lower T_3 generation, aims to regulate, at a lower level, the energetic metabolism in order to compensate the reduced intake of food.

Basal oxygen consumption and heart rate decline, nitrogen balance returns toward normal, and peripheral steroid metabolism shifts toward the pattern seen in hypothyroidism. Thyroid dysfunctions may be one of the essential reasons for lipid metabolism disorder in AN.

The abnormal T_3 and rT_3 concentrations in serum are quickly restored to normal by administrations of small quantities (200kcal) of carbohydrates. Similar quantities of protein have no effect on the serum T_3 level, but may lower the serum rT_3 level. Calories given as fat are ineffective [52]. During weight gain, increases in T_3 are associated with increases in resting energy expenditure, which is independent of reduced fat-free mass, which is considered to be the strongest determinant of REE [53].

Among other factors influencing HPT, we can also consider leptin, which may be the link between weight status and thyroid hormones. Many reports suggest that leptin may modify hypothalamic production of TSH. Amongst others, the synthesis of TSH is also regulated by leptin, which innervates hypophysiotropic TRH neurons [54]. Furthermore, there is a synchronicity between the secretion of leptin and TSH [55]. Moreover, leptin concentrations have not been found to respond to short-term re-feeding, in contrast to long-term weight gain in patients with AN [56].

Furthermore, it is known that in man, serum serotonin levels correlate positively with T_3 levels. It is possible that the low serum levels of thyroid hormones in AN subjects result in low serum serotonin and its product, melatonin [57]. Finally, an important role in the physiopathology of low T_3 syndrome is attributed to cytokines, in analogy comparison with other situations, such as stress or excess of physical training [45].

It is well established that there is a relationship between AN and depressive symptoms, and there is increased prevalence of primary affective disorders in the relatives of the anorexic patients. Thyroid disorders clearly are associated with affective disturbances and, at times, may persist even after appropriate substitution [58]. On the other hand, abnormalities of the thyroid axis have been observed in euthyroid patients with affective disorders, as well as in AN patients. For instance, a blunted and delayed TSH response to exogenously administrated TRH has been reported in normal-weight patients with depressive illness and in about 25% to 50 % of AN patients [59]. In AN patients, TSH can be stimulated by a TRH prohormone, which has no stimulatory effect in healthy subjects or in subjects with systemic illness [60]. However, the potential effect was not investigated in patients with affective disorders. Although controversial, exogenous administration of TSH or T_3 previously has been reported to accelerate the antidepressive effect of imipramin, whereas TRH has been reported to possess a direct antidepressant effect [61].

In general, there is evidence that AN and affective disorders are associated with a common hypothalamic-pituitary-thyroid axis dysfunction. It is not known whether the thyroid atrophy may have clinical significance beyond that of thyroid function assessed by the biochemical findings. Thyroid atrophy in AN patients, most likely, is secondary to the emaciation and low IGF-1 levels. Once initiated, it still could play a role in a vicious circle maintaining anorexic or depressive symptomatology.

5. Hypothalamic-Pituitary-Adrenal Axis (HPA)

There is a great effort in literature to evaluate the role of the hypothalamic-pituitary-adrenal (HPA) axis as a relevant factor capable of influencing the onset and the course of an eating disorder (ED) and to evaluate the prognosis of the disease. On the other hand, other studies have suggested that the onset of an ED is often preceded by severe life events, and that chronic stress is associated with the persistence of these disorders. As the biological response to stress is the activation of the HPA axis, it needs to be extensively described.

The central control areas of the so-called "stress system" are located in the hypothalamus and the brain stem. They include two main centers: the parvocellular neurons of the paraventricular nuclei of the hypothalamus, secreting corticotrophin-releasing hormone (CRH) and arginine vasopressin (AVP), and the locus coeruleus/norepinephrine (LC-NE) system (central sympathetic system). The HPA axis and the efferent sympathetic/ adrenomedullary system represent the effector limbs, via which the brain influences all the body organs during exposure to the threatening stimuli [62].

CRH is the main regulating hormone of the HPA axis, which is quickly activated after exposure to an acute or chronic stressor, whatever it is. CRH stimulates the secretion of adrenocorticotropic hormone (ACTH) from the anterior pituitary, which, in turn, stimulates secretion by the adrenal cortex of glucocorticoid hormones, mainly cortisol in humans. AVP, together with CRH, is a potent synergistic factor in stimulating ACTH secretion. Furthermore, it appears that there is a reciprocal positive interaction between CRH and AVP at the level of the hypothalamus, with each neuropeptide stimulating the secretion of the other [63].

In non-stressful situations, both CRH and AVP are secreted in the portal system (the vascular connection between hypothalamus and pituitary) in a pulsatile fashion, with a frequency of about two to three secretory episodes per hour. The amplitude of the CRH and AVP pulses increase in the early morning hours, resulting in ACTH and cortisol secretory bursts in the general circulation, generating a circadian rhythm. These diurnal variations are perturbed by changes in light cycle, feeding habits, and activity, and are disrupted by stress. During acute stress, the amplitude and synchronization of the CRH and AVP pulsations markedly increase, resulting in augmented ACTH and cortisol secretory episodes. Other factors such as AVP of magnocellular neuron origin, angiotensin II and various cytokines, and lipid mediators of inflammation are secreted, and act on hypothalamic, pituitary, or adrenal components of the HPA axis, potentiating its activity in accordance with the kind of stress [62].

The adrenal cortex is the main target organ of pituitary- derived circulating ACTH, which is the key regulator of glucocorticoid secretion by this gland. Other hormones or cytokines, either originating from the adrenal medulla or coming from the systemic circulation, as well as neuronal information from the autonomic innervations of the adrenal cortex, may also participate in the regulation of cortisol secretion [64]. Glucocorticoids are the final effectors of the HPA axis and participate in the control of whole body homeostasis and the organism response to stress. Furthermore, glucocorticoids have a key regulatory role in the basal control of HPA axis activity and in the termination of the stress response by acting on extrahypothalamic regulatory centers, such as the hippocampus and frontal cortex, the paraventricular nucleus of the hypothalamus, and the pituitary gland [65]. The inhibitory glucocorticoid feedback on the ACTH secretory response acts to limit the duration of the total tissue exposure to glucocorticoids, minimizing the catabolic, lipogenic, antireproductive, and immunosuppressive effects of these hormones [66]. Moreover, there are mutual interactions of the central stress stations with three higher brain control areas that influence affect and anticipatory phenomena (mesocortical/ mesolimbic systems); the initiation, propagation, and termination of stress system activity (amygdala/hippocampus complex); and the setting of the pain sensation (arcuate nucleus). In summary, glucocorticoids exert a great number of physiological and behavioral effects and participate in the different mechanisms that control HPA axis activation and integrate the stress response [66].

The central neuronal areas regulating food intake and energy expenditure, mainly in the hypothalamus, as above described, are potently influenced by various components of the stress system. It is a common observation that acute stressful situations are usually associated with the onset of anorexia and subsequent restriction of food consumption. Indeed, increases in the central CRH secretion acutely stimulate the POMC neurons of the arcuate nucleus, which, in turn, elicit anorexic signals via the just-mentioned MSH release, and increase thermogenesis. In addition, the stimulation of NPY by ARC concomitantly enhances the CRH release, probably in order to counter-regulate its own actions, and also inhibits the locus coeruleus/norepinephrine sympathetic system and activates the parasympathetic system, in order to decrease thermogenesis and enhance the digestion and storage of nutrients. Stress-induced suppression of NPY secretion is also likely to be involved in the anorexic phase during acute stress [67]. Notably, this circuitry also receives significant input from stimuli originating in the periphery, such as leptin and cortisol: leptin inhibits the secretion of hypothalamic NPY, and, hence, CRH, while it stimulates arcuate nucleus POMC neurons. Additionally, at the level of the adrenal gland, leptin directly suppresses the production of glucocorticoids; conversely, the acute elevations of the glucocorticoid levels stimulate the adipocyte expression of leptin, resulting in transient increases in the leptin plasma concentrations [68]. Lastly, the increase in circulating glucocorticoid concentrations enhances the intake of carbohydrates and fat, suppressing CRH and stimulating NPY hypothalamic secretion [66]. Considering the complexity of the aforementioned interactions that represent the way to ensure optimal chances of survival under different stressful conditions, an intricate circuitry of centrally acting neuropeptides and hormones, exhibiting synergistic or antagonistic actions, regulates the equilibrium of the body's energy intake and expenditure. Thus, it can be hypothesized that acute stress induces HPA axis activation, which aims primarily, through CRH, to temporarily inhibit the immediate energy-consuming activities related to finding, ingesting, and digesting food; conversely, the activation of the HPA axis under conditions of chronic stress tends to heighten the relatively more prolonged central actions of glucocorticoids in the appetite centers, which are collectively orexigenic and stress relieving [68]. The relationship between cortisol and food intake in humans may also involve the effects of glucocorticoids on opioids and endocannabinoids. The activation of the HPA axis elicits—among other neurotransmitter system effects—the release of endogenous opioids. There is strong evidence suggesting that opioid release is part of an organism's powerful defense mechanism against the detrimental effects of stress. The opioids decrease the activity of the HPA axis on different levels, in order to attenuate and terminate the stress response, providing a negative feedback control mechanism. The opioid release increases the palatable food intake, and palatable food sustains the opioid release. Thus, food intake resembles a powerful tool to shut down stress-induced HPA axis activation. If stress becomes chronic and eating is learned to be an effective coping behavior, highly palatable food may appear to be "addictive," via the neurobiological adaptations mentioned above [66]. Many studies have investigated the functioning of the three main components of the HPA axis (hypothalamus, pituitary, and adrenal cortex) both in basal condition and after a pharmacological challenge (stimulation or suppression tests).

Plasma and cerebrospinal fluid (CSF) CRH levels indicate basal hypothalamus function, while plasma ACTH levels have a relationship to pituitary function in the same condition.

The combined administration of CRH and arginine vasopressin (CRH/AVP test) helps to investigate the activity of the HPA axis by measuring both the response of cortisol (adrenal) and ACTH (pituitary) to a stressor. The dexamethasone suppression test (DST), which is the most widely used method, explores the whole HPA axis functioning. The dexamethasone suppressed corticotrophin-releasing hormone stimulation test (DST-CRH test) explores pituitary and adrenal functioning by measuring ACTH and cortisol levels after a low-dose dexamethasone suppression test and subsequent stimulation with CRH. The ACTH stimulation test also explores adrenal activity by measuring cortisol levels. The adrenal activity is evaluated by plasma, salivary, urinary, and CSF cortisol levels, both basal and after stimuli [66].

The main alterations of HPA in AN can be summarized as follows: although the diurnal variation is maintained, there is a persistent hypersecretion of cortisol throughout the day; normal or low ACTH levels and urinary cortisol metabolites, secondary to reduction in cortisol metabolism; hypercortisolemia partially suppressed with DST; prolonged cortisol half-life and decreased metabolic clearance, correlated with malnutrition; changes in cortisol metabolism, probably related to low plasma T_3 levels; changes in cortisol-binding globulin affinity and decreased glucocorticoid receptor function; a blunted ACTH response to CRH that persists after short-term weight restoration and disappears after long-term weight restoration; CRH released continuously regardless of plasma cortisol concentrations, then the negative feedback response is normal at the pituitary level but not at the hypothalamic level, indicating possible hypothalamic dysfunction in this disease and disturbances of the feedback mechanism; DDAVP (1-deamino-8D-arginine vasopressin, potent secretagogue for ACTH) does not stimulate ACTH and cortisol, due to a down-regulation of hypophyseal VV3 receptors; all of these disturbances may have a role in mechanism of amenorrhea [66].

Many authors studied HPA axis functioning during different phases of the disease. In the past years, some studies reported decreased cortisol production and excretion and a normalization of CRH levels and pituitary-adrenal function [69,70] in anorexic patients after weight recovery. More recently, other authors suggested that hypercortisolemia is a direct consequence of under-nutrition, whereas weight recovery is associated with a significant decrease in the number of cortisol secretory bursts [71], and with the normalization of cortisol response to AVP and to the DST/CRH test [72]. Putignano et al. [73] reported less pronounced HPA axis alterations, although still statistically significant, in treated patients suffering from AN. On the other hand, Schweitzer et al. [74] did not find a consistent relationship between the normalization of the DST response and weight gain in AN patients.

In AN, the main difficulty is to establish whether the HPA axis abnormalities are related to starvation and weight loss or to AN itself. In fact, patients who have other forms of serious protein-caloric malnutrition have elevated levels of plasma cortisol and diminished rates of cortisol metabolism. In 1986, Fichter and Pirke [75] studied five healthy female subjects participating in a starvation experiment, causing a loss of about eight kg in a three-week complete food abstinence; thereafter, they recovered to their original body weight, which remained stable for more than four weeks. Half of DST tests in the fasting phase showed insufficient suppression, while, in the following weight-gain phase, the cortisol suppression was generally restored. Twenty-four-hour plasma cortisol patterns during fasting showed a significant increase, as well as increased cortisol half-life, increased time in secretory activity, and an increased number of secretory episodes. These results suggest that HPA axis is influenced by weight loss, reduced caloric intake, and catabolic state in normal subjects [75].

Since AN represents a model of functional hypercortisolism that shares similar pathophysiological mechanisms with the other causes of pseudo-Cushing's-syndrome states, other dynamic tests were performed as reviewed [66]: DST-CRH test (combination of dexamethasone-induced suppression of HPA axis function and subsequent stimulation with CRH) did not induced increases in plasma ACTH or cortisol levels. However, weight gain was associated with blunting of the endocrine response to the DST-CRH test, which may have been related to the rising estrogen levels. In one study [72], an AVP challenge test was also performed, showing a cortisol response to AVP reduced by 138% in the active AN group, suggesting an impairment in pituitary sensitivity to AVP, which began to normalize with weight gain. Thus, unlike previous studies, where centrally directed AVP levels in underweight patients with AN were found to be abnormally increased [76], upregulated AVP activity or enhanced pituitary sensitivity to AVP in AN, which could increase the response to CRH in AN, was not observed [72]. Misra et al. [71] reported that the frequency of nocturnal secretory bursts, total nocturnal pulsatile cortisol secretion, and total cortisol secretion were significantly higher in women with AN than in healthy controls. Furthermore, weight recovery has been associated with a significant decrease in the number of secretory bursts. Only one study [74] failed to report a consistent relationship between normalization of the DST response and weight gain. In fact, unlike patients with pure malnutrition, a number of weight-restored anorexic patients continue to show or return to non-suppression. It could be hypothesized that the reversion to a positive DST result might reflect a stress response in patients who failed to achieve weight stabilization. Furthermore, it seems that patients who did not normalize their DST responses are at higher risk of a poor outcome [77].

The CRH hypersecretion etiology in patients with AN remains unclear, but some data support the hypothesis that hypercortisolemia could be an intrinsic abnormality of the disorder, not necessarily secondary to starvation and/or malnutrition. It must be taken into account, however, that other factors, such as the common presence of major affective disorders and other psychological or behavioral symptoms, could be responsible for these abnormalities [78]. Most of the authors, nevertheless, found that these abnormalities do not correlate with depressive symptoms or clinical measures of nutritional status, such as body weight and body mass index (BMI) (see review, ref. 66). Moreover, the hyperactivity of the HPA axis differs in depression and AN, with a greater involvement of AVP in depressive disorder and perhaps more reliance on CRH to drive the axis in AN [72]. Therefore, most authors proposed malnutrition as the main determinant responsible for HPA axis alterations.

In conclusion, the involvement of the HPA axis in AN is a main characteristic, not related to the occurrence of comorbid concurrent pathology. Furthermore, in AN patients, HPA axis arousal, an increased secretion of cortisol under basal conditions or after stress stimuli, and reduced or absent suppression at DST have been observed. These findings seem to be directly associated with weight loss. The relative influence of AN and malnutrition on HPA function is uncertain, as data observed in different studies reported discordant results. However, alterations seem to be more relevant as the severity of the illness becomes higher (e.g., untreated and severely underweight patients) and when weight recovery does not normalize HPA functions. Further studies are needed in order to detect the possible causal relationship between HPA alterations and the different biopsychological features of AN.

6. Hypothalamic-Pituitary-Gonadal Axis (HPG)

The most important alterations in AN occur in the reproductive system. The alterations of hypothalamic-pituitary-gonadal axis are the most interesting by clinical and biological points of view. They cause amenorrhoea without loss of secondary sexual characteristics. The persistence and the evidence of pubic and axillary hairs, associated sometimes to diffuse lanugo, instead represents a characteristic semiotic element important in the differential diagnosis with hypogonadotropic hypogonadism of pituitaric origin. By a physiopathological point of view, the alterations of gonadotropic secretion are characterized by a "regression" (or "arrest" in adolescent patients) of the regulation of hypothalamus-gonadotropins system at puberal age.

The circulating concentration of LH is decreased and the FSH levels are at the lower limit of normal values, with an augmented FSH/LH ratio. The secretory pulsatility of LH, typical of woman in fertile era, is replaced by variations linked to sleep-wake rhythm, as characteristic in fact of puberal period. The gonadotropin response to administration of GnRH is also abnormal, with decreased secretion of LH and late-onset and exaggerated of FSH, as occurs during puberal age.

In some patients, there is also the loss of the counter regulation positive mechanism of estrogen, with absence of response to clomiphene administration.

The regression of the regulation of hypothalamus-pituitary-gonads axis causes anovulation and the presence of multiple follicular cysts, with an anatomic, functional, and ecographic patterns similar to those observed in puberal years. The altered gonadotropinic secretory pattern has a relative importance in clinical practice, but is very interesting in the biological field. According to the hypothesis formulated by Frisch and Revelle, the menarche would coincide with the achievement of a "critical weight" and a "critical ratio between adipose tissue and body weight." The achievement of these critical levels would represent the trigger moment of the puberal phenomena through an increase of steroid metabolism in the adipose tissue and a modification of hypothalamic responsiveness to gonadal steroids. In the patients with anorexia nervosa, the loss of weight and fat mass under "critical levels" would trigger the "regression" of secretory regulation of gonadotropins as occurs typically in first steps of puberty [79].

However, the mechanisms are far more complex; due to its importance, this topic is particularly addressed in Chapter 3.

7. Other Pituitary Hormones

There are no descriptions about relevant alterations of PRL secretion. However, the changes in prolactin secretion are almost the same in male and female patients. Studies performed in different periods confirm this normality in PRL [80-82].

Some interesting data concern neurohypophysis, the posterior lobe of pituitary gland, site of production of vasopressin (antidiuretic hormone, ADH) and oxytocin (OX); it is a problem with clinical relevance since in about one-third of the cases, there is a partial insipid diabetes, which can be corrected by ADH administration.

AN patients frequently show defects in osmoregulation and urinary concentration or dilution with inappropriate secretion of antidiuretic hormone, which may be due to intrinsic defects in the neurohypophysis or to abnormalities of its regulatory afferent neurons [83].

The group of Demitrack [84] has demonstrated peripheral osmoregulatory defects in underweight anorexics, coupled with hypersecretion of AVP into the cerebrospinal fluid (CSF). Conversely, a relative reduction of CSF OX is seen in underweight anorexics. Speculatively, these reciprocal changes in neurohypophyseal peptides in the underweight anorexic may enhance the observed neuroendocrine and cognitive abnormalities. In addition, the alterations in CSF OX may occur as a consequence of the abnormal gastrointestinal function present during the acute stages of anorexia nervosa. An augmented cerebrospinal fluid level of AVP was confirmed in further studies [85].

Conflicting results suggest also that the disorder may be related to hypothalamic dysfunction and/or a primary renal defect. Particularly, AN patients are characterized by abnormal osmoregulation at baseline and a lack of reactivity of ADH with a significant urinary concentrating defect after water deprivation. The origin of these defects in AN patients is probably multifactorial, but the duration of the disease and the prescription of antidepressants, which are increasingly prescribed in AN patients, could play a role [86]. Other studies hypothesised that hypothalamic-pituitary-adrenal (HPA) axis hyperactivity in anorexia nervosa (AN) is associated with: (a) elevated arginine vasopressin (AVP) activity, and (b) enhanced pituitary sensitivity to AVP, as it is in depressive illness; thus, contrary to the hypotheses, these studies did not find: (a) evidence of upregulated AVP activity, or (b) enhanced pituitary sensitivity to AVP in AN. Probably these findings suggest that the mechanism of HPA axis hyperactivity differs in depression and AN, with greater involvement of AVP in depressive disorder and perhaps more reliance on CRH to drive the axis in AN. Underweight patients with anorexia nervosa have abnormally high levels of centrally directed AVP and reduced OX levels. These modifications could enhance the retention of cognitive distortions of aversive consequences of eating [87].

Moreover [88], magnetic resonance imaging (MRI) of the brain was used to examine the morphology and dimensions of the pituitary gland in 18 patients with eating disorders (eight anorexics and ten bulimics), in comparison with 13 healthy volunteers; measurements revealed that the anorexics and bulimics had smaller pituitary gland cross-sectional areas ($p < 0.05$) and smaller pituitary gland heights, compared with healthy controls. These preliminary findings in anorexics and bulimics could be suggestive of pituitary atrophy secondary to nutritional or endocrine alterations rather than a primary pituitary pathology.

It has been identified [89] that a majority of patients with AN and bulimia nervosa (BN), as well as some control subjects, display autoantibodies (autoAbs) reacting with alpha-melanocyte-stimulating hormone (alpha-MSH) or adrenocorticotropic hormone, melanocortin peptides involved in appetite control and the stress response. In addition to previously identified neuropeptide autoAbs, further study revealed the presence of autoAbs reacting with OX or AVP in both patients and controls. Analysis of serum levels of identified autoAbs showed an increase of IgM autoAbs against alpha-MSH, OX, and AVP, as well as of IgG autoAbs against AVP in AN patients when compared with BN patients and controls. Further, it has been found that there are significantly altered correlations between alpha-MSH autoAb levels and the total Eating Disorder Inventory-2 score, as well as most of its subscale dimensions in AN and BN patients vs. controls. Remarkably, these correlations were opposite in AN vs. BN patients. In contrast, levels of autoAbs reacting with adrenocorticotropic hormone, OX, or AVP had only few altered correlations with the Eating Disorder Inventory-2 subscale dimensions in AN and BN patients. Thus, these data seem to reveal that core psychobehavioral abnormalities characteristic for eating disorders correlate with the levels of autoAbs against alpha-MSH, suggesting that AN and BN may be associated with autoAb-mediated dysfunctions of primarily the melanocortin system.

8. LEPTIN

Due to its importance both in appetite regulation and in reproductive systems, we mainly describe this hormone, also called adipocytokine, for its source and chemical structure. Other adipocytokines are described in Chapter 2.

Leptin is a proteic hormone synthesized by adipose tissue, involved in the regulation of food intake and energy expenditure; its primary target is the hypothalamus [5]. Leptin, acting at this level, causes a decrease in appetite, which, in turn, results in weight loss and activation of the gonadal axis by stimulation of GnRH secretion.

Leptin physiology and action has been recently reviewed [90]. Leptin mRNA is expressed in white adipose tissue, stomach, placenta, and mammary gland, and encodes a 167 amino acid protein, that is a member of the longchain helical cytokine family. Leptin circulates in plasma both in the free and bound form; its levels show a significant circadian and ultradian variation. Serum leptin levels are closely associated with the amount of adipose stores as well as short-term energy balance. Apart from the composition of the diet, hormonal factors regulate leptin levels, too: insulin levels increase; activation of the adrenergic system reduces leptin mRNA expression and circulating levels; the effect of glucocorticoids remains controversial. Moreover, several cytokines, such as tumor necrosis factor α (TNFα) and interleukins 1 and 6, alter serum leptin levels. Finally, women have higher leptin levels than men, because of either their different body fat distribution or the inducing effects of estrogen/progesterone combined with the suppressive effect of androgens. Leptin acts by binding to specific leptin receptors in the brain and activating the JAK-STAT system (JAK-signal transducer and activator of transcription), which results in altered expression of many hypothalamic neuropeptides. Altered expression of neuropeptide Y (NPY), and possibly other neuropeptides, by leptin results in changes of energy homeostasis and activation of several neuroendocrine axes, including the hypothalamic-pituitary-gonadal axis. The fact that leptin receptors are also expressed in peripheral tissues, including ovaries, has been interpreted as a suggestion of a direct effect of leptin in the gonads, but the physiologic significance of gonadal leptin receptors has not yet been fully elucidated.

Different reports have been published on leptin in eating disorders (see review, ref. 91). Serum leptin levels in anorexia nervosa and nonspecific eating disorders are low but similar to those of healthy subjects with comparable BMI. However, patients with anorexia nervosa appear to have more efficient transport of leptin to the CSF at lower serum leptin concentrations and have normalization of the CSF and serum leptin levels before the BMI returns to normal. These findings may explain the difficulty patients with anorexia nervosa have in gaining weight and may provide the underlying mechanism for the neuroendocrine abnormalities seen in patients with anorexia nervosa or strenuously exercising women.

Mutational analysis of the coding region and part of the promoter region of the leptin gene in patients with AN has yielded negative results, suggesting that involvement of this gene in the etiology of AN is unlikely (see review, ref. 6).

Effects of leptin on hypothalamic-pituitary gonadal axis are described in Chapter 3.

9. INSULIN

Insulin, produced by beta-cells of pancreatic islets, is the main hormone regulating glucose metabolism, promoting both its oxidation to produce energy and storage in the liver and muscle glycogen. It is also fundamental for tissue aminoacid uptake and protein synthesis. Since it is stimulated by glucose, aminoacids, and gastrointestinal hormones, it is not strange that its circulating levels are low in AN. Fat mass is related with insulin levels (as well as leptin) [92].

However, data on insulin sensitivity (IS) are conflicting. Original data showed an impaired glucose tolerance after oral glucose test [93]. Then, different studies reported normal [94], enhanced [95,96], or decreased [97] insulin-stimulated glucose disposal. These discrepancies can be due to the method employed for evaluating insulin sensitivity. By hyperinsulinemic-euglycemic clamp, glucose disposal has been reported normal [94], varied [98], or decreased [99]; using a minimal model by frequently sampled intravenous glucose tolerance test, an increased insulin-sensitivity has been hypothesized [95]. The simple index HOMA (homeostasis model assessment) suggested an increased insulin sensitivity in most studies [100-103]. A recent study showed a negative correlation between insulin and adiponectin (Apn) (an adipocytokine, see Chapter 2), suggesting that hyperadiponectinemia can be responsible for this phenomenon. This hypothesis is supported by data in mice, showing an insulin-sensitizing effect of adiponectin administration [104], even if, on the other side, it has been shown that in vitro, Apn gene expression is reversibly down-regulated by insulin [105]. Other authors hypothesized that hyperadiponectinemia might represent a compensatory mechanism for the reduced insulin-stimulated glucose metabolism [99].

However, the extremely low fat mass in AN may alter the expected correlations between fat mass, insulin, HOMA index and adiponectin [106]. Other factors causing an uncoupling between Apn and insulin-mediated glucose metabolism include some cytokines, such as TNF-α [107].

When considering oxidative and non-oxidative glucose metabolism, as in the cited study of Panacciulli [99], using hyperinsulinemic-euglycemic glucose clamp together with indirect calorimetry during the last 60 minutes of the insulin clamp, interesting data were obtained. In fact, a prevalent impairment of non-oxidative glucose metabolism (which represents more than 90% storage of glucose as glycogen in muscle) was shown, according to the data of lower glycogen concentration in muscle of AN patients [108]. Therefore, we can maintain the concept of a reduced insulin sensitivity referring to non-oxidative pathway, as commonly observed in starvation. Such an insulin resistance could be compensatory for energy deprivation, directing glucose toward immediate utilization rather than storage.

Other possible factors influencing IS are: the activity of sympathoadrenal system [109] through the up- or down-regulation of Apn production; the increased activity was shown in vivo in subcutaneous abdominal adipose tissue of AN [110]; an excess of growth hormone and cortisol may also account for the altered glucose tolerance.

10. Conclusions

The complex interplay between orexigenic and anorexigenic transmitters and hormones is surely altered in AN, but it is difficult to establish the etiological role of this phenomenon. Similarly, different hormonal alterations, including hypogonadotropic hypogonadism, hypercortisolemia, growth hormone resistance, "sick euthyroid syndrome," and low leptin and insulin secretion, are observed as consequences of starvation, but can play a role in a vicious circle that can cause progressive malnutrition until the final stage of cachexia, and ultimately, death for damage of multiple organ and systems, if a therapeutic approach is not started.

References

[1] Walsh, Timothy B., Eating disorders. In: Braunwald, E; Fauci, AS; Kasper, DL; Hauser, SL; Longo, DL; Jameson, JL, Editors. *Harrison's Principles of Internal Medicine,* 15th ed. New York: McGraw-Hill, 2001, 486-490.

[2] Krassas, GE. Endocrine abnormalities in anorexia nervosa. *Pediatr Endocrinol Rev,* 2003, 1, 46-54.

[3] Burt, AM. Autonomic nervous system and hypothalamus. In: Burt, AM, editor. *Textbook of neuroanatomy*. Philadelphia: W.B. Saunders Company, 1993.

[4] Manni, E. Diencefalo. In: Rindi, G.; Manni, E; editors. Fisiologia umana. Torino: *UTET,* 2001, 280-282.

[5] Valassi, E; Scacchi, M; Cavagnini, F., Neuroendocrine control of food intake. *Nutr Metab Cardiovasc Dis,* 2008, 18, 158-168.

[6] Munoz, MT & Argente, J. Anorexia nervosa in female adolescents: endocrine and bone mineral density disturbances. *Eur J Endocrinol,* 2002, 147, 275-286.

[7] Gerald, C; Walker, AW; Criscione, L; Gustaffson, EL; Batzl-Hartman, C; Smith, E; Vaysse, P; Durkin, MM; Laz, TM; Linemeyer, DL; Schaffhauser, AO; Whitebre, AD; Hofbauer, KG; Taber, RI; Branchek, TA, Weinshank, RL. A receptor subtype involved in neuropeptide-Y induced food intake. *Nature,* 1996, 382, 168-171.

[8] Rosenkranz, K; Hinney, A; Ziegler, A; von Prittwitz, S; Barth, N; Roth, H; Mayer, H; Siegfried, W; Lehmkuhl, G; Poutska, F; Schmidt, M, Schafer H, Remschmidt, H, Hebebrand, J. Screening for mutations in the neuropeptide YY5 receptor gene in cohorts belonging to different weight extremes. *Int J Obes Rel Metab Dis,* 1998, 22, 157-163.

[9] Sakurai, T; Amemiya, A; Ishii, M; Matsuzaki, T; Chemelli, RM; Tamaka, H; Williams, SC; Richardson, JA; Kozlowski, GP; Wilson, S; Arch, JR; Buckingham, RE; Haynes, AC; Carr, SA; Annan, RS; McNulty, DE; Liu, WS; Terrett, JA; Elshourbagy, NA; Bergsma, DJ; Yanagisawa, M. Orexins and orexin receptors: a family of hypothalamic

neuropeptides and G protein-coupled receptors that regulate feeding behavior. *Cell,* 1998, 92, 573-585.

[10] Fan, W; Boston, B; Kesterson, R; Hruby, V; Cone, R. Role of melanocortinergic neurons in feeding and the agouti obesity syndrome. *Nature,* 1997, 385, 165-168.

[11] Hinney, A; Schmidt, A; Nottebom, K; Heibitt, O; Becker, I; Ziegler, A; Gerber, G; Sina, M; Gorg, T; Mayer, H; Siegfried, W; Fichter, M; Remschmidt, H, Hebebrand, J. Several mutations in the melanocortin-4 receptor gene including a nonsense and frame shift mutation associated with dominantly inherited obesity in humans. *J Clin Endocrinol Metab,* 1999, 84, 1483-1486.

[12] Hinney, A; Remschmidt, H; Hebebrand, J. Candidate gene polymorphism in eating disorders. *Eur J Pharmacol,* 2000, 410, 147-159.

[13] Kaye, WH & Weltzin, T. Serotonin activity in anorexia nervosa and bulimia nervosa. Relationship to the modulation of feeding and mood. *J Clin Psychiatry,* 1991, 52 (Suppl), 41-48.

[14] Halford, JC & Blundell, JE. Separate systems for serotonin and leptin in appetite control. *Ann Med* 2000, 32, 222-232.

[15] Collier, DA; Arranz, MJ; Li, T; Mupita, D; Brown, N; Treasure, J. Association between 5-HT2A gene promoter polymorphism and anorexia nervosa. *Lancet,* 1997, 350, 412.

[16] Enoch, MA; Kaye, WH; Rotondo, A; Greenberg, BD; Murphy, DL; Goldman, D. 5-HT2A promoter polymorphism-1438 G/A, anorexia nervosa, and obsessive-compulsive disorder. *Lancet,* 1998, 351, 1785-1786.

[17] Ziegler, A; Hebebrand, J; Gorg, T; Rosenkranz, K; Fichter, M; Herpertz-Dahlamam, B; Remschmidt, H; Hinney, A. Further lack of association between the 5-HT2A gene promoter polymorphism and susceptibility to eating disorders and a meta-analysis pertaining to anorexia nervosa. *Mol Psychiatr,* 1999, 4, 410-412.

[18] Nacmias, B; Ricca, V; Tedde, A; Mezzani, B; Rotella, C.M; Sorbi, S. 5-HT2A receptor gene polymorphism in anorexia nervosa and bulimia nervosa. *Neurosci Lett,* 1999, 277, 134-136.

[19] Aubert, R; Betonlla, D; Herbeth, B; Siest, G.; Fumaron, F. 5-HT2A receptor gene polymorphism is associated with food and alcohol intake in obese people. *Int J Obes Rel Metab Dis*, 2000, 24, 920-924.

[20] Spigset, O; Andersen, T; Hagg, S; Mjondal, T. Enhanced platelet serotonin 5-HT2A receptor binding in anorexia nervosa and bulimia nervosa. *Eur Neuropsychopharmacol,* 1999, 9, 469-473.

[21] Baranowska, B; Wolinska-Witort, E; Wasilewska-Dziubinska, E; Roguski, K; Martynska, L; Chmielowska, M. The role of neuropeptides in the disturbed control of appetite and hormone secretion in eating disorders. *Neuroendocrinol Lett,* 2003, 24, 431-434.

[22] Zakrzewska, KE; Cusin, I; Sainsbury, A; Rohner-Jeansenaud, F; Jeansenaud, B. Glucocorticoids as contraregulatory hormones of leptin: towards an understanding of leptin resistance. *Diabetes,* 1997, 46, 717-719.

[23] Schwartz, MW; Seeley, RJ; Campfeld, LA; Burn, P; Baskin, DG. Cerebral nervous system control of food intake. *Nature,* 2000, 404, 661-671.

[24] Kaye, WH; Berrettini, NH; Gwirstmann, HE; Gold, PW; Jimerson, DC; Ebert, MH. Contribution of CNS neuropeptide (NPY, CRH and beta-endorphin) alterations to

psychophysiological abnormalities in anorexia nervosa. *Psychopharmacol Bull,* 1989, 25, 433-438.

[25] Naisberg, Y; Modai, I; Weizman, A. Metabolic bioenergy homeostatic disruption: a cause of anorexia nervosa. *Med Hypotheses,* 2001, 56, 454-461.

[26] Usdan, LS; Khaodhiar, L; Apovian, CM. The endocrinopathies of anorexia nervosa. *Endocr Pract,* 2008, 14, 1055-1063.

[27] Jimerson, DC & Wolfe, BE. Neuropeptides in eating disorders. *CNS Spectr*, 2004, 9, 516-522.

[28] Morpurgo, PS; Sartorio, A; Travaglini, P. Patologia della massa grassa. In: Faglia G., editor. *Malattie del Sistema Endocrino e del Metabolismo.* Milano: McGraw-Hill, 2002, 499-522.

[29] Scacchi, M; Pincelli, AI; Cavagnini, F. Nutritional status in the neuroendocrine control of growth hormone secretion: the model of anorexia nervosa. *Front Neuroendocrinol,* 2003, 24, 200-224.

[30] Scacchi, M; Pincelli AI; Caumo, A; Tomasi, P; Delitala, G; Baldi, G; Cavagnini, F. Spontaneous nocturnal growth hormone secretion in anorexia nervosa. *J Clin Endócrinol Metab,* 1997, 82, 3225-3229.

[31] Argente, J; Caballo, N; Barrios, V; Munoz, MT; Pozo, J; Chowen, JA, Morandé, G; Hernandez, M. Multiple endocrine abnormalities of the growth hormone and insulin-like growth factor axis in patients with anorexia nervosa: effect of short- and long-term weight recuperation. *J Clin Endocrinol Metab,* 1997, 82, 2084-2092.

[32] Stoving, RK; Veldhuis, JD; Flyvbjerg, A; Vinten, J; Hangaard, J; Koldkjaer, OG; Kristiansen, J; Hagen, C. Jointly amplified basal and pulsatile growth hormone (GH) secretion and increased process irregularity in women with anorexia nervosa: indirect evidence for disruption of feedback regulation within the GH-insulin-like growth factor I axis. *J Clin Endocrinol Metab,* 1999, 84, 2056-2063.

[33] Genazzani, AD; Petraglia, F; Gastaldi, M; Gamba, O; Corazza, F; D'Ambrogio, G; Genazzani, AR. Growth hormone (GH)-releasing hormone-induced growth hormone-induced GH response in hypothalamic amenorrhea: evidence of altered central neuromodulation. *Fertil Steril,* 1996, 65, 935-938.

[34] De Marinis, L; Folli, G; D'amico, C; Mancini, A; Sambo, P; Tofani, A; Oradei, A; Barbarino, A. Differential effects of feeding on the ultradian variation of the growth hormone (GH) response to GH-releasing hormone in normal subjects and patients with obesity and anorexia nervosa. *J Clin Endocrinol Metab,* 1988, 66, 598-604.

[35] De Marinis, L; Mancini, A; D'amico, C; Zuppi, P; Tofani, A; Della Casa, S; Saporosi, A; Sambo, P; Fiumara, C; Calabrò, F; Barbarino, A. Influence of naloxone infusion on prolactin and growth hormone response to growth hormone-releasing hormone in anorexia nervosa. *Psychoneuroendocrinology,* 1991, 16, 499-504.

[36] Nussbaum, MP; Blethen, SL; Chasalow, FL; Jacobson, MS; Shenker, IR; Feldman, J. Blunted growth hormone responses to clonidine in adolescent girls with anorexia nervosa. Evidence for an early hypothalamic defect. *J Adolesc Health Care,* 1990, 11, 145-148.

[37] Scacchi, M; Invitti, C; Pincelli, AI; Pandolfi, C; Dubini, A; Cavagnini, F. Lack of growth hormone response to acute administration of dexamethasone in anorexia nervosa. *Eur J Endocrinol,* 1995, 132, 152-158.

[38] Giusti, M; Foppiani, L; Ponzani, P; Cuttica, CM; Falivene, RM; Valenti, S. Hexarelin is a stronger GH-releasing peptide than GHRH in normal cycling women but not in anorexia nervosa. *J Endocrinol Invest,* 1997, 20, 257-263.

[39] Gianotti, L; Lanfranco, F; Ramunni, J; Destefanis, S; Ghigo, E; Arvat, E. GH/IGF-I axis in anorexia nervosa. *Eat Weight Disord,* 2002, 7, 94-105.

[40] Mancini, A; De Marinis, L; Fabrizi, ML; Conte, G; Iacona, T; La Rosa, C; Daini, S. Correlation of growth hormone dynamics and personality or affective patterns in anorexia nervosa: preliminary data. In: Cuzzolaro, M; Caputo, G; Guidetti, V; Ripa di Meana, G, Editors. Advances in Diagnosis and Treatment of Anorexia, Bulimia and Obesity. *Firenze: Promo Leader Service,* 1993, 415-419.

[41] Cummings, E; Purnell, JQ; Frayo, SR; Schmidova, K; Wisse, BE; Weigle, DS. A pre-prandial rise in plasma ghrelin levels suggests a role in meal initiation in humans. *Diabetes,* 2001, 50, 1714-1719.

[42] Otto, B; Cuntz, U; Fruehauf, E; Wawaarta, R; Folwaczny,,C; Riepl, RL; Heiman, ML; Lehnert, P; Fichter, M; Tschop, M. Weight gain decreases elevated plasma ghrelin concentrations of patients with anorexia nervosa. *Eur J Endocrinol,* 2001, 145, 669-673.

[43] Plata-Salaman, R. Leptin, anorexia nervosa, and anorexia of acute and chronic disease. *Nutrition,* 1999, 15, 943-945.

[44] Hashizume, K; Suzuki, S; Komatsu, A; Hiramatsu, K; Mori, J; Yamazaki, M; Takeda, T; Kakizawa, T; Miyamoto, T; Koizumi, Y; Ichikawa, K. Administration of recombinant human growth hormone normalizes GH-IGF1 axis and improves malnutrition-related disorders in patients with anorexia nervosa. *Endocr J,* 2007, 54, 319-327.

[45] De Groot, LJ. "Non-thyroidal illness syndrome" is a manifestation of hypothalamic-pituitary dysfunction, and in view of current evidence, should be treated with appropriate replacement therapies. *Critical Care Clinical,* 2006, 22, 57-86.

[46] Kiyohara, K; Tamai, H; Takaichi, Y; Nakagawa, T; Kumagai, LF. Decreased thyroidal triiodothyronine secretion in patients with anorexia nervosa: influence of weight recovery. *Am J Clin Nutr,* 1989, 50, 767-772.

[47] Méndez JP, Garcia E, Salinas JL, Pérez-Palacios G, Ulloa-Aguirre A. Anorexia nervosa: endocrine function during the phases of body weight loss and recovery. *Rev Invest Clin*, 1989, 41, 337-344.

[48] Leslie, RD; Isaacs, AJ; Gomez, J; Raggat, PR; Bayliss, R. Hypothalamo-pituitary-thyroid function in anorexia nervosa: influence of weight gain. *Br Med J,* 1978, 2, 526-528.

[49] Støving, RK; Bennedbaek, FN; Hegedüs, L; Hagen, C. Evidence of diffuse atrophy of the thyroid gland in patients with anorexia nervosa. *Int J Eat Disord,* 2001, 29, 230-235.

[50] Cheung, NW & Boyages, SC. The thyroid gland in acromegaly: an ultrasonographic study. *Clin Endocrinol,* 1997, 46, 545-549.

[51] Takahashi, S; Conti, M; Prokop, C; Van Wyk, JJ; Earp, HS 3rd. Thyrotropin and insulin-like growth factor I regulation of tyrosine phosphorylation in FRTL-5 cells. Interaction between cAMP-dependent and growth factor-dependent signal transduction. *J Biol Chem,* 1991, 266, 7834-7841.

[52] Mathieson, RA; Walberg, JL; Gwazdauskas, FC; Hinkle, DE; Gregg, JM. The effect of varying carbohydrate content of a very-low-caloric diet on resting metabolic rate and thyroid hormones. *Metabolism,* 1986, 35, 394-398.

[53] Krahn, DD; Rock, C; Dechert, RE; Nairn, KK; Hasse, SA. Changes in resting energy expenditure and body composition in anorexia nervosa patients during re-feeding. *J Am Diet Assoc,* 1993, 93, 434-438.

[54] Ortiga-Carvalho, TM; Oliveira, KJ; Soares, BA; Pazos-Moura, CC. The role of leptin in the regulation of TSH secretion in the fed state: in vivo and in vitro studies. *J Endocrinol,* 2002, 174, 121-125.

[55] Mantzoros, CS; Ozata, M; Negrao, AB; Suchard, MA; Ziotopoulou, M; Caglayan, S; Elashoff, RM; Cogswell, RJ; Negro, P; Liberty, V; Wong, ML; Veldhuis, J; Ozdemir, IC; Gold, PW; Flier, JS; Licinio, J. Synchronicity of frequently sampled thyrotropin (TSH) and leptin concentrations in healthy adults and leptin-deficient subjects: evidence for possible partial TSH regulation by leptin in humans. *J Clin Endocrinol Metab,* 2001, 86, 3284-3291.

[56] Pauly, RP; Lear, SA; Hastings, FC; Birmingham, CL. Resting energy expenditure and plasma leptin levels in anorexia nervosa during acute re-feeding. *Int J Eat Disord,* 2000, 28, 231-234.

[57] Escobar, L; Freire, JM; Espinosa, R; Pajares, M; Girón, JA; Vázquez, JM; Chover, A; Carrasco, M; Ortero, J; Gavilán, I; Segura, E; Aguilar, M. Determination of insulin, leptin and neuropeptide y by radioimmunoanalysis in patients with morbid obesity and anorexia nervosa after therapeutic intervention. *Rev Esp Med Nucl,* 2002, 21, 3-11.

[58] Boswell, EB; Anfinson, TJ; Nemeroff, CB. Depression associated with endocrine disorders. In: Robertson MM; Katona CLE, editors. *Depression and physical illness.* Chichester: Wiley; 1997, 2255-2292.

[59] Kiriike, N; Nishiwaki, S; Izumiya, Y; Maeda, Y; Kawakita, Y. Thyrotropin, prolactin, and growth hormone responses to thyrotropin-releasing hormone in anorexia nervosa and bulimia. *Biol Psychiatry,* 1987, 22, 167-176.

[60] Mori, M; Murakami, M; Satoh, T; Miyashita, K; Iriuchijima, T; Yamada, M; Inukai, T; Kobayashi, I. A possible direct precursor of thyrotropin-releasing hormone, pGlu-His-Pro Gly, stimulates prolactin secretion in anorexia nervosa. *J Clin Endocrinol Metab,* 1990, 71, 252-255.

[61] Joffe, RT. The use of thyroid supplements to augment antidepressant medication. *J Clin Psychiatry,* 1998, 59 (Suppl 5), 26-29.

[62] Tsigos, C & Chrousos, GP. Hypothalamic-pituitary-adrenal axis, neuroendocrine factors and stress. *J Psychosom Res,* 2002, 53, 865–871.

[63] Kyrou, I; Chrousos, GP; Tsigos, C. Stress, visceral obesity, and metabolic complications. *Ann N Y Acad Sci,* 2006, 1083, 77–110.

[64] Kyrou, I & Tsigos, C. Stress mechanisms and metabolic complications. *Horm Metab Res,* 2007, 39, 430–438.

[65] Pasquali, R; Vicennati, V; Cacciari, M; Pagotto, U. The hypothalamic-pituitary-adrenal axis activity in obesity and the metabolic syndrome. *Ann N Y Acad Sci,* 2006, 1083, 111–128.

[66] Lo Sauro, C; Ravaldi, C; Cabras, PL; Faravelli, C; Ricca, V. Stress, Hypothalamic-Pituitary-Adrenal Axis and Eating Disorders. *Neuropsychobiology,* 2008, 57, 95–115.

[67] Mastorakos, G & Zapanti, E. The hypothalamic-pituitary-adrenal axis in the neuroendocrine regulation of food intake and obesity: the role of corticotropin releasing hormone. *Nutr Neurosci,* 2004, 7, 271–280.

[68] Charmandari E, Tsigos C, Chrousos G. Endocrinology of the stress response. Annu Rev Physiol, 2005, 67, 259-284.

[69] Wals, BT; Katz, JL; Levin, J; Kream, J; Fukushima, DK; Weiner, H; Zumoff, B. The production rate of cortisol declines during recovery from anorexia nervosa. *J Clin Endocrinol Metab,* 1981, 53, 203–205.

[70] Gwirtsman, HE; Kaye, WH; George, DT; Jimerson, DC; Ebert, MH; Gold, PW. Central and peripheral ACTH and cortisol levels in anorexia nervosa and bulimia. *Arch Gen Psychiatry,* 1989, 46, 61–69.

[71] Misra, M; Miller, KK; Almazan, C; Ramaswamy, K; Lapcharoensap, W; Worley, M; Neubauer, G; Herzog, DB; Klibanski, A. Alterations in cortisol secretory dynamics in adolescent girls with anorexia nervosa and effects on bone metabolism. *J Clin Endocrinol Metab,* 2004, 89, 4972–4980.

[72] Connan, F; Lightman, SL; Landau, S; Wheeler, M; Treasure, J; Campbell, IC. An investigation of hypothalamic-pituitary-adrenal axis hyperactivity in anorexia nervosa: the role of CRH and AVP. *J Psychiatr Res,* 2006, 41, 131–143.

[73] Putignano, P; Dubini, A; Toja, P; Invitti, C; Bonfanti, S; Redaelli, G; Zappulli, D; Cavagnini, F. Salivary cortisol measurement in normal-weight, obese and anorexic women: comparison with plasma cortisol. *Eur J Endocrinol,* 2001, 145, 165–171.

[74] Schweitzer, I; Szmukler, GI; Maguire, KP; Harrison, LC; Tuckwell, V; Davies, BM. The dexamethasone suppression test in anorexia nervosa: the influence of weight, depression, adrenocorticotrophic hormone and dexamethasone. *Br J Psychiatry,* 1990, 157, 713–717.

[75] Fichter, MM & Pirke, KM. Effect of experimental and pathological weight loss upon the hypothalamo-pituitary-adrenal axis. *Psychoneuroendocrinology,* 1986, 11, 295–305.

[76] Scantamburlo, G; Ansseau, M; Legros, JJ. Role of the neurohypophysis in psychological stress. *Encephale,* 2001, 27, 245–259.

[77] Herpertz-Dahlmann, B & Remschmidt, H. The prognostic value of the dexamethasone suppression test for the course of anorexia nervosa – comparison with depressive diseases. *Z Kinder Jugendpsychiatr*, 1990, 18, 5–11.

[78] Walsh, BT; Roose, SP; Katz, JL; Dyrenfurth, I; Wright, L; Vande Wiele, R; Glassman, AH. Hypothalamic-pituitary-adrenal-cortical activity in anorexia nervosa and bulimia. *Psychoneuroendocrinology,* 1987, 12, 131–140.

[79] Cantalamessa, E; Baldini, M. Malattie ipotalamo-ipofisarie. In: Rugarli, C; Editor. *Medicina interna sistematica,* IV ed. Milano: Masson, 2000, 1021-1053.

[80] Hasegawa, K. Endocrine and reproductive disturbances in anorexia nervosa and bulimia nervosa. *Nippon Rinsho,* 2001, 59, 549-553.

[81] Codaccioni, JL; Roulier, R; Conte-Devolx, B; Berliner, A. The endocrine status in anorexia nervosa. *Acta Psychiatr Belg,* 1980, 80, 505-526.

[82] De Marinis, L; Mancini, A; D'Amico, C; Passeri, M; Sambo, P; Zuppi, P; Barbarino, A. Plasma prolactin response to GRF 1-44 in acromegaly and anorexia nervosa. In: Molinatti, GM; Martini, L; Editors. *Endocrinology 1985*. Amsterdam: *Excerpta Medica,* 1986, 315-318.

[83] Evrard, F; da Cunha, MP; Lambert, M; Devuyst, O. Impaired osmoregulation in anorexia nervosa: a case-control study. *Nephrol Dial Transplant,* 2004, 19, 3034-3039.

[84] Demitrack, MA; Lesem, MD; Brandt, HA; Pigott, TA; Jimerson, DC; Altemus, M; Gold, PW. Neurohypophyseal dysfunction: implications for the pathophysiology of eating disorders. *Psycopharmacol Bull,* 1989, 25: 439-443.

[85] Frank, GK; Kaye, WH; Altemus, M; Greeno, CG. CSF oxytocin and vasopressin levels after recovery from bulimia nervosa and anorexia nervosa, bulimic subtype. *Biol Psychiatry,* 2000 48, 315-318.

[86] Connan, F; Lightman, SL; Landau, S; Wheeler, M; Treasure, J; Campbell, IC. An investigation of hypothalamic-pituitary-adrenal axis hyperactivity in anorexia nervosa: the role of CRH and AVP. *J Psychiatr Res,* 2007, 41, 131-143.

[87] Gibbs DM. Vasopressin and oxytocin: hypothalamic modulators of the stress response:a review. *Psychoneuroendocrinology*, 1986, 11, 131-139.

[88] Doraiswamy, PM; Krishnan, KR; Figiel, GS; Husain, MM; Boyko, OB; Rockwell, WJ; Ellinwood, EH Jr. A brain magnetic resonance imaging study of pituitary gland morphology in anorexia nervosa and bulimia. *Biol Psychiatry,* 1990, 28, 110-116.

[89] Fetissov, SO; Harro, J; Jaanisk, M; Järv, A; Podar, I; Allik, J; Nilsson, I; Sakthivel, P; Lefvert, AK; Hökfelt, T. Autoantibodies against neuropeptides are associated with psychological traits in eating disorders. *Proc Natl Acad Sci,* 2005, 102, 14865-14870.

[90] Mantzoros, CS. Role of leptin in reproduction. *Ann N Y Acad Sci,* 2000, 900, 174-183.

[91] Heberbrand, J; Blum, W; Barth, N; Coners, H; Englaro, P; Juul, A; Ziegler, A; Warnke, A; Rascher, W; Remschmidt, H. Leptin levels in patients with anorexia nervosa are reduced in the acute stage and elevated upon short-term weight restoration. *Mol Psychiatry,* 1997, 2, 330–334.

[92] Kadowaki T, Yamauchi T, Kubota N, Hara K, Ueki K, Tobe K. Adiponectin and adiponectin receptors in insulin resistance, diabetes and the metabolic syndrome. *J Clin Invest,* 2006, 116: 1784-1792.

[93] Franssila-Kallunki, A; Rissanen, A; Ekstrand, A; Eriksson, J; Saloranta, C; Widen, E; Schalin-Jantti, C; Goop, L. Fuel metabolism in anorexia nervosa and simple obesity. *Metabolism,* 1991, 40, 689-694.

[94] Castillo, M; Scheen, A; Lefebvre, PJ; Luyckx, AS. Insulin-stimulated glucose disposal is not increased in anorexia nervosa. *J Clin Endocrinol Metab,* 1985, 60, 311-314.

[95] Fukushima, M; Nakai, Y; Taniguchi, A; Imura, H; Nagata, I; Tokuyama, K. Insulin sensitivity, insulin secretion, and glucose effectiveness in anorexia nervosa: a minimal model analysis. *Metabolism,* 1993, 42, 1164-1168.

[96] Kubota, S; Tamai, H; Ishimoto-Goto, J; Nozaki, T; Kobayashi, N; Matsubayashi, S; Nakagawa, T; Aoki, TT. Carbohydrate oxidation rates in patients with anorexia nervosa. *Metabolism,* 1993, 42, 1164-1168.

[97] Gniuli D, Liverani E, Capristo E, Greco AV, Mingrone G. Blunted glucose metabolism in anorexia nervosa. *Metabolism Clin Exper*, 2001, 50, 876-881.

[98] Kiriike, A; Nishiwaki, S; Nagata, T; Okuno, Y; Yamada, J; Tanaka, S; Fujii, A; Kawakita, Y. Insulin sensitivity in patients with anorexia nervosa and bulimia. *Acta Psychiatr Scand,* 1990, 81, 236-239.

[99] Panacciulli, N; Vettor, R; Milan, G; Granzotto, M; Catucci, A; Federspil, G; De Giacomo, P; Giorgino, R; De Pergola, G. Anorexia nervosa is characterized by

increased adiponectin plasma levels and reduced nonoxidative glucose metabolism. *J Clin Endocrinol Metab,* 2003, 88, 1748-1752.

[100] Delporte, ML; Brichard, SM; Hermans, MP; Beguin, C; Lambert, M. Hypoadiponectinemia is associated with ischemic cerebrovascular disease. *Arterioscler Thromb Vasc Biol,* 2005, 25: 821-826.

[101] Misra, M; Miller, KK; Almazan, C; Ramaswamy, K; Aggarwal, A; Herzog, DB; Neubauer, G; Breu, J; Klibanski, A. Hormonal and body composition predictors of soluble leptin receptor, leptin and free leptin index in adolescent girl with anorexia nervosa and controls and relation to insulin sensitivity. *J Clin Endocrinol Metab,* 2004, 89, 3486-3495.

[102] Housova, J; Anderlova, K; Krizova, J; Haluzikova, D; Kremen, J; Kumstyrova, T; Papezova, H; Haluzik, M. Serum adiponectin and resistin concentrations in patients with restrictive and binge/purge form of anorexia nervosa and bulimia nervosa. *J Clin Endocrinol Metab,* 2005, 90, 1366-1370.

[103] Dostalova, I; Smitka, K; Papezova, H; Kvasnickova, H; Nedvidkova, J. Increased insulin sensitivity in patients with anorexia nervosa: The role of adipocytokines. *Physiol Res,* 2007, 56, 587-594.

[104] Yamauchi, T; Kamon, J; Waki, H; Terauchi, Y; Kubota, N; Hara, K; Mori, Y; Ide, T; Murakami, K; Tsuboyama-Kasaoka, N; Ezaki, O; Akanuma, Y; Gavrilova, O; Vinson, C; Reitman, ML; Kagechika, H; Shudo, K; Yoda, M; Nakano, Y; Tobe, K; Nagai, R; Kimura, S; Tomita, M; Froguel, P; Kadowaki, T. The fat-derived hormone adiponectin reverses insulin resistance associated with both lipoatrophy and obesity. *Nat Med,* 2001, 7, 941-946.

[105] Fasshauer, M; Klein, J; Neumann, S; Eszlinger, N; Paschke, R. Hormonal regulation of adiponectin gene expression in 3T3-L1 adipocytes. *Biochem Biophys Res Commun,* 2002, 290, 1084-1089.

[106] Misra, M; Miller, KK; Cord, J; Prabhakaran, R; Herzog, DB; Goldstein, M; Katzman, DK; Klibanski, A. Relationships between serum adipokines, insulin levels, and bone density in girls with anorexia nervosa. *J Clin Endocrinol Metab,* 2007, 92, 2046-2052.

[107] Hotamisligil, GS; Shargill, NS; Spiegelman, BL. Adipose expression of tumor necrosis factor-α: direct role in obesity-linked insulin resistance. *Science,* 1993, 259, 87-91.

[108] Hoffer LJ. Starvation. In: Shils ME; Young VR, editors. *Modern nutrition in health and disease*. Philadelphia: Lea & Febiger, 1988, 774-794.

[109] Fasshauer, M; Klein, J; Neumann, S; Eszlinger, N; Paschke, R. Adiponection gene expression is inhibited by beta-adrenergic stimulation via protein-kinase A in 3T3-L1 adipocytes. *FEBS Lett,* 2001, 507, 142-146.

[110] Bartak, V; Vybiral, S; Papezova, H; Dostalova, I; Pacak, K; Nedvidkova, J. Basal and exercise-induced sympathetic nervous activity and lipolysis in adipose tissue of patients with anorexia nervosa. *Eur J Clin Invest,* 2004, 34:, 371-377.

In: Anorexia Nervosa: A Multi-Disciplinary Approach ISBN: 978-1-60876-200-2
Editors: A. Mancini, S. Daini, L. Caruana, pp. 31-49

Chapter 2

ANOREXIA NERVOSA AND CYTOKINES

***A. Mancini*[1], *E. Leone*[1], *V. Di Donna*[1], *R. Festa*[2]**
[1]Division of Endocrinology, Catholic University of the Sacred Heart, Rome, Italy
[2]Institute of Clinical Pathology, University "Politecnica delle Marche," Ancona, Italy

ABSTRACT

Cytokines, produced by the immunocompetent system, exhibit strong relationships with nervous and endocrine systems. Therefore, they are object of many studies on eating disorders, in order to establish their causative role or, at least, an involvement in symptoms and clinical course of the disease. Especially IL-1, IL-6, and TNFα are found in increased amounts, but this could reflect a consequence of malnutrition. Other than these molecules, other bioactive molecules synthesized in adipose tissue, acting with endocrine and paracrine ways, and therefore called "adipocytokines," have been investigated. This chapter particularly focuses on adiponectin, which has anti-diabetic, anti-inflammatory, and anti-atherogenic properties. It is surprisingly elevated in anorexia nervosa, despite the low amount of fat tissue, and may contribute to increase insulin sensitivity, though it could have a role in weight loss and hematological complications of the disease.

1. INTRODUCTION

In eating disorders, strong interrelations among the endocrine, nervous, and immune systems do exist. Moreover, it has been postulated that pro-inflammatory cytokines, such as IL-1, IL-6, TNFα, and IFNγ, may play a key role in the pathogenesis of eating disorders [1]. Therefore, this topic is focused upon in this chapter.

Cytokines are peptides produced by many cellular types (above all, by circulating cells of the immune system, such as lymphocytes and activated macrophages, after contacting foreigner pathogens, but also endothelial, epithelial and connectival cells). They are able to exert "hormonal" actions on distant target cells after blood transportation, interacting with specific receptors. Among these activities, a fundamental role is exerted on pituitary-adrenal axis, mainly by interaction with the hypothalamus, in the context of coordinated autonomic, endocrine and behavioural components of the response to acute stimulation. Therefore, neuroimmunology is a term referred to the discipline that studies the interaction between immune and nervous systems [2].

Cytokines produced by mononuclear phagocytes are often called monokines, while those produced by activated lymphocytes are called lymphokines. Moreover, both monocytes and macrophages produce cytokines, as colony-stimulating factors (CSF), stimulating the immature leucocytes growth of the bone marrow. The interleukins (IL) are a wide family of cytokines produced by hemopoietic cells and act, above all, on leucocytes. The chemokines are cytokines able to stimulate the motility (chemokinesis) and the oriented movement (chemotaxis) of leucocytes and are particularly important in inflammation. Many classic growth factors act as cytokines, and, on the other side, many cytokines are able to stimulate the cellular proliferation [3].

2. Cytokines and Eating Disorders

An increased and chronic production of cytokines, such as IL-1, IL-6, TNFα and IFNγ, may favor the catabolic reactions and cachexia observed in cancerous states [4]. Physiopathologist parallels have been made between the role of cytokines in cancerous cachexia and their putative involvement in the undernourished states observed in anorexia nervosa (AN). In fact, in experimental animals, peripherally and centrally secreted or injected IL-1, IL-6 and TNFα induce changes in neurochemical, behavioral and physiological parameters, which are the same also observed in AN [5]. TNFα, which is known as cachectin, also mediates weight loss in rats and has been proposed as a mediator of appetite suppression [6]. Holden and Pakula have proposed a model based on a bio-clinical relationship between stress, anxiety state and AN, grounded on a continuum of the same cytokine profile. The biological response common to each of these disorders could be an up-regulation of IL-1 and TNFα and a down-regulation of the major type-1 cytokines (IFNγ, IL-2) [7].

Mechanisms of Cytokine-induced Anorexia

A growing body of evidence suggests that pro-inflammatory cytokines have direct and indirect effects on the central nervous system (CNS) involved in eating behavior (see review, ref.1).

IL-1, TNFα and IFNγ affect the hypothalamic neurons implicated in the regulation of eating behavior and appetite. Excessive local production of IL-1 in specific brain areas could be responsible for decreased food intake. IL-1 and TNFα alter the firing rate of glucose-sensitive neurons in the lateral hypothalamus [5] and may affect peripheral signals to the feeding centers.

IL-1β activates the hypothalamo-pituitary-adrenocortical (HPA) axis and also activates norepinephrine and dopamine metabolism and serotonin catabolism in the anterior hypothalamus in rats [8]. The resulting increase in plasma levels of catecholamines may thereby result in food-intake suppression. As described in Chapter 1, a fundamental role in appetite control is exerted by serotonin, norepinephrine and the proopiomelanocortin (POMC)-derived peptides, β-endorphin and ACTH, which even interact with the immune function, and the cytokines network. Several pro-inflammatory cytokines, the most noteworthy of which are IFNγ, IL-1, Il-6 and TNFα, stimulate glucocorticoid secretion and interact with the POMC-related peptides [1]. Vasoactive intestinal peptide (VIP), another peptide involved in the course of anorexia nervosa, is known to up-regulate the production of pro-inflammatory cytokines through the inhibition of IL-2 and IL-4 [9].

Clinical Research into Cytokine Production in Eating Disorders

Cytokine Levels in CSF

Excess local production of IL-1 in specific brain areas could account for decreased food intake; pro-inflammatory cytokines (IL-1,IL-6) are known to stimulate ACTH production [10].

Circulating Levels of Cytokines in Anorexia Nervosa

Some studies report increased circulating levels of IL-1, Il-6 or TNFα [11,12], whereas others found no differences compared to controls [13,14]. Decreased serum levels of IL-2 have been reported [14]. Significantly diminished serum levels of TGFβ-2 have also been described [15], while Pomeroy et al. [11] found significantly increased levels of TGFβ in anorexic patients that were reversible after weight gain.

Defective granulopoiesis has been noted in anorexic patients with a deficiency of granulocyte-macrophage colony stimulating factors (GM-CSF) [16]. This might be one of the putative causes of the tendency to mild leukopenia and/or anemia observed in anorexia. Because IL-6 might contribute to the pathogenesis of post-menopausal osteoporosis, the deregulation of the IL-6 system [17] may also contribute to the complications of anorexia nervosa, including osteoporosis.

The discrepancy in findings could be related to the particularity of each sample or to the methods used to measure cytokines (enzyme-linked immuno-sorbent assay ELISA, radioimmunoassay RIA, bioassay). Bioassays might reflect biological activity, whereas immunoassays might reflect levels of cytokines. Then, anorexia nervosa may be associated with enhanced activity of the pro-inflammatory cytokines, without concomitantly increased serum levels of these cytokines [1]. However, an analysis of the results in terms of circulating levels of cytokines remains complex. Cytokines derive primarily from heterogeneous synthetic sources: the immune system, the CNS and also the adipose tissue [17].

Cytokine Receptors

The measurement of cytokine receptors may, therefore, be critically important in the interpretation of circulating levels of cytokines. Much attention has been paid to IL-2 and its soluble receptor (sIl-2r) and to TNFα and its two TNFα receptors (sTNFRI, an agonist receptor, and sTNFRII, an antagonist receptor that suppresses the TNF-mediated inflammatory response) [1].

The levels of sIl-2r are affected by the nutritional state, the HPA axis and CNS [18]. Monteleone et al. [19] found increased levels of soluble cytokine receptor proteins, such as leukemia inhibitory factor receptor (LIF-R) and a cytokine protein receptor (gp130), which are involved in the transduction of pro-inflammatory cytokines signals. These two receptors exhibit significant negative correlation with body mass index, suggesting a direct link with the severity of being underweight, whereas plasma levels of LIF-R were enhanced within the restrictive group of anorexics, and inversely correlated with the plasma levels of 17β-estradiol. These authors have mentioned a compensatory mechanism, secondary to a reduced production of cytokines, which might be due either to under-nutrition or to the altered gonadal steroid milieu of anorexics or to a deregulation of the pro-inflammatory/anti-inflammatory balance in eating disorders.

Cytokines and the Neuroendocrine System

The POMC-derived peptides, β-endorphin and ACTH interact with the immune function and the cytokines network. As indicated above, several pro-inflammatory cytokines, the most noteworthy of which are IFN, IL-1 and TNF, induce alterations of the POMC-related peptides and stimulate glucocorticoid secretion. The HPA axis has certainly been the most documented in eating disorders. Extreme weight loss is accompanied by hypercortisolism with an overdrive of the HPA axis, as described in Chapter 1. In anorexic patients, no difference for the T-lymphocyte proliferating responses are reported, while there were higher basal levels of ACTH and cortisol compared to health subjects. The hyperactivity of the HPA system in anorexia nervosa does not interfere with immune function and may be the result of an increased production of pro-inflammatory cytokines. It could be also related to some compensatory endocrine mechanisms due to reduced CRH and cortisol-receptor sensitivity on the T-lymphocyte [1].

Immunity in Eating Disorders

Malnutrition is one of the most common causes of secondary immunodeficiency. Despite their undernourished status, anorexics are relatively free of infection, at least until they enter the advanced stages of debilitation. The maintenance of an intact functional cell-mediated immune system in anorexics, in contrast to other diseases related to malnourishment, suggests that compensatory mechanisms, involving the endocrine system, psychopathological factors and/or a relatively preserved protein-caloric intake, are working to protect such patients [1].

3. Nutritional Status and Cytokine Production

Deregulation of cytokines in anorexia nervosa could reflect a primary disorder or might result from starvation. Diet (protein-energy balance and fat and carbohydrate intake) is known to play an important role in the immune system. Several lines of evidence indicate that malnutrition or chronic hypocaloric nutrition is responsible for impaired production of cytokines [20-22]; on the other hand, obese patients exhibit higher levels of circulating pro-inflammatory cytokines [17,23]. Adipose tissue has been found to secrete various biologically active adipocytokines such as TNFα and IL-6 [17]. Partial links have been noted between excess weight gain or body fat mass and increased levels of circulating cytokines such as IL-6 and TNFα [23]. In anorexia nervosa, re-feeding is frequently associated with the recovery of cytokine production [11, 18, 24]. Marcos et al. [25] noted that an anorexic diet, although deficient in carbohydrates and fat, is relatively sufficient in protein, which could explain the maintenance of an intact functional immune system compared to the case of protein-energy malnutrition. Thus, anorexia nervosa may be distinguished from other conditions of nutritional deprivation that are associated with severe immunosuppression. Then, plasma from anorexics has sufficient nutrients to sustain a normal lymphocyte transformation response. Protein deficiency reduces the ability of monocytes to produce cytokines [26]. In patients with malnutrition, impaired capacity to produce IL-1, IL-6 and TNF improved after nutrition rehabilitation [22, 27]; in malnourished anorexics, TNFα and IL-1β levels are higher and return to normal after re-feeding or when nutritional status becomes less critical [24]. Vaisman and Hahn [21] also observed that TNF production was higher in anorexic patients than in patients subject to chronic under-nutrition. It remains to be seen whether elevated levels of TNFα and pro-inflammatory cytokines contribute to the pathogenesis of anorexia nervosa or whether there is a compensatory mechanism in undernourished anorexic patients, which could be associated with favored TNFα production. This might be related less to a primary etiologic role involving specific cytokines than to a compensatory mechanism due to a relatively better-preserved consumption of protein [1].

In conclusion, several authors consider that the regulation of cytokines and defective natural cytotoxicity in anorexia nervosa is related to a semi-starvation state and not to a primary etiological role of cytokines. The fact that some cytokines are elevated rather than depleted in eating disorders, while there is relative protein energy malnutrition, may also be considered as secondary to a physiological compensatory mechanism leading to a transitory, enhanced production of cytokines [1].

4. Adipocytokines

It has been recently recognized that adipose tissue is not only a store of fuels and excess energy, but also a source of hormones involved in the control of metabolism, control of appetite and energy balance. The biologically active molecules, synthesized in adipocytes and active by both endocrine and paracrine mechanisms, are collectively indicated as "adipocytokines;" they include classically considered cytokines (such as IL-6 and TNF-α), acylation-stimulating protein (ASP), plasminogen activator inhibitor-1 (PAI-1), adiponectin, and resistin, but the most important is leptin. Leptin is considered to be a fundamental signal of satiety to the brain and has a variety of actions, ranging from interference with sympathetic activity to hematopoiesis and reproductive function [28]. It is extensively treated in Chapter 1.

ASP increases triglyceride synthesis by increasing adipocyte glucose uptake, activating diacylglycerol-acyl-transferase and inhibiting hormone-sensitive lipase [29]. Overproduction of TNF-α by adipose tissue is involved in insulin resistance in obesity [17], and PAI-1 is a well-recognized causative factor for vascular thrombosis.

More recently, resistin has been identified as a novel adipose-specific, cysteine-rich protein with a capacity to impair insulin sensitivity and glucose tolerance in murine models [30]. Resistin was originally proposed to be a link between obesity and insulin resistance/diabetes. However, some authors [31] have previously demonstrated that fat resistin mRNA expression is severely reduced in morbidly obese *ob/ob* mice [32]. Despite decreased fat mRNA expression, circulating resistin levels are increased in *ob/ob* mice relative to lean animals and, thus, could contribute to insulin resistance phenotype. In contrast, the role of resistin in human physiology is currently unclear and probably different from that in mice [31]. There are generally a lot of contradictory data regarding resistin levels in humans, some reports showing a positive correlation with BMI and increased levels in obesity while others do not, and with no change in the groups with different degrees of adiposity [33, 34].

Adiponectin (Apn) is a recently discovered adipocytokine, also referred to as gelatin-binding protein-28 [35]. It is a 244-amino acid protein, the product of the apM1 gene, which is specifically and highly expressed in human adipose cells. This cytokine is a collagen-like protein that belongs to the soluble defense collagen superfamily and has structural homology with collagen VIII and X and complement factor C1q [36-38]. Apn is abundant in human plasma, with concentrations ranging from 5 to 30 mg/mL, thus accounting for approximately 0.01% of total plasma protein [39]. This concentration is three orders of magnitude higher than concentrations of most other hormones. A physiological role for Apn has not been fully established; however Apn, leptin, and resistin are specific fat-derived hormones that affect human fuel homeostasis and insulin action and may also be involved in haematopoiesis and immunity. Serum leptin levels correlated positively with BMI and body fat content and were inversely related to serum soluble leptin receptor and Apn levels. Serum soluble leptin receptor levels correlated positively with serum Apn and were inversely related to BMI, insulin, and leptin levels. Serum Apn levels correlated positively with serum soluble leptin receptor levels and were inversely related to BMI, body fat content, serum leptin levels, and blood glucose concentrations. In contrast, serum resistin levels were not significantly related to any of other parameters studied [31]. We focus our attention on Apn, since it has been implicated both in pathogenesis and complications observed in AN. In summary, Apn increases insulin sensitivity by stimulating fatty acid oxidation, decreases plasma triglycerides and improves glucose metabolism. Apn levels are inversely related to the degree of adiposity. Anorexia nervosa and type 1 diabetes are associated with increased plasma Apn levels and higher insulin sensitivity. Decreased plasma Apn levels were reported in insulin-resistant states, such as obesity and type 2 diabetes, and in patients with coronary artery disease. Activity of Apn is associated with leptin, resistin and with steroid and thyroid hormones, glucocorticoids, NO and others. Furthermore, reduced adipose tissue apM1 gene expression and reduced plasma levels of Apn have been implicated in the pathogenesis of obesity and type 2 diabetes mellitus [40]. Mice lacking Apn have been found to display insulin resistance in some conditions [41].

Moreover, experimental data suggest that Apn may have anti-atherogenic [42] and anti-inflammatory [43] properties. Apn suppresses expression of extracellular matrix adhesive proteins in endothelial cells and atherosclerosis-favoring cytokines. Very recent data have shown that Apn-deficient mice have severe neo-intimal thickening and increased proliferation of vascular smooth muscle cells in mechanically injured arteries [41, 44]. Anti-atherogenic and anti-inflammatory properties of Apn and the ability to stimulate insulin sensitivity have made Apn an important object for physiological and pathophysiological studies with the aim of potential therapeutic applications. Therefore, numerous experimental studies have been performed in the last years and are partly summarized in the following paragraph.

Animal Studies

Experimental data obtained on some animal models suggest that a reduction of Apn expression is associated with obesity and insulin resistance [45]. The expression of Apn may be activated during adipogenesis, but a feedback inhibition on its production may be involved in the development of obesity. It was demonstrated that the expression of adipogenic genes was suppressed during the development of obesity and diabetes mellitus in mice. These observations suggest the existence of a feedback inhibitory pathway [46]. The decrease in plasma Apn levels preceded the development of insulin resistance and diabetes in rhesus monkeys, suggesting that low plasma Apn may contribute to the pathogenesis of insulin resistance and diabetes mellitus in animals. Apn knock-out mice showed delayed clearance of free fatty acid from plasma and low levels of fatty acid transport protein 1 mRNA in muscles. There was no evidence of insulin resistance when Apn knock-out mice were fed a regular diet. Taken together, these observations indicate that Apn deficiency contributes to the induction of insulin resistance and that Apn may play a protective role against insulin resistance [48]. Administration of recombinant Apn in pharmacological studies reduced serum glucose in normal and diabetic rodents without stimulation of insulin secretion. A full-length Apn molecule produced in mammalian cells in culture is more effective in enhancing insulin sensitivity than that produced in bacterial cells. This could be attributed to post-transcriptional modifications of endogenous Apn in eukaryotic cells. Apn receptor 1 (AdipoR1) is abundantly expressed in skeletal muscle, whereas Apn receptor 2 (AdipoR2) is predominantly expressed in the liver; it has been supposed that receptors serve for globular (AdipoR1) and full-length (HMW) Apn molecules (AdipoR2 binds both). Experimentally activated expression, or suppression of AdipoR1/R2, support the conclusion that they mediate increased AMP kinase and PPAR ligands activities, as well as fatty-acid oxidation and glucose uptake by Apn [49]. The mechanism responsible for the control of Apn synthesis has not been determined in detail, so far. Among factors that suppress Anp, we remember: TNF-α, insulin, β-adrenergic agonists and glucocorticoid. TNF-α significantly reduces the expression and secretion of Apn from adipocytes [50]. TNF-α is one of the candidate molecules responsible for causing insulin resistance; TNF-α is a key modulator of adipocyte metabolism, with a direct role in several insulin-mediated processes, including glucose homeostasis and lipid metabolism, and is a major contributor to the development of adipose tissue insulin resistance. Insulin, which reduces the level of Apn mRNA in a dose- and time-dependent fashion [50], β-adrenergic agonists [51] and glucocorticoid are reported to inhibit Apn gene expression and secretion, suggesting that decreased Apn production could play a role in catecholamine- or glucocorticoid-induced insulin resistance. Finally, the stomach-derived peptide, ghrelin, inhibits Apn gene expression [52]. On the other hand, other factors increase Apn gene expression: Peroxisome proliferator-activated nuclear receptor-γ (PPARγ) and liver receptor homolog-1 (LRH-1) play significant roles in the transcriptional activation of Apn gene via the peroxisome proliferator-activated receptor gamma response element (PPRE) and the LRH-RE in its promoter. The PPARs are nuclear receptor isoforms, with key roles in the regulation of lipid and glucose metabolism. PPARγ and PPARα, and probably also PPARδ, have the effect of promoting insulin sensitization in the context of obesity. PPARγ and PPARα have anti-inflammatory effects and reduce the progression of atherosclerosis in animals (α, γ) or in humans (α). Apn is induced by PPARγ agonists. Synthetic PPARγ agonist administered to differentiated adipocytes cultured in vitro increased

Apn mRNA [53]. PPARγ abundant in fat tissue induces adipocyte differentiation, and it is also an insulin sensitizer in vivo. It was thought that the effects of PPARγ in adipose tissue are crucial in explaining its role in insulin sensitization. More recent studies have highlighted the contribution of the other tissues [33]. The upregulation of the Apn pathway by PPARγ may play a role in the increasing β-oxidations of lipids, leading to decreased triglycerides from the liver and muscle [54]. According to these data, from a pharmacological point of view, thiazolidinediones (TZD), PPAR-γ agonists, enhanced the expression and release of mediators of insulin resistance originating in adipose tissue (e.g., increased free fatty acids, decreased Apn) in a way that results in net improvement of insulin sensitivity in the muscle and liver [55]. TZD normalized or increased Apn mRNA expression and Apn secretion in adipose tissue of obese mice [54]. TZD also enhanced Apn promotor activity and restored the inhibitory effect of TNF-α on this promotor [56]. The carboxy-terminal globular structure of Apn, through its use of gC1q receptor found in mitochondria of the thyroid, could be a regulator of thyroid hormone production [57]. Additional evidence for a role of thyroid hormones in the regulation of Apn expression comes from a recent study showing increased Apn levels in mice exposed to cold [58]. It was postulated that Apn could regulate body temperature and basal metabolic rate in response to changing environmental conditions. It was then concluded that Apn might play a role in thermogenesis. These data suggest that thyroid and adrenal activity modulate Apn expression, and Apn possesses anti-atherogenic and anti-inflammatory properties. A recent study has shown that estradiol is negatively and indirectly associated with Apn, whereas there is no association between serum Apn and leptin, cortisol, or free testosterone levels [59]. However, Nishizawa et al. [60] observed that testosterone leads to a reduction in plasma Apn.

Human Studies [45]

A clear relationship exists between Apn and fat mass in humans. Apn release is positively correlated with fat cell size and negatively correlated with body mass index (BMI). Apn release is significantly lower in omentum than in subcutaneous adipose tissue [61]. In contrast to leptin, Apn levels are significantly reduced not only in obese subjects [62], but also in patients with some of the disease states associated with obesity, such as type 2 diabetes [63] and coronary artery disease [64]. The trend towards increased Apn on a high-fat diet in more insulin-sensitive subjects is suggestive of increased capacity for fat oxidation and may be protective against development of type 2 diabetes [65]. Apn serum concentrations were negatively correlated with the increase in muscle intracellular lipids after dietary lipid challenge. Suppression of lipid oxidation by hyperinsulinaemia prevents effects of Apn on muscle intracellular lipid stores. Apn promotes lipid oxidation in humans [66]. The HMW (high-molecular weight) protein affects hepatic gluconeogenesis through improved insulin sensitivity, and LMW (low-molecular weight) Apn stimulates β-oxidation in muscle. Pajvani et al. [67] showed that the ratio, and not the absolute amounts, between two Apn molecular forms (HMW to LMW) is crucial in determining the insulin sensitivity. Apn was inversely associated with insulin resistance in non-diabetic subjects, independent of age, blood pressure, adiposity and serum lipids [68]. Another study performed in subjects with normal weight has shown that plasma Apn is negatively correlated with BMI, systolic and diastolic blood pressure, fasting plasma glucose, insulin, insulin resistance, total and LDL-cholesterol, triglycerides and uric acid; and it is positively correlated with HDL-cholesterol [69]. Serum Apn was positively associated with HDL-cholesterol in both diabetic and non-diabetic subjects. On the contrary, plasma Apn concentrations are significantly increased in type 1 diabetic patients compared with healthy controls [70].

Experimental evidence suggests that Apn may play a protective role against atherosclerosis, with a role in blood pressure and fibrinolysis. Hyperinsulinaemia caused a significant decrease of Apn plasma levels under euglycaemic conditions, while hypoadiponectinemia might at least partly be a link between hyperinsulinemia and vascular disease in metabolic syndrome [56]. Apn concentrations seem to be gender-dependent, being higher in women than in men [69]. Apn exerts vascular actions by direct stimulation of NO production in endothelial cells using phosphatidylinositol 3-kinase pathways involving phosphorylation of endothelial NO synthase (eNOS) by AMP-activated protein kinase (AMPK) and stimulating new blood vessel growth and taking part in vasodilator actions and increasing blood flow. Thus, Apn mimics vascular as well as metabolic actions of insulin. The fact that insulin and Apn regulate activation of eNOS by slightly different mechanisms suggests that therapies designed to increase Apn levels may be beneficial in treatment of insulin resistance, diabetes, vascular complications and atherosclerosis [71].

As circulating Apn levels were found to be suppressed fivefold in patients with severe insulin resistance due to dominant-negative PPARγ mutations, it has been suggested that Apn may be a biomarker of in vivo PPARγ activation. Similar to the animal models, TZD treatment should enhance endogenous Apn production in humans [54]. TZD increases circulating Apn levels in normal subjects and in obese and type 2 diabetic patients. Plasma Apn levels in diabetic patients were increased more than twofold after three months of rosiglitazone therapy and remained elevated after six months of the same therapy. There was a tendency towards an increase in Apn mRNA expression after 24-hour incubation of human adipose tissue with either rosiglitazone or pioglitazone. The results may suggest that in humans, TZD affects Apn at the transcriptional level [72].

Finally, Apn is a novel determinant of bone mineral density and visceral fat. This peptide also stimulates angiogenesis by promoting cross-talk between AMP-activated protein kinase and other signaling pathways in endothelial cells [73].

In summary, Apn is a fat-derived hormone with antidiabetic properties. The ability of Apn to increase insulin sensitivity in conjunction with its anti-inflammatory and anti-atherogenic properties have made this novel adipocytokine a promising therapeutic tool for the future, with potential applications in states associated with low plasma Apn levels [45].

5. Adipocytokines in Anorexia Nervosa

AN is associated with altered glucose and lipid metabolism, multiple endocrine perturbations and other dysfunctions such as haematological and immune defects. Some of these abnormalities may be linked to altered adipocytokine production. Whether Apn is altered in anorexic patients with low body fat is still unsettled. Unlike other adipocytokines, Apn is paradoxically decreased in human obesity [61]. On the other hand, its circulating level is strongly reduced in patients with generalized lipodystrophy who exhibit marked adipose tissue depletion [74].

Although Apn is secreted only by adipocytes, plasma concentrations of this adipose-specific factor were higher in low-weight anorexic patients than in controls [75]. This difference was further amplified when Apn levels were expressed by "secretion unit" (i.e., normalized for BMI, as surrogate for fatness). This paradoxical increase appears to be the mirror image of hypoadiponectinaemia in obesity [62].

At least three metabolic features of anorexia nervosa could potentially contribute to up-regulate Apn. First, reduced fatness per se. Plasma Apn increased following body weight loss in obese patients, a finding that was, after multivariate analysis, primarily explained by fatness reduction [76]. In agreement with this observation, adipose tissue may synthesize a factor that destabilizes Apn mRNAs as shown by in vitro experiments conducted in human cultured adipose explants [77]. Thus, in vivo and in vitro evidence indicates that fat mass may exert a negative feedback on its own Apn production. The lack of such negative feedback could contribute to hyperadiponectinaemia in AN. However, this does not rule out the possibility that under a critical (and presumably extremely low) fatness threshold, Apn production might ultimately plummet. Such extremely low levels, life-threatening during severe starvation, may be observed in rare cases of generalized lipodystrophy, characterized by intrinsic and profound defects of adipocyte function [74].

Second, enhanced insulin sensitivity, although controversial, has been documented in AN (see Chapter 1). Several studies in nonhuman primates or in humans have shown relationships between insulin sensitivity modulation and plasma Apn levels. Prospective longitudinal studies in rhesus monkeys, which spontaneously develop obesity and type 2 diabetes, have revealed that plasma Apn levels decreased at an early phase of obesity in parallel with reduced insulin sensitivity [63]. Similarly, in Caucasians and in Pima Indians, a population with a high propensity for obesity and type 2 diabetes, decreased Apn levels were closely related to the degree of insulin resistance [78]. Conversely, reversal of insulin resistance by thiazolidinediones administered to glucose-intolerant or type 2 diabetic subjects resulted in increased plasma Apn levels [54]. Taken together, these epidemiological and experimental data establish a link between insulin sensitivity and Apn in nonhuman primates and in humans. It is, therefore, tempting to speculate that besides being a potential effect, increased insulin sensitivity could also be a causative factor of hyperadiponectinaemia in man.

Third, other metabolic or hormonal contributors might contribute to up-regulate Apn. The altered sympathetic nervous tone, which is decreased in AN, may be one of these. This abnormality may up-regulate Apn as catecholamines do, in fact, decrease Apn mRNA and secretion [79]. Apn levels were strongly related to several lipid parameters in healthy controls but not in anorexic subjects. Apn is also inversely related to total cholesterol and LDL-cholesterol. There were no correlations with plasma lipid parameters in AN. Slightly elevated cholesterol levels, primarily composed of LDL-cholesterol, are found frequently in AN despite very low cholesterol intake [80]. This may result from abnormal catabolism: a decrease in biliary cholesterol excretion and a defect in cellular cholesterol uptake have been incriminated. Impaired activity of lipoprotein lipase and subsequent altered catabolism of very low density lipoprotein (VLDL) triglyceride particles have also been reported [80]. In general, lipid metabolism is abnormal in AN. This abnormality may disrupt the relationships that otherwise occur between circulating Apn and plasma lipids in controls. Whether hyperadiponectaemia may be implicated in the pathogenesis of some metabolic or other dysfunctions of AN is still unsettled. Hyperadiponectinaemia could also potentially contribute to weight loss, by analogy to weight reduction in mice caused by prolonged administration of the cytokine [81]. However, basal metabolic rate is reduced in AN, whereas Apn administration to mice resulted in increased thermogenesis [49]. Like leptin, Apn is emerging as a pleiotropic cytokine, linked not only to metabolic events but also to other fundamental body functions such as hematopoiesis and immunity. However, unlike leptin, which stimulates these last two functions, Apn is found to be inhibitory. Thus, Apn inhibits the growth of myelomonocytic progenitors, blocks B-lymphopoiesis and suppresses mature macrophage functions in vitro [82]. The fact that plasma Apn levels in hemodialysis patients are increased after erythropoietin treatment, seemingly as a result of a negative feedback on Apn triggered by improved hematological status, supports in vivo the possible involvement of this adipocytokine in hematopoiesis [83]. Anorexic patients frequently suffer from mild anemia and moderate leucopoenia accompanied by defective in vitro granulopoiesis (reduction of both granulocyte-macrophage colony-forming cells and colony-stimulating factor) and are prone to severe infections [83]. High Apn might thus potentially contribute to these hematological and infectious complications, although further studies are warranted to firmly establish its direct implication in such disorders. In conclusion, plasma Apn levels are increased in anorexia nervosa. This may, at least in part, be due to the lack of a negative feedback exerted by fat mass on Apn production and/or to enhanced insulin sensitivity. Hyperadiponectinaemia could, in turn, contribute to maintain a state of enhanced insulin sensitivity and possibly exacerbate hematological and infectious complications of anorexia nervosa [75].

Some studies compared cytokine levels in different forms of AN [31]. The restrictive form of AN represents an extreme example of psychosomatic-based malnutrition induced by chronically decreased food intake, caused by inappropriate fear of obesity and distorted body image. In the binge/purge form of AN, the reduction of food intake is combined with periods of binge eating and/or purging. As a result, the body fat content of patients with the binge/purge form is usually less severely decreased than in patients with the restrictive form of AN. The above-described subtypes of eating disorders affect nutritional status very differently.

Circulating leptin concentrations were markedly decreased in restrictive AN patients and less so in binge/purge AN patients, relative to control group; Serum soluble leptin receptor levels were significantly higher in restrictive and binge/purge AN groups relative to both control groups. Serum Apn concentrations in patients with both restrictive and binge/purge forms of AN were higher than the control group. In contrast to marked differences in serum leptin and Apn levels between malnourished patients with AN and control and bulimia nervosa subjects, serum resistin concentrations in patients with binge/purge and restrictive forms of AN did not differ from those of control and bulimia nervosa groups, respectively [31]. Leptin and Apn levels in patients with restrictive and binge/purge types of AN were strongly related to nutritional status, whereas resistin levels were not [31]. This finding may be explained in part by the fact that although leptin and Apn are produced almost exclusively by adipocytes, the main source of resistin in humans is immunocompetent cells in the adipose tissue [85]. Numerous studies have previously found that leptin levels in malnourished patients are severely decreased, reflecting lowered body fat content [86]. In contrast, serum soluble leptin receptor levels in these patients were reported to be increased. This increase may represent a protective mechanism that decreases free leptin bioavailability and thus further facilitates energy conservation. Serum leptin levels in patients with the binge/ purge form of AN are higher than in the restrictive form, but lower than in the control group [30].

It must be underlined that studies focused on serum Apn levels in AN patients brought rather contradictory results. Even if most authors found increased Apn levels in AN [87,88], in contrast, Iwahashi et al. [89] did not observe any difference in Apn levels between AN patients and healthy women. Tagami et al. [90] found even decreased Apn levels in AN patients. Housova et al. [31] found results similar to Delporte et al. [87] and Pannacciulli et al. [88] that indicated increased Apn levels in AN patients, demonstrating that there was a gradual rise in Apn levels related to the nutritional status of AN patients. Less severely malnourished patients with the binge/purge form of AN had a relatively modest increase in circulating Apn, whereas a more prominent rise in this parameter was found in severely malnourished restrictive AN patients. The finding of increased Apn levels in patients with AN may have interesting etiopathogenetic consequences. It has been recently demonstrated in mice that intracerebroventricular administration of Apn decreased body weight [91]. It is tempting to speculate that hyperadiponectinaemia could be a contributing etiopathogenetic factor in patients with AN. However, a more likely possibility is that increased Apn levels are, rather, the consequence of severely decreased body fat and/or other metabolic changes in anorexic patients. Finally, it has been hypothesized that elevated circulating Apn concentrations in patients with AN might represent a compensatory mechanism for the reduced insulin-stimulated glucose metabolism [88].

In contrast to leptin and adiponectin, circulating resistin levels did not significantly differ in the groups studied herein, despite huge distinctions in BMI and body fat content [31]. We, therefore, suggest that neither malnutrition nor changes in eating patterns is an important factor affecting circulating resistin levels in patients with eating disorders. Thus, resistin does not appear to be a contributing factor in the etiopathogenesis of either anorexia. In conclusion, circulating levels of leptin and Apn in patients with different eating disorders are primarily determined by their nutritional status. In contrast, resistin levels were unrelated to either anthropometric or insulin sensitivity variables. So, increased Apn levels could contribute to metabolic changes and/or decreased food intake in AN patients, whereas resistin does not appear to be involved in this process.

In conclusion, advances in physiopathology of adipose tissue could add more information to the nutritional and metabolic status of patients with AN and furnish useful tools for treatment of this condition. But further studies could also help to give an unequivocal picture and a clearer definition of interplay between peripheral signals and central regulation of appetite, both in normal subjects and in eating disorders.

REFERENCES

[1] Corcos, M; Guilbaud, O; Paterniti, S; Moussa, M; Chambry, J; Chaouat, G; Consoli, SM; Jeammet, P. Involvement of cytokines in eating disorders: a critical review of the human literature. *Psychoneuroendocrinology*, 2003, 28, 229-249.

[2] Cone, RD; Low, MJ; Elmquist, JK; Cameron, JL. Neuroendocrinology. In: Reed Larsen, P; Kronenberg, HM; Melmed, S; Polonsky, KS, Editors. *Williams Textbook of Endocrinology 10th edition.* Philadelphia: WB Saunders, 2003, 81-176.

[3] Collins, T. Acute and chronic inflammation. In: Cotran, RS; Kumar, V; Collins, T, Editors. Robbins. *Pathological basis of diseases*, 6th edition. Philadelphia: WB Saunders, 1999, 25-46.

[4] Espat, NJ; Moldawer, LL; Copeland, EM. Cytokine-mediated alterations in host metabolism prevent nutritional repletion in cachetic cancer patients. *J Surg Oncol,* 2005, 55, 77-82.

[5] Plata-Salaman, CR. Cytokines and anorexia nervosa: a brief overview. *Semin Oncol,* 1995, 25 (Suppl 1), 64-72.

[6] Langstein, HN; Doherty, GM; Fraker, DL; Buresh, CM; Norton, JA. The roles of gamma-interferon and tumor necrosis factor alpha in an experimental rat model of cancer cachexia. *Cancer Res,* 1991, 51, 2302-2306.

[7] Holden, RJ & Pakula, IS. The role of tumor necrosis factor-alpha in the pathogenesis of anorexia and bulimia nervosa, cancer cachexia and obesity. *Med Hypotheses,* 1996, 52, 156-162.

[8] Dunn, AJ; Wang, J; Ando T. Effects of cytokines on cerebral neurotransmission Comparison with the effects of stress. *Adv Exp Med Biol,* 1999, 461, 117-127.

[9] Sun, L & Ganea, D. Vasoactive intestinal peptide inhibits interleukin (IL-) IL-2 and IL-4 production through different molecular mechanisms in T cells activated via the T cell receptor/CD3 complex. *J Neuroimmunol,* 1993, 48, 59-69.

[10] Dantzer, R; Bluthè, RM; Kent, S; Goodall, G. Behavioral effects of cytokine: an insight into mechanisms of sickness behavior. *Methods Neurosci,* 1993, 17, 130-150.

[11] Pomeroy, C; Eckert, E; Shuxian, H; Eiken, B; Mentik, M; Crosby, RD; Chao, CC. Role of interleukine-6 and transforming growth factor-α in anorexia nervosa. *Soc Biol Psychiatry,* 1994, 36, 836-839.

[12] Nakai, Y; Hamagaki, S; Tagaki, R; Taniguchi, A; Kurimoto, F. Plasma concentrations of tumor necrosis factor α (TNF α) and soluble TNF receptors in patients with anorexia nervosa. *J Clin Endocrinol Metab,* 1999, 84, 1226-1228.

[13] Brambilla, F; Monti, D; Franceschi, C. Plasma concentrations of interleukin-1-beta, interleukin-6 and tumor necrosis factor-alpha, and of their receptors and receptor antagonist in anorexia nervosa. *Psychiatry Res,* 2001, 103, 107-114.

[14] Corcos, M; Guilbaud, O; Chaouat, G; Cayol, V; Speranza, M; Chambry, J; Paterniti, S; Moussa, M; Flament, M; Jeammet, PH. Cytokines and anorexia nervosa. *Psychosom Med,* 2001, 63, 502-504.

[15] Licinio, J; Altemus, ME; Wong, M; Gold, PW. Circulating levels of interleukin-2 in patients with anorexia nervosa. *Biol Psychiatry,* 1991, 29 (Suppl 9), 56 A.

[16] Nagata, T; Tobitani, W; Kiriike, N; Iketani, T; Yamagami, S. Capacity to produce cytokines during weight restoration in patients with anorexia nervosa. *Psychosom Med,* 1999, 61, 371-377.

[17] Hotamisligil, GS; Shargill, NS; Spiegelman, BM. Adipose expression of tumor necrosis factor-α: direct role in obesity-liked insulin resistance. *Science,* 1993, 259, 87-91.

[18] Nagata, T; Kiriike, N; Tobitani, W; Kawarada, Y; Matsunaga, H; Yamagami, S. Lymphocyte subset, lymphocyte proliferative response, and soluble interleukin-2 receptors in anorexic patients. *Biol Psychiatry,* 1996, 45, 471-474.

[19] Monteleone, P; Maes, M; Fabrazzo, M; Tortorella, A; Lin, A; Bosmans, E; Kenis, G; Maj, M. Immunoendocrine findings in patients with eating disorders. *Neuropsychobiology*, 1999, 40, 115-120

[20] Bhaskaram, P; Sivakumar, B. Interleukin-1 in malnutrition. *Arch Dis Child,* 1986,182-185.

[21] Vaisman, N; Hahn, T. Tumor necrosis factor-α and anorexia-cause or effect? *Metabolism,* 1991, 40, 720-723.

[22] Munoz, C; Arevalo, M; Lopez, M; Schlesinger, L. Impaired interleukin-1 and tumor necrosis factor production in protein-caloric malnutrition. *Nutr Res*, 1994, 14, 347-352.

[23] Kern, PA; Ranganathan, S; Li, C; Wood, L; Ranganathan, G. Adipose tissue tumor necrosis factor and interleukin-6 expression in human obesity and insulin resistance. *Am J Physiol Endocrinol Metab*, 2001, 280, E745-E751.

[24] Allende, LM; Corell, A; Manzanares, J; Madruga, D; Marcos, A; Madromo, A; Lopez-Goyanes, A; Garcia-Perez, MA; Moreno, JM; Rodrigo, M; Sanz, F; Arnaiz-Villena, A. Immunodeficiency associated with anorexia nervosa is secondary and improves after re-feeding. *Immunology,* 1998, 94, 543-551.

[25] Marcos, A; Varela, P; Toro, O; Nova, E; Lopez-Vidriero, I; Morande, G. Evaluation of nutritional status by immunologic assessment in bulimia nervosa: influence on body mass index and vomiting episodes. *Am J Clin Nutr,* 1997, 66, 491S-497S.

[26] Grimble, RF. Nutrition and cytokine action. *Nutr Res Rev,* 1990, 3, 193-210.

[27] Dohertyr, JF; Golden, MHN; Remick, DG; Griffin, GE. Production of interleukin-6 and tumor necrosis factor-alpha in vitro is reduced in whole blood of severely malnourished children. *Clin Sci,* 1994, 86, 347-351.

[28] Mantzoros, CS. The role of leptin in human obesity and disease: a review of current evidence. *Ann Int Med,* 1999, 130, 651–657.

[29] Murray, I; Sniderman, AD; Havel, PJ; Cianflone, K. Acylation stimulating protein (ASP) deficiency alters postprandial and adipose tissue metabolism in male mice. *J Biol Chem,* 1999, 274, 36219–36225.

[30] Steppan, CM; Bailey, ST; Bhat, S; Brown, EJ; Banerjee, RR; Wright, CM; Patel, HL; Ahima, RS; Lazar, MA. The hormone resistin links obesity to diabetes. *Nature,* 2001, 409, 307–312.

[31] Housova, J; Anderlova, K; Krizová, J; Haluzikova, D; Kremen, J; Kumstyrová, T; Papezová, H; Haluzik, M. Serum adiponectin and resistin concentrations in patients with restrictive and binge/purge form of anorexia nervosa and bulimia nervosa. *J Clin Endocrinol Metab,* 2005, 90, 1366-1370.

[32] Ma, K; Cabrero, A; Saha, PK; Kojima, H; Li, L; Chang, BH; Paul, A; Chan, L. Increased β-oxidation but no insulin resistance or glucose intolerance in mice lacking adiponectin. *J Biol Chem,* 2002, 277, 34658–34661.

[33] Yamauchi, T; Kamon, J; Waki, H; Terauchi, Y; Kubota, N; Hara, K; Mori, Y; Ide, T; Murakami, K; Tsuboyama-Kasaoka, N; Ezaki, O; Akanuma, Y; Gavrilova, O; Vinson, C; Reitman, ML; Kaqechika, H; Shudo, K; Yoda, M; Nakano, Y; Tobe, K; Nagai, R; Kimura, S; Tomita, M; Froguel, P; Kadowaki, T. The fat-derived hormone adiponectin reverses insulin resistance associated with both lipoatrophy and obesity. *Nat Med,* 2001, 7, 941–946.

[34] Picard, F & Auwerx, J. Ppar-γ and glucose homeostasis. *Ann Rev Nutr,* 2002, 22, 167–197.

[35] Nakano, Y; Tobe, T; Choi-Miura, NH; Mazda, T; Tomita, T. Isolation and characterization of GBP28, a novel gelatin-binding protein purified from human plasma. *J Biochem,* 1996, 120, 803–812.

[36] Maeda, K; Okubo, K; Shimomura, I; Funahashi, T; Matsuzawa, Y; Matsubara, K. C-dna cloning and expression of a novel adipose specific collagen-like factor, apm1 (adipose most abundant gene transcript 1). *Biochem Biophys Res Commun,* 1996, 221, 286–289.

[37] Scherer, PE; Williams, S; Fogliano, M; Baldini, G; Lodish, HF. A novel serum protein similar to c1q, produced exclusively in adipocytes. *J Biol Chem,* 1995, 270, 26746–26749.

[38] Takahashi, M; Arita, Y; Yamagata, K; Matsukawa, Y; Okutomi, K; Horie, M; Shimomura, I; Hotta, K; Kuriyama, H; Kihara, S; Nakamura, T; Yamashita, S; Funahashi, T; Matsuzawa, Y. Genomic structure and mutations in adipose specific gene, adiponectin. *Int J Obes Relat Metab Disord,* 2000, 24, 861–868.

[39] Arita, Y; Kihara, S; Ouchi, N; Takahashi, M; Maeda, K; Miyagawa, J: Hotta, K; Shimomura, I; Nakamura, T; Miyaoka, K; Kuriyama, H; Nishida, M; Yamashita, S; Okubo, K; Matsubara, K; Maraguchi, M; Ohmoto, Y; Funahashi, T; Matsuzawa, Y. Paradoxical decrease of an adipocyte specific protein, adiponectin, in obesity. *Biochem Biophys Res Commun,* 1999, 257, 79–83.

[40] Statnick, MA; Beavers, LS; Conner, LJ; Corominola, H; Johnson, D; Hammond, CD; Rafaeloff-Phail, R ; Seng, T ; Suter, TM ; Sluka, JP ; Ravussin, E ; Gadski, RA ; Caro, JF. Decreased expression of apM1 in omental and subcutaneous adipose tissue of humans with type 2 diabetes. *Int J Reprod Diab Res,* 2000, 1, 51–58.

[41] Maeda, N; Shimomura, I; Kishida, K; Nishizawa, H; Matsuda, M; Nagaretani, H; Furuyama, N; Kondo, H; Takahashi, M; Arita, Y; Komuro, R; Ouchi, N; Kihara, S; Tochino, Y; Okutomi, K; Horie, M; Takeda, S; Aoyama, T; Funahashi, T; Matsuzawa, Y. Diet-induced insulin resistance in mice lacking adiponectin/ACRP30. *Nat Med,* 2002, 8, 731–737.

[42] Ouchi, N; Kihara, S; Arita, Y; Maeda, K; Kuriyama, H; Okamoto, Y; Hotta, K; Nishida, M; Takahashi, M; Nakamura, T; Yamashita, S; Funahashi, T; Matsuzawa, Y. Novel modulator for endothelial adhesion molecules: adipocyte-derived plasma protein adiponectin. *Circulation,* 1999, 100, 2473–2476.

[43] Yokota, T; Oritani, K; Takahashi, I; Ishikawa, J; Matsuyama, A; Ouchi, N; Kihara, S; Funahashi, T; Tenner, AJ; Tomiyama, Y; Matsuzawa, Y. Adiponectin, a new member of the family of soluble defense collagens, negatively regulates the growth of myelomonocytic progenitors and the functions of macrophages. *Blood,* 2000, 96, 1723–1732.

[44] Matsuda, M; Shimomura, I; Sata, M; Arita, Y; Nishida, M; Maeda, N; Kumada, M; Okamoto, Y; Nagaretani, H; Nishizawa, H; Kishida, K; Komuro, R; Ouchi, N; Kihara, S; Nagai, R; Funahashi, T; Matsuzawa, Y. Role of adiponectin in preventing vascular stenosis. The missing link of adipo–vascular axis. *J Biol Chem,* 2002, 277, 37487–37491.

[45] Nedvídková, J; Smitka, K; Kopský, V; Hainer, V. Adiponectin, an adipocyte derived protein. *Physiol Res,* 2005, 54, 133-140.

[46] Nadler, ST; Stoehr, JP; Schueller, KL; Tanimoto, G; Yandell, BS; Attie, AD. The expression of adipogenic genes is decreased in obesity and diabetes mellitus. *Proc Natl Acad Sci USA*, 2001, 97, 11371-11376.

[47] Hotta, K; Funahashi, T; Bodkin, NL; Ortmeyer, HK; Arita, Y; Hansen, BC; Matsuzawa, Y. Circulating concentrations of the adipocyte protein adiponectin are decreased in parallel with reduced insulin sensitivity during the progression to type 2 diabetes in rhesus monkeys. *Diabetes*, 2001, 50, 1126-1133.

[48] Matsuzawa Y, Funahashi T, Kihara S, Shimomura I. Adiponectin and metabolic syndrome. *Arterioscler Thromb Vasc Biol*, 2004, 24: 29-33.

[49] Yamauchi, T; Kamon, J; Ito, Y; Tsuchida, A; Yokomizo, T; Kita, S; Sugiyama, T; Miyagishi, M; Hara, K; Tsunoda, M; Murakami, K; Ohteki, T; Uchida, S; Takekawa, S; Waki, H; Tsuno, NH; Shibata, Y; Terauchi, Y; Froguel, P; Tobe, K; Koyasu, S; Taira, K; Kitamura, T; Shimizu, T; Nagai, R; Kadowaki, T. Cloning of adiponectin receptors that mediate antidiabetic metabolic effects. *Nature*, 2003, 423, 762-769.

[50] Fasshauer, M; Klein, J; Lossner, U; Paschke, R. Negative regulation of adipose-expressed galectin 12 by isoproterenol, tumor necrosis factor α, insulin and dexamethasone. *Eur J Endocrinol*, 2002, 147, 553-559.

[51] Zhang, Y; Matheny, M; Zolotukhin, S; Tumer, N; Scarpace, PJ. Regulation of adiponectin and leptin gene expression in white and brown adipose tissues: influence of β3 adrenergic agonists, retinoic acid, leptin and fasting. *Biochem Biophys Acta*, 2002, 1584: 115-122.

[52] Ott, V; Fasshauer, M; Dalski, A; Meier, B; Perwitz, N; Klein, HH; Tschop, M; Klein, J. Direct peripheral effects of ghrelin include suppression of adiponectin expression. *Horm Metab Res*, 2002, 34, 640-645.

[53] Chineti, G; Zawadski, C; Fruchart, JC; Staels, B. Expression of adiponectin receptors in human macrophages and regulation by agonist of the nuclear receptors pparα, pparγ, and LXR. *Biochem Biophys Res Commun*, 2004, 314, 151-158.

[54] Maeda, N; Takahashi, M; Funahashi, T; Kihara, S; Nishizawa, H; Kishida, K; Nagaretani, H; Matsuda, M; Komuro, R; Ouchi, N; Kuriyama, H; Hotta, K; Nakamura, T; Shimomura, I; Matsuzawa, Y. pparγ ligands increase expression and plasma concentrations of adiponectin, an adipose derived protein. *Diabetes*, 2001, 50, 2094-2099.

[55] Stumvoll, M. Thiazolidinediones – some recent developments. *Exp Opin Invest Drugs*, 2003, 12, 1179-1187.

[56] Diez, JJ & Iglesias, P. The role of the novel adipocyte-derived hormone adiponectin in human disease. *Eur J Endocrinol*, 2003, 148, 293-300.

[57] Soltys, BJ, Kang, D; Gupta, RS. Localization of P32 protein (gc1q-R) in mitochondria and at specific extramito-chondrial locations in normal tissues. *Histochem Cell Biol*, 2000, 114, 245-255.

[58] Yoda, M; Nakano, Y; Tobe, T; Shioda, S; Choi-Miura, NH; Tomita, M. Characterization of mouse GBP28 and its induction by exposure to cold. *Int J Obes Relat Metab Disord*, 2001, 25, 75-83.

[59] Gavrila, A; Chan, JL; Yinnakouris, A; Kontogianni, M; Miller, LC; Orlova, C; Mantzoros, CS. Serum adiponectin levels are inversely associated with overall and central fat distribution but are not directly regulated by acute fasting or leptin

administration in humans: cross-sectional and interventional studies. *J Clin Endocrinol Metab,* 2003, 88, 4823-4831.

[60] Nishizawa, H; Shimomura, I; Kishida, K; Maeda, N; Kuriyama, H; Nagaretani, H; Matsuda, M; Kondo, H; Furuyama, N; Kihara, S; Nakamura, T; Tochino, Y; Funahashi, T; Matsuzawa, Y. Androgens decrease plasma adiponectin, an insulin-sensitizing adipocyte derived protein. *Diabetes,* 2002, 51, 2734-2741.

[61] Johnson, J; Flancbaum, L; Albu, J. Adiponectin release in deep subcutaneous abdominal and visceral tissue depots. *Obes Res,* 2003, 11, A 34.

[62] Arita, Y; Kihara, S; Ouchi, N; Takahashi, M; Maeda, K; Miyagawa, J; Hotta, K; Shimomura, I; Nakamura, T; Miyaoka, K; Kuriyama, H; Nishida, M; Yamashita, S; Okubo, K; Matsubara, K; Muraguchi, M; Ohmoto, Y; Funahashi, T; Matsuzawa, Y. Paradoxical decrease of an adipocyte specific protein, adiponectin, in obesity. *Biochem Biophys Res Commun,* 1999, 257, 79-83.

[63] Hotta, K; Funahashi, T; Arita, Y; Takahashi, M; Matsuda, M; Okamoto, Y; Iwahashi, H; Kuriyama, H; Ouchi, N; Maeda, K; Nishida, M; Kihara, S; Sakai, N; Nakajima, T; Hasegawa, K; Muraguchi, M; Ohmoto, Y; Nakamura, T; Yamashita, S; Hanafusa, T; Matsuzawa, Y. Plasma concentration of a novel adipose specific protein, adiponectin, in type 2 diabetic patients. *Artherioscler Tromb Vasc Biol,* 2000, 20, 1595-1599.

[64] Ouchi, N; Kihara, S; Arita, Y; Maeda, K; Kuriyama, H; Okamoto, Y; Hotta, K; Nishida, M; Takahashi, M; Nakamura, T; Yamashita, S; Funahashi, T; Matsuzawa, Y. Novel modulator for endothelial adhesion molecules: adipocyte-derived plasma protein adiponectin. *Circulation,* 1999, 100, 2473-2476.

[65] Berk, E; Kovera, A; Boozer, C; Pi-Sunyer, FX; Johnson, J; Albu, J. Adiponectin levels and insulin sensitivity during low and high fat diets in obese, premenopausal, non-diabetic women. *Obes Res,* 2003, 11, A 34.

[66] Thamer, C; Machann, J; Tschritter, O; Haap, M; Wietek, B; Dahl, D; Bachmann, O; Fritsche, A; Jacob, S; Stumvoll, M; Schick, F; Haring, Hu. Relationship between serum adiponectin concentration and intramyocellular lipid stores in humans. *Horm Metab Res,* 2003, 34, 646-649.

[67] Pajvani, UB; Hawkins, M; Combs, TP; Rajala, MW; Doebber, T; Berger, JP; Wagner, JA; Wu, M; Knopps, A; Xiang, AH; Utzschneider, KM; Kahn, SF; Olefsky, JM, Buchanan, TA, Scherer, PE. Complex distribution, not absolute amount of adiponectin, correlates with thiazolidine-mediated improvement in insulin sensitivity. *J Biol Chem,* 2004, 279, 12152-12162.

[68] Matsubara, M; Katyose, S; Maruoka, S. Decreased plasma adiponectin concentrations in nondiabetic women with elevated homeostasis model assessment ratios. *Eur J Endocrinol,* 2003, 148, 343-350.

[69] Yamamoto, Y; Hirose, H; Saito, I; Tomita, M; Taniyama, M; Matsubara, K; Okazaki, Y; Ishii, T; Nishikai, K; Saruta, T. Correlation of the adipocyte derived protein adiponectin with insulin resistance index serum high-density lipoprotein-cholesterol in the Japanese population. *Clin Sci,* 2002, 103, 137-142.

[70] Imagawa, A; Funahashi, T; Nakamura, T; Moriwaki, M; Tanaka, S; Nishizawa, H; Sayama, K; Uno, S; Iwahashi, H; Yamagata, K; Miyagawa, J; Matsuzawa, Y. Elevated serum concentration of adipose derived factor, adiponectin, in patients with type 1 diabetes. *Diabetes Care,* 2002, 25, 1665-1666.

[71] Chen, H; Montagnani, M; Funahashi, T; Shimomura, I; Quon, MJ. Adiponectin stimulates production of nitric oxide in vascular endothelial cells. *J Biol Chem*, 2003, 278, 45021-45026.

[72] Lihn, A; Yunk-Wook, KK; Bruun, J; Pedersen, S; Richelsen, B. Human in vitro and in vivo effects of thiazoledinediones on adiponectin. *Obes Res*, 2003, 11, A 35.

[73] Ouchi, N; Kobayashi, H; Kihara, S; Kumada, M; Sato, K; Inoue, T; Funahashi, T; Walsh, K. Adiponectin stimulates angiogenesis by promoting cross-talk between AMP-activated protein kinase and Akt signaling in endothelial cells. *J Biol Chem*, 2004, 279, 1304-1309.

[74] Haque, WA; Shimomura, I; Matsuzawa, Y; Garg, A. Serum adiponectin and leptin levels in patients with lipodystrophies. *J Clin Endocrinol Metab*, 2002, 87, 2395-2398.

[75] Delporte, ML; Brichard, SM; Hermans, MP; Beguin, C; Lambert, C. Hyperadiponectinaemia in anorexia nervosa. *Clin Endocrinol*, 2003, 58, 22–29.

[76] Yang, WS; Lee, WJ; Funahashi, T; Tanaka, S; Matsuzawa, Y; Chao, CL; Chen, CL; Tai, TY, Chuang, LM. Weight reduction increases plasma levels of an adipose-derived anti-inflammatory protein, adiponectin. *J Clin Endocrinol Metab*, 2001, 86, 3815-3819.

[77] Halleux, CM; Takahashi, M; Delporte, ML; Detry, R; Funahashi, T; Matsuzawa, Y; Brichard, SM. Secretion of adiponectin and regulation of apm1 gene expression in human visceral adipose tissue. *Biochem Biophys Res Commun*, 2001, 288, 1102-1107.

[78] Weyer, C; Funahashi, T; Tanaka, S; Hotta, K; Matsuzawa, Y; Pratley, RE; Tataranni, PA. Hypoadiponectinemia in obesity and type 2 diabetes: close association with insulin resistance and hyperinsulinemia. *J Clin Endocrinol Metab*, 2001, 86, 1930-1935.

[79] Fasshauer, M; Klein, J; Neumann, S; Eszlinger, M; Paschke, R. Adiponectin gene expression is inhibited by beta-adrenergic stimulation via protein kinase A in 3T3-L1 adipocytes. *FEBS Letters*, 2001, 507, 142-146.

[80] Feillet, F; Feillet-Coudray, C; Bard, JM; Parra, HJ; Favre, E; Kabuth, B; Fruchart, JC Vidailhet, M. Plasma cholesterol and endogenous cholesterol synthesis during re-feeding in anorexia nervosa. *Clin Chim Acta*, 2000, 294, 45-56.

[81] Fruebis, J; Tsao, T.S; Javorschi, S; Ebbets-Reed, D; Erickson, M.R; Yen, FT; Bihain, BE; Lodish, HF. Proteolytic cleavage product of 30-kda adipocyte complement-related protein increases fatty acid oxidation in muscle and causes weight loss in mice. *Proc Nat Acad Sci USA*, 2001, 98, 2005-2010.

[82] Yokota, T; Meka, CS; Medina, KL; Igarashi, H; Comp, PC; Takahashi, M; Nishida, M; Oritani, K; Miyagawa, J; Funahashi, T; Tomiyama, Y; Matsuzawa, Y; Kincade, PW. Paracrine regulation of fat cell formation in bone marrow cultures via adiponectin and prostaglandins. *J Clin Invest*, 2002, 109, 1303-1310.

[83] Zoccali, C; Mallamaci, F; Tripepi, G; Benedetto, FA; Cutrupi, S; Parlongo, S; Malatino, LS; Bonanno, G; Seminara, G; Rapisarda, F; Fatuzzo, P; Buemi, M; Nicocia, G; Tanaka, S; Ouchi, N; Kihara, S; Funahashi, T; Matsuzawa, Y. Adiponectin, metabolic risk factors, and cardiovascular events among patients with end-stage renal disease. *J Am Soc Nephrol*, 2002, 13, 134-141.

[84] Devuyst, O; Lambert, M; Rodhain, J; Lefebvre, C; Coche, E. Haematological changes and infectious complications in anorexia nervosa: a case-control study. *Q J Med*, 1993, 86, 791-799.

[85] Patel, L; Buckels, AC; Kinghorn, IJ; Murdock, PR; Holbrook, JD; Plumpton, C; Macphee, CH, Smith SA. Resistin is expressed in human macrophages and directly regulated by PPAR -activators. Biochem Biophys Res Commun, 2003, 300, 472–476.

[86] Kilic, M; Taskin, E; Ustundag, B; Aygun, AD. The evaluation of serum leptin level and other hormonal parameters in children with severe malnutrition. *Clin Biochem,* 2004, 37, 382–387.

[87] Delporte, ML; Brichard, SM; Hermans, MP; Beguin, C; Lambert, M. Hyperadiponectinaemia in anorexia nervosa. Clin Endocrinol (Oxf), 2003, 58, 22–29.

[88] Pannacciulli, N; Vettor, R; Milan, G; Granzotto, M; Catucci, A; Federspil, G; De Giacomo, P; Giorgino, R; De Pergola, G. Anorexia nervosa is characterized by increased adiponectin plasma levels and reduced nonoxidative glucose metabolism. *J Clin Endocrinol Metab,* 2003, 88, 1748–1752.

[89] Iwahashi, H; Funahashi, T; Kurokawa, N; Sayama, K; Fukuda, E; Okita, K; Imagawa, A; Yamagata, K; Shimomura, I; Miyagawa, JI; Matsuzawa, Y. Plasma adiponectin levels in women with anorexia nervosa. *Horm Metab Res,* 2003, 35, 537–540.

[90] Tagami, T; Satoh, N; Usui, T; Yamada, K; Shimatsu, A; Kuzuya, H. Adiponectin in anorexia nervosa and bulimia nervosa. *J Clin Endocrinol Metab*, 2004, 89, 1833–1837.

[91] Qi, Y; Takahashi, N; Hileman, SM; Patel, HR; Berg, AH; Pajvani, UB; Scherer, PE; Ahima, RS. Adiponectin acts in the brain to decrease body weight. *Nat Med,* 2004, 10:524–529.

In: Anorexia Nervosa: A Multi-Disciplinary Approach
Editors: A. Mancini, S. Daini, L. Caruana, pp. 51-73
ISBN: 978-1-60876-200-2

Chapter 3

AMENORRHEA IN ANOREXIA NERVOSA

E. Giacchi, E. Leone, V. Di Donna and A.Mancini
Center for Study and Research on Natural Fertility Regulation and Division of Endocrinology, Catholic University of the Sacred Heart, Rome, Italy

ABSTRACT

The diagnostic criteria for Anorexia Nervosa (AN), according to the American Psychiatric Association, includes amenorrhea among the most important features of AN. Gonadotropin secretion in anorexic women exhibits a typical prepubertal pattern that is similar to other forms of hypothalamic anovulation, with prevalent FSH secretion in comparison to LH and low estradiol levels. Different factors, such as weight loss, decreased body fat, abnormal eating attitudes and behaviors, exercise and psychological stressors, are involved. Endocrine mechanisms influencing the pituitary-gonadal axis are the hyperactivation of pituitary-adrenal axis (the "stress" system), the low levels of insulin and leptin and the GH-resistance. The consequences of prolonged amenorrhea are not entirely reversible with weight gain; therefore, underlying the importance of this phenomenon it is not a simple symptom but an epiphenomenon of the complex psychophysical interface of AN.

1. INTRODUCTION

The diagnostic criteria for Anorexia Nervosa (AN), according to the American Psychiatric Association, includes amenorrhea among the most important features of AN. In postmenarchal females, amenorrhea is defined as absence of at least three consecutive menstrual cycles, with exclusion of drug-induced menses.

The etiology of amenorrhea is multifactorial and is the result of a complex interplay of many factors including weight loss, decreased body fat, abnormal eating attitudes and behaviors, exercise and psychological stressors [1]. Hormone environment modifications are involved as the main mechanism underlying the action of such factors.

As described in Chapter 1, gonadotropin secretion in anorexic women exhibits a prepubertal pattern similar to other forms of hypothalamic anovulation. Typical patterns of LH secretion and normal or supranormal response to LHRH are seen when there are moderate degrees of weight recovery. Anovulation can persist in up to 50% of anorexic patients, even after achieving normal weight. Moreover, anorexic patients exhibit hyperactivation of the hypothalamus-pituitary system. Although the diurnal variation is maintained, there is a persistent hypersecretion of cortisol throughout the day. Cushingoid features (clinical symptoms due to inappropriate cortisol secretion, like in Cushing's syndrome), however, are not present, in part because of mild hypercortisolemia and also because of a reduction of peripheral glucocorticoid receptors. Levels of both CRH and β-endorphin are increased in the central nervous system [2].

A mention of the maturation of the hypothalamic-pituitary-ovarian axis (HPO) and the physiology of the normal menstrual cycle is essential in order to understand the mechanism of amenorrhea in AN.

2. Hypothalamic-Pituitary-Ovarian Axis (HPO)

Gonadotropin secretion in AN exhibits a prepubertal pattern, similar to that in other forms of hypothalamic anovulation (lack of ovulation due to dysfunction in central nervous system); in fact, adolescents with AN have hypothalamic hypogonadism with impaired gonadotropin-releasing hormone (GnRH) secretion by the hypothalamus and low serum levels of luteinizing hormone (LH), follicular-stimulating hormone (FSH), and estradiol [3].

The HPO axis becomes active, in a human fetus, during the second trimester of pregnancy. Gonadotropin levels peak at mid gestation and decline at term because of a negative feedback by placental hormones. A mild secondary peak in gonadotropin levels occurs after birth, caused by the withdrawal of placental steroids, but since 1–2 years of age, levels of gonadotropins remain low until puberty begins. They are suppressed by circulating sex hormones primarily produced by the adrenals and mediated via the negative feedback loop [4]. Prepubertal children have low levels of LH, with minimal variation during all 24 hours. The onset of puberty is a centrally driven process, the detailed mechanisms of which are not entirely known. It is translated into an increased activity of the hypothalamic "GnRH pulse generator." The hypothalamus becomes less sensitive to circulating gonadal hormones. Pulses of GnRH increase in amplitude and frequency and are followed by pulses of LH and FSH. Augmented secretion of both LH and FSH is more prominent during sleep [5]. Onset of puberty is associated with a greater increase in LH pulse amplitude than frequency and a much greater increase in LH and FSH; moreover, a progressive increase in daytime pulsatility occurs, with a gradual reduction of sleep-entrained amplification.

In response to rising LH and FSH levels, the ovary produces estrogen, which initiates sexual maturation, heralded by breast development (telarche). There is a normal progression of pubertal development in both boys and girls. The physiological modifications have been divided into five stages by Tanner and Whitehouse [6]. In girls, the first appearance of menses (menarche) usually occurs during Tanner stage four of breast development and usually within two and a half to three years after thelarche. Once menarche has occurred, it takes approximately five to seven years for the HPO axis to mature and regular menstrual cycles to establish. The interval from the first menstrual period to the second period can be quite long, but subsequent cycles usually vary from 21 to 45 days, with few cycles falling out of this range. In the first year after menarche, approximately 50% of cycles are anovulatory, but 80% still fall within the range of 21 to 45 days' duration. By the third year after menarche, 95% of menstrual cycles fall into this range. In general, anovulatory cycles occur most frequently during the first two years after menarche.

Reports have shown that adolescents with AN display a prepubertal or early pubertal pulsatile secretion pattern of LH. Boyar et al. [7] demonstrated age-inappropriate 24-hour LH secretion patterns in females ages 17 to 23 years, with AN and primary or secondary amenorrhea. These findings suggest that females with AN have a regression of the hypothalamic-pituitary ovarian axis, with an associated arrest in normal menstrual functioning.

Marshal et al. studied patients affected by anorexia nervosa to determine whether gonadotropin-releasing hormone (GnRH) administration could induce the hormonal changes that occur during normal puberty. All the studied patients were prepubertal, as evidenced by immature LH and FSH responses to a standard GnRH test and the absence of spontaneous LH peaks both during the day and during sleep. The results demonstrate a normal pituitary responsiveness to physiological administration of GnRH and a changing pattern of FSH and LH secretion similar to those seen during normal puberty in girls and during the follicular phase of the menstrual cycle of adult women [3].

3. Factors Involved in Amenorrhea

Body Weight

The role of decreased body weight is underlined by various studies on recovery of menses after weight gain. Golden et al. [8] demonstrated that a weight approximately 90% of standard body weight was the average one at which resumption of menses occurred and is a reasonable treatment goal weight, because 86% of patients who achieved this goal resumed menses within six months. Resumption of menses required restoration of HPO function, since serum estradiol levels at follow-up best assesses resumption of menses (with a required limit >110 pmol/L).

According to Swenne [9], the weight level required for return of menstruation is highly individual but can be predicted by the weight at which menstruations cease. The considerable overlap in the weight of amenorrhoic girls with those who menstruate further emphasizes the need for such an individual prediction. The tight correlation between weight at return and weight at loss of menstruations, and its linearity throughout a wide weight range, further support the view that a substantial proportion of girls with eating disorders need attain a weight or BMI above the population average to menstruate. A target weight at or below the population mean is thus both too low and too generalized to allow prediction in individuals with sufficient precision, as showed by the growth curves commonly used in clinical practice [15]. However, it should be remembered that the weight at which a menstruation returns is only a minimal requirement. In order to establish regular and ovulatory menstrual cycles and to restore lean body mass and general physical health, further weight gain may be needed.

Then, Swenne demonstrated that the return of menses was achieved when patients reached a weight consistent with their prepubertal growth trajectory. This group suggested that target weight should be based on a patient's individual pre-illness growth curve percentile (i.e., their inborn genetic potential), as opposed to population norms of weight for height, since there are a proportion of adolescent females who need to achieve a weight or BMI above the population average in order to menstruate [10].

The use of pelvic ultrasound has demonstrated its usefulness in determining the return of the normal menstrual cycle. In underweight and hypoestrogenic adolescents with AN, the ovaries are small and amorphous, and the uterus is regressed to a prepubertal size with a very thin or undetectable endometrium. As adolescents with AN gain weight, the ovaries develop small multifollicular features and the uterus increases in size [16]. Return to normal menstrual function correlates with the appearance of a dominant ovarian follicle and ovarian and uterine maturity. The observation of a dominant ovarian follicle has been demonstrated to be correlated with premorbid weight, not simply BMI [17].

Key et al. [18] showed that 88% of adolescents with AN required a weight-to-height ratio of 100% (BMI=20), as determined by Tanner–Whitehouse British Standards, to achieve reproductive maturity according to pelvic ultrasound pattern. In this study, only 11% of patients attained ovarian and uterine maturity at 90% ideal body weight (IBW), and a significant percent remained amenorrheic without achieving full reproductive maturity. Therefore, persistent amenorrhea may reflect the fact that an adolescent with AN is not truly "weight recovered" despite being at a weight within the normal range for her age and height.

Fat Mass

Already in 1974, Frisch and McArthur [14] proposed the critical weight or fat mass hypothesis for the onset of menarche or resumption of menses, suggesting that the minimum or threshold weight for height for menarche is at approximately 17% fat as a percentage of body weight. Additionally, the authors reported that an average of 26% to 28% fat achieved at the completion of normal growth and that a minimum weight representing 22% body fat is required for the maintenance or resumption of menses in females greater than 16 years of age. According to Frish [15], the percentage of body fat in women may influence reproductive ability directly: [1] as fat is an extragonadal source of estrogen by enzymatic mechanism (aromatization of androgen to estrogen); [2] by addressing estrogen metabolism toward more potent or less potent forms; or [3] by changes in the binding properties of sex-hormone-binding globulin (SHBG, a protein that vehiculates estrogen in the general circulation). Indirect signals may be of abnormal control of temperature and changes in energy metabolism, which accompany excessive leanness.

Recently, Misra et al. [16] compared menses-recovered AN subjects with amenorrhoic AN and controls, showing different hormonal milieu in the first group (higher baseline cortisol levels and greater increases in leptin in menses recovered subject) related to greater increase in fat mass than women of other groups. They demonstrated that high baseline cortisol levels predicted increases in body fat and that the last, in turn, predicted recovery of menses in adolescents with AN.

Miller et al. [17] observed that, although amenorrhea due to acquired GnRH deficiency is nearly universal in AN, a subset of patients maintains menses despite low weight. The two groups were similar in body mass index, percent ideal body weight, duration of eating disorder, age of menarche, and exercise. As expected, eumenorrheic patients had a higher mean estradiol level and higher mean percent body fat, total body fat mass, and truncal fat than amenorrheic patients. Patients with eumenorrhea had more body fat and higher levels of nutritionally dependent hormones, including leptin and IGF-I, than their amenorrheic counterparts of similar weight. Moreover, reduced bone density was observed in both groups, but was less severe at the spine, but not the hip, in women with under-nutrition and preserved menstrual function than in amenorrheic women of similar weight. Therefore, fat mass may be important for preservation of normal menstrual function in severely undernourished women, and this may be in part mediated through leptin secretion (see below). In addition, nutritional intake and normal hormonal function may be independent contributors to maintenance of trabecular bone mass in low-weight women.

Alimentary Habits

In as many as two-thirds of patients with AN, absence of menses precedes significant weight loss [18]. This suggests that factors other than significant weight loss contribute to the amenorrhea of AN. For instance, in many young women with AN, disordered eating behaviors, particularly caloric restriction, precede the attainment of low weight. The effect of disordered eating per se on the menstrual cycle has been investigated in women without an eating disorder [25,26]. Loucks et al. [25] showed that low serum LH in exercising women is caused by low energy availability rather than by exercise. Similarly, Warren and Perlroth [26] (26) reported that the primary cause of GnRH suppression in athletes is caloric restriction. These conclusions are further supported by work done in woman with functional hypothalamic amenorrhea (FHA) [27], who reported significantly more symptoms of disordered eating than eumenorrheic women or women with organic amenorrhea. Schneider et al. [28] also looked at FHA and its relationship with grehlin, a hormone secreted by the stomach in response to hunger, and disordered eating. Both ghrelin and eating behaviors (as measured by the Eating Attitudes Test) are significantly elevated in FHA, even in light of normal caloric intake. There is evidence that ghrelin acts as a restraining metabolic signal preventing the return of regular menses in women with both disordered eating and FHA.

Exercise

Excessive exercise is commonly seen in patients with AN [23]. Excessive exercise in non–eating-disordered athletes has been associated with menstrual irregularities. Exercise-induced amenorrhea has an incidence of 5% to 25%, depending on the type and level of activity, and is due to hypothalamic dysfunction associated with a decrease in pulse frequency of GnRH, with ensuing low levels of LH, FSH, and estradiol [24]. When combined with malnutrition and weight loss, exercise increases the likelihood of amenorrhea developing sooner and for a longer time. Litt and Glader [25] compared exercising and sedentary females with AN and found that exercisers with AN had a greater degree of menstrual dysfunction and took longer to resume menses following weight gain. The "female athlete triad" is defined as the combination of disordered eating, amenorrhea, and osteoporosis, as reviewed by Golden and Carlson [26]. The female athlete triad results from an imbalance between energy intake and energy expenditure [19,20]. This, in turn, stimulates compensatory mechanisms, such as weight loss or energy conservation, subsequently causing a central suppression of reproductive function and concomitant hypoestrogenism.

Psychological Stressors

As mentioned previously, menstrual dysfunction in adolescents with eating disorders is a complex phenomenon. Persistent amenorrhea may reflect the fact that young people with AN are not actually "weight recovered" or that weight may not be the sole factor contributing to the amenorrhea. For instance, psychological recovery has been shown to be an important feature contributing to resumption of menses in AN. One study followed a cohort of women for one-year post treatment for AN [27]. Those patients who were weight-recovered but amenorrheic tended to have eating attitudes and behaviors consistent with AN. For example, these young women restricted their fat intake, were concerned with food and a thin, ideal body, had fears of becoming fat, and had a distorted body image to a greater extent than those with return of menses. In addition, affective and/or anxiety disorders occur in 33% to 73% of young women with AN [28]. Major depression, anxiety, and stress are associated with increased cortisol secretion and resistance to the negative feedback of cortisol on cortisol-releasing hormone (CRH), resulting in inhibition of GnRH secretion [29]. When depression, anxiety, or stress occur concurrently with an eating disorder, the effect of weight loss on the hypothalamic-pituitary-gonadal (HPG) axis may be compounded and contribute to amenorrhea.

4. Hormones Affecting HPO Axis

Growth Hormone

As Growth Hormone (GH), obligatory for growth and development, is also involved in the processes of sexual differentiation and pubertal maturation and participates in gonadal steroidogenesis, gametogenesis and ovulation, the alterations of GH-Igf-1 axis in anorexia nervosa (exaggerated GH secretion and reduced IGF-I levels, suggesting a peripheral GH resistance for impairment of the negative IGF-I feedback action on GH secretion; enhanced somatotroph responsiveness to GHRH and impaired GH response to most central nervous system-mediated stimuli; resistance to cholinergic manipulation, suggesting a somewhat specific alteration in the somatostatin-mediated cholinergic influence on GH secretion; paradoxical GH responses to glucose load, thyrotropin releasing hormone and GnRH; increased ghrelin, as reviewed in Chapter 1) have a role in mechanism of amenorrhea. Moreover, the hypoestrogenism that accompanies amenorrhea could be involved in the alterations in GH secretion; it has been suggested that malnutrition underlies the increase in the amount of GH secreted in each pulse and that hypoestrogenism is responsible for the increased pulse frequency.

So it is important to focus on the concept that GH is an important modulator of female reproduction in order to understand this role in the mechanism of amenorrhea in anorexia nervosa.

GH has numerous gonadotrophic roles in female reproduction and is additionally progestational, mammogenic and galactopoietic. These actions may reflect direct endocrine actions of pituitary GH or be mediated by its induction of hepatic or local IGF-I production. However, as GH is also produced in gonadal, placental and mammary tissues, it may act in paracrine or autocrine ways to regulate local processes that are strategically regulated by pituitary GH.

The actions of GH are generally progonadal at physiological concentrations and antigonadal at pharmacological concentrations and in pathophysiological excess, deficit or resistance.

A significant amount of literature supports a role for GH in the production of viable gametes, since GH modulates gonadotropin-independent early folliculogenesis and gonadotrophin-dependent late folliculogenesis by increasing cell proliferation and inhibiting atresia. GH also increases oocyte fertility by enhancing nuclear and cytoplasmic maturation and facilitating ovulation. Ovarian and hepatic IGF-I appear to be involved in some, but not all, of these actions in some species. As a result of these gametogenic and folliculogenic actions, GH has been shown to influence fertility. An extensive review is presented by Hull and Harvey [30], to which we remand for specific references.

Folliculogenesis

The relative number of small, medium and large follicles varies over the course of the ovarian cycle. As the cycle proceeds, the growth of a dominant follicle is associated with a reduction in the number of small- and medium-sized follicles. The growth and development of follicles larger than two mm is dependent upon pituitary hormones, as shown in animal experiments (hypophysectomy in sheep results in follicular atresia and cessation of small follicle growth). The resumption of normal follicular development requires the administration of gonadotropins and GH; thus, GH may be permissive for gonadotropin-induced follicular development. This effect may be dependent on IGF-I, because follicular growth and IGF-I increase in a coordinated fashion. Conversely, GH stimulates the proliferation of human luteinized granulosa cells via an FSH and IGF-I-independent mechanism. GH-induced development of preantral follicles in immature mice is similarly independent of IGF-I but is dependent on FSH, and this effect of GH is blocked by other proteic hormones usually implicated in FSH regulation (folliculostatin, which binds and inactivates activin). Activin can also stimulate follicle growth; therefore, GH may augment early follicular development by increasing ovarian activin production. Thus, the mechanism by which GH stimulates follicular development appears to be species-specific and to vary over the ovarian cycle [30].

Oocyte Maturation

As the follicle matures, nuclear and cytoplasmic events within the oocyte are required before it can be successfully fertilized. Nuclear events include the completion of meiosis and the extrusion of the first polar body, and an accelerated rate of nuclear maturation is associated with enhanced zygote formation. Indeed, the beneficial effect of GH on female fertility noted in some studies in vivo may reflect the stimulatory effect of GH on the kinetics of nuclear maturation. Experimental studies have shown that GH-treated bovine oocytes complete meiosis I faster and undergo zygote cleavage and blastocyst formation more frequently than untreated oocytes. GH stimulates nuclear maturation by IGF-I-independent actions mediated through cumulus cells, probably via changes in intracellular cAMP, even if different events could be involved in various animal species. GH incubation increases the proportion of bovine oocytes manifesting the characteristics of both cytoplasmic maturation and nuclear maturation. Thus, GH may enhance the co-ordination between nuclear and cytoplasmic maturation [31].

Ovulation

GH plays a non-essential but facilitory role in ovulation. For instance, although GH alone fails to cause ovulation in sheep, pigs or rabbits, gonadotropin-induced ovulation in perifused rabbit ovaries is significantly improved by GH co-administration (see for review ref 30). Moreover, fertility is reduced but not abolished in models of animals with an absence of GH receptor (GHR-knockout mice) [32], and egg production and fertility are not impaired in GH-resistant sex-linked dwarf chickens. In such cases, other GH-like hormones, particularly prolactin, may compensate for the lack of GH action. GH may facilitate ovulation by increasing sensitivity to gonadotropins and by reducing the incidence of apoptosis in preovulatory ovarian follicles. The increased number of corpora lutea and reduced numbers of atresic follicles in the ovaries of mice transgenically expressing GH supports this view [33]. This action of GH is thought to be IGF-I mediated (33). GH may also facilitate ovulation by increasing tissue plasminogen activator synthesis, which activates the enzymes (serine protease) required for rupture of the ovarian capsule. The timing of ovulation may also be GH-dependent, since it is delayed in normal female mice paired with GHR-knockout mice [32].

Female Infertility

Reproductive dysfunctions in some women have been associated with partial GH deficiencies [34]. The possible use of GH as an adjunct to human menopausal gonadotrophin (hMG) for ovulation induction has been the focus of extensive research [35]. Clinical studies have shown that GH may be therapeutically useful in some, but not all, infertile women. In particular, GH administration to hypogonadotropic anovulatory women significantly reduces the dosage and duration of hMG treatment required for ovulation induction and increases the percentage of successfully treated patients. GH therapy may also be used in assisted reproductive techniques to enhance the hyperovulatory response to hMG. Numerous clinical studies have demonstrated that the addition of GH to the hMG treatment regimen improves oocyte recovery and the rate of successful fertilization and pregnancies, particularly in women with polycystic ovary syndrome [36]. However, owing to the heterogeneous causes of female infertility, GH therapy does not always enhance gonadotrophin responsiveness. Blumenfeld et al. [37] reported that GH secretion was impaired in most women who responded to GH–hMG co-treatment. Thus, the infertility in responders may result, in part, from relative GH deficiency, whereas other dysfunctions are causal in the infertility of non-responders. However, normal fertility does not always require a normal GH axis. Indeed, GH-deficient [34] and GH-resistant [38] women usually have normal pubertal development and menstrual cycles and conceive normally.

Steroidogenesis

The actions of GH in ovarian function are partly mediated by changes in ovarian steroidogenesis, as indicated by the partial progesterone deficiency in GHR-deficient cattle. Numerous mammalian studies have demonstrated an increase in ovarian steroid production after GH administration in vivo, for example, in pigs, or in vitro, for example, in cattle. However, in different studies, GH is ineffective or inhibitory, for example, in pigs and in women. GH may induce steroidogenesis directly or by potentiating gonadotropin action. One hypothesis is that GH upregulates LH receptors, thus enhancing LH-induced luteinization and the acquisition of progesterone synthetic ability. This possibility is supported by the inability of GH to induce progesterone production in the absence of gonadotropins in rats. However, GH is effective in women and other species in the absence of gonadotropins, and so GH must also act independently. Early studies assumed that IGF-I was the sole mediator of GH action in the ovary, since IGF-I or GH enhance steroid production to the same extent in rats, and GH usually increases follicular–luteal IGF-I in cows. Moreover, Hutchinson et al. observed that IGF-I antibodies significantly inhibit GH effects on FSH-induced progesterone secretion in rat ovaries. However, Wathes et al. did not detect IGF-I in the follicular fluid of GH-treated bovine follicles, despite increased progesterone release. In addition, IGF-I antibodies cannot completely block GH-induced progesterone synthesis in pig granulosa cells or androgen synthesis by rat thecal–interstitial cells. Therefore, GH may stimulate ovarian steroidogenic enzymes by direct and IGF-I-mediated mechanisms. GH may activate some enzymes by cAMPdependent mechanisms that involve de novo protein synthesis (perhaps IGF-I), but other enzymes independent of both cAMP and protein synthesis. However, the steroidogenic action of GH may also reflect its induction of cellular proliferation or the differentiation of follicular cells, since the conversion of rat follicular cells into granulosa luteal cells is associated with increased progesterone synthesis and aromatase activity. All these experiments are reviewed in ref. 30.

Gonadal Minihypophysis

Since the gonads are highly vascularized, many of the gonadal actions of exogenous GH are likely to reflect the endocrine actions of pituitary GH. However, as some gonadal cells (germ cells, granulosa cells in females and the correspondent cells in males, Sertoli cells, at adluminal compartments) in the ovary and testis are avascular or physically separated from systemic circulation by a barrier, some of the steroidogenic and gametogenic actions of GH may reflect the actions of GH produced locally. Indeed, the entire GH gene family (comprising GH, placental GH (hGH-V) and placental lactogens) is transcribed in the human testes and ovary [39], with hGH-V being the most active gene transcriptionally. "Hypothalamic" GH-regulating hormones may regulate gonadal GH synthesis in a similar manner to pituitary GH synthesis, since a mini hypothalamic–hypophyseal axis is also present in male and female reproductive tracts. GH-releasing hormone (GHRH) [40] and somatostatin (SRIF) [41] are synthesized in the male and female gonad and bind to gonadal receptors. However, the importance of ovarian GHRH and SRIF in ovarian and testicular GH synthesis is unclear, since GH synthesis in non-pituitary sites is often independent of traditional GH secretagogues [42]. Moreover, these factors have been shown to have other local roles unrelated to GH regulation. Instead, gonadal GH synthesis may be modulated by locally relevant factors, although this possibility has yet to be assessed.

Finally, numerous actions on uterus and oviduct have been described, but they overcome the purpose of this chapter [30].

Leptin

Adequate nutrition and energy reserves are required for fertility and pregnancy. Their effects on reproductive function have long been suspected to be mediated by metabolic signal(s) that link adipose stores with neuroendocrine function. The discovery of leptin, and recent data suggesting that this hormone may influence reproduction, provided the biochemical basis of the communication that exists between fat stores and the brain. Leptin appears to be the link between nutrition/energy reserves and reproductive function. In addition to regulating body weight and energy homeostasis, leptin stimulates a wide variety of biologic responses, including reproductive development and function. We refer to the excellent review of Mantzoros [43].

Leptin in Childhood–Puberty

According to the above-reported hypothesis of Frisch and McArthur [14] that the percentage of body fat can be a signal to the brain for the onset of puberty, it has been proposed that leptin may serve as such signal for the brain, indicating the critical amount of fat stores necessary for initiation of puberty and maintenance of menstrual cycles and reproductive ability. This hypothesis is in agreement with the hypogonadotropic hypogonadism of leptin deficient ob/ob mice and the fact that leptin treatment corrects the reproductive system defects of these mice [44] independently of its effect on decreasing body weight. In addition, animal experiments have consistently shown that leptin administration to prepubertal mice and nonhuman primates accelerates puberty [45]. In normal children, leptin levels rise before puberty as body fat mass increases, and they reach their peak at the onset of puberty, suggesting that leptin may trigger the initiation of puberty in humans, too [46]. By contrast, subjects with inactivating mutations of the leptin receptor remain prepubertal and have hypogonadotrophic hypogonadism similar to that of the ob/ob mouse model of obesity [47]. Leptin, therefore, appears to provide a necessary signal to the brain regarding the amount of energy stores that would be necessary to successfully carry a pregnancy to term. However, whether leptin acts directly on the hypothalamic–pituitary–gonadal axis or whether leptin acts only as a permissive factor to allow reproductive pubertal maturation to proceed if and only when metabolic resources are adequate for pregnancy remains to be demonstrated. Recent evidence demonstrates that leptin acts on hypothalamic cells to release LHRH, thereby regulating the release of gonadotropins [48]. The subsequent stimulation of gonadal steroid secretion leads to development of the reproductive tract and induction of puberty. The exact mechanism by which leptin regulates LHRH secretion and the function of the hypothalamic–pituitary–gonadal axis, as well as the potential indirect effects of leptin on the reproductive system, are currently the subject of intensive research efforts.

Leptin in Normal Reproductive Function : leptin is secreted in a pulsatile manner, and its circulating levels display a distinct circadian rhythm in humans. Moreover, minute-to-minute variations in serum leptin levels are significantly related to minute-to-minute changes in ACTH and cortisol levels in normal human subjects. More importantly, minute-to-minute variations of serum leptin levels are also significantly associated with serum luteinizing hormone (LH) and estradiol levels in normal women [49], indicating that leptin may contribute to physiologic levels and rhythmicity of reproductive hormones. Interestingly, leptin pulse amplitude is higher in women than in men, indicating that the strongest distinction between the sexes is not at the level of organization or oscillation frequency, but rather in the amount of leptin released per unit time. Animal experiments have shown that rats treated intracerebroventricularly with leptin antiserum have impaired LH pulsatility consistent with a direct role of leptin in regulating LHRH and LH pulsatile secretion.

Leptin in Relation to the Reproductive Abnormalities in Response to Starvation

It has been suggested that leptin may have primarily evolved as an adaptive mechanism to starvation. Thus, one of leptin's main roles would be to conserve energy by decreasing thyroid hormone levels and to mobilize energy stores by increasing the secretion of glucocorticoids, while at the same time suppressing gonadal function during periods of starvation, when the energy demands of pregnancy and lactation cannot be met. This hypothesis was proved on the basis of animal physiology experiments and recent "experiments of nature" [50]. More specifically, leptin administration to starving mice restores the neuroendocrine changes induced by falling leptin levels due to food deprivation, including the suppressed gonadal axis. This effect is, at least in part, NPY mediated [51]. In addition, experiments of nature recently demonstrated that the foregoing observations are also part of human physiology. "Functional leptin deficiency" due to mutations of the leptin receptor gene results in abnormalities of the hypothalamic–pituitary–gonadal axis [47]. Furthermore, leptin deficiency associated with anorexia nervosa, a disease model of starvation, is also characterized by reproductive abnormalities. Based on the foregoing observations, it can reasonably be claimed that leptin is the hormone that signals to the brain the state of starvation and thus results in teleologically appropriate changes of the reproductive system that would limit procreation under conditions of limited energy availability.

Amenorrhea in these women may indicate that fat content is sensed via leptin; and in low leptin states, that is, in women who do not have an adequate amount of nutritional reserves, ovulation is inhibited [14]. In addition, it was recently shown that increasing serum-luteinizing hormone levels in response to re-feeding in women with anorexia nervosa track very closely their increase in serum leptin level. Thus, low leptin levels appear to cause amenorrhea in women with anorexia nervosa, and normalization of leptin levels should be a necessary factor for the resumption of menses in these patients [52].

A leptin level less than 2μg/L has been proposed as the critical threshold value for amenorrhea [53]. In a comparison of 43 underweight females and 63 females with anorexia nervosa, only leptin predicted a lifetime occurrence of amenorrhea, whereas BMI, fat mass, and percent body fat did not predict the lifetime occurrence of amenorrhea [54]. Fasting leads to decreased leptin levels before the onset of weight loss and may explain why, in some patients, amenorrhea occurs before the onset of weight loss. Exogenous administration of recombinant human leptin has been shown to improve reproductive function in women with hypothalamic amenorrhea. Welt et al. [55] administered twice-daily recombinant human leptin over three months to eight women with hypothalamic amenorrhea due to strenuous exercise or low weight (within 15% IBW) who did not have active eating disorders. These subjects were compared to six controls with hypothalamic amenorrhea who did not receive recombinant human leptin. Treatment with recombinant human leptin increased mean LH level and LH pulse frequency and increased maximal follicular diameter, the number of dominant follicles, ovarian volume and estradiol levels. Three of these patients achieved an ovulatory menstrual cycle, which was higher than the expected rate of spontaneous ovulation of 10 percent. Like other mentioned factors, the return of normal leptin levels is not by itself sufficient for the return of normal menstrual function. Like most neuroendocrine hormones, leptin works in concert with other factors contributing to the menstrual dysfunction observed in patients with AN. This is underscored by one study on eumenorrheic and amenorrheic weight-recovered patients with AN, whose leptin levels were normal; however, women with amenorrhea have low levels of estradiol and GH [56]. Since low levels of leptin are correlated with low levels of IGF-I in women with AN, we may conclude that, other than leptin levels, nutritional status, IGF-1 levels and even insulin secretion contribute to menstrual dysfunction in AN. Insulin can exert effects on folliculogenesis acting on both its own receptor and receptors for IGF-1 [57]; moreover, insulin can influence leptin secretion [58] and finally modify SHBG levels. Therefore, the low insulin levels, related to reduced fuel introduction, can contribute to ovarian dysfunction in AN. Some studies suggest a condition of insulin resistance in AN, while other do not confirm this hypothesis. Studies reporting a degree of insulin sensitivity (IS) in AN provided rather contradictory results; hyperadiponectinemia in patients with AN could play a role in increased insulin sensitivity (see Chapter 1).

Pituitary-adrenal Axis

The hypothalamic-pituitary-adrenal axis exerts deep, multilevel inhibitory effects on the female reproductive system. Corticotropin-releasing hormone (CRH) and CRH-induced pro-opiomelanocortin peptides inhibit hypothalamic gonadotropin-releasing hormone secretion, whereas glucocorticoids suppress pituitary luteinizing hormone and ovarian estrogen and progesterone secretion and make target tissues resistant to estradiol. The hypothalamic-pituitary-adrenal axis is thus responsible for the "hypothalamic" amenorrhea caused by stress, which is also seen in melancholic depression, malnutrition, eating disorders, chronic active alcoholism, chronic excessive exercise, and the hypogonadism of the Cushing's syndrome, the illness mentioned due to multiple conditions of cortisol excess. Conversely, estrogen directly stimulates the CRH gene promoter and the central noradrenergic system, which may explain adult women's slight hypercortisolism, preponderance of affective, anxiety, and eating disorders, and mood cycles and vulnerability to autoimmune and inflammatory disease, both of which follow estradiol fluctuations. Several components of the hypothalamic-pituitary-adrenal axis and their receptors are present in reproductive tissues as "autacoid" (biological factors that act as local hormones, with brief duration) regulators. These include ovarian and endometrial CRH, which may participate in the inflammatory processes of the ovary (ovulation and luteolysis) and of endometrium (blastocyst implantation and menstruation). The placental CRH may participate in the physiology of pregnancy and the timing of labor and delivery. The hypercortisolism of the latter half of pregnancy can be explained by high plasma levels of placental CRH. This hypercortisolism causes a transient postpartum adrenal suppression that, together with estrogen withdrawal, may partly explain the depression and autoimmune phenomena of the postpartum period [59].

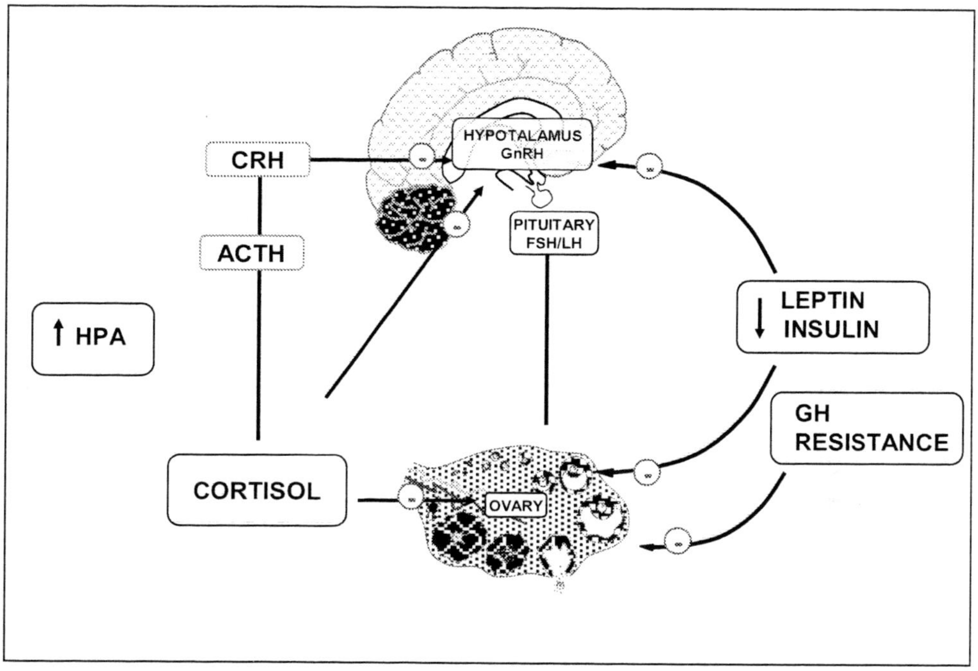

Figure 1. Mechanisms influencing the hypothalamic-pituitary-gonadal axis: an activation of the hypothalamic-pituitary-adrenal axis (CRH-ACTH-cortisol), as stress-response, exerts negative effects at various levels of the axis; low levels of leptin contribute to maintain low the activity of the system. Low insulin levels and low IGF-1, due to GH-resistance, have a direct negative impact on gonadal function.

The hypothalamic-pituitary-adrenal axis, together with the arousal and autonomic nervous systems, constitutes the stress system. This system is activated during stress and produces the clinical phenomenology described by Hans Selye as the stress syndrome [60]. Indeed, during stress, several changes take place in the central and peripheral nervous system of mammals, changes that help to preserve the individual and the species. These include the mobilizing of adaptive behaviors and peripheral functions and the inhibiting of biologically costly behaviors and vegetative functions, such as reproduction, feeding, and growth.

The principal molecular regulators of the hypothalamic-pituitary-adrenal axis are corticotropin-releasing hormone (CRH), a 41-amino acid peptide, and the nonapeptide arginine-vasopressin, both of which are secreted by parvicellular neurons of the paraventricular nucleus of the hypothalamus into the hypophyseal portal system [60]. They synergistically stimulate pituitary adrenocorticotropic hormone (ACTH) secretion and, consequently, cortisol secretion by the adrenal cortex. The noradrenergic brainstem neurons that regulate the central arousal (locus ceruleus) and systemic sympathetic-adrenomedullary systems are reciprocally connected and stimulate the parvicellular hypothalamic CRH and arginine-vasopressin neurons of the paraventricular nucleus.

An excellent example of the effect of stress on the female reproductive system is the so-called stress-induced or "functional hypothalamic amenorrhea" (the FHA mentioned above) [61]. Indeed, the prevalence of sustained secondary amenorrhea in normal young women is about 2%. This rate increases markedly in proportion to chronic stress, all the way up to 100%

in prisoners before execution. Thus, severe enough stress can completely inhibit the female reproductive system. During her reproductive life, a normal woman is exposed to a monthly fluctuation of circulating estradiol and progesterone that may affect her behavior, mood, immune and other functions. Indeed, epidemiologic data underscore the effect of gonadal function on nonreproductive female processes [62]. Thus, suicide attempts and allergic bronchial asthma attacks correlate with the phase of the menstrual cycle, with fourfold increases in prevalence seen when the plasma estradiol level is at its lowest (that is, in the late luteal and menstruation phases). Other studies have suggested that the period of peak estradiol secretion in the state immediately before ovulation is associated with elevations in mood, a phenomenon that might contribute to fecundity.

The hypothalamic-pituitary-adrenal axis, when activated by stress, has an inhibitory effect on the reproductive system; teleologically, this makes sense. Indeed, the hypothalamic CRH neurons innervate and inhibit directly or indirectly, through proopiomelanocortin neurons, the hypothalamic control center of the gonadal axis [63]. In addition, glucocorticoids secreted from the adrenal cortex act at the levels of the hypothalamic, pituitary, gonadal, and target tissues to suppress the gonadal axis. On the other hand, estradiol exerts a negative, although indirect, effect on the activity of the gonadotropin-releasing hormone neuron, which has no detectable estrogen receptor (Figure 1).

The interaction between the hypothalamic-pituitary-adrenal and gonadal axes at the level of the hypothalamus was directly examined in rhesus monkeys [64]. Insulin-induced hypoglycemia caused an increase in cortisol levels and a decrease in plasma luteinizing hormone levels associated with reduced electrical activity measured directly at the gonadotropin-releasing hormone neuron. When a CRH antagonist was given intracerebroventricularly, the effect of insulin hypoglycemia on electrical activity at the gonadotropin-releasing hormone pulse generator was greatly attenuated; this finding suggests that CRH has a direct effect on the hypothalamic neurons that secrete gonadotropin-releasing hormone. Glucocorticoids inhibit gonadal axis function at the hypothalamic, pituitary, and uterine levels [65-67]. Sakakura and colleagues studied women who had received prednisolone for various indications for 1.5 to five months in daily doses ranging from 10 mg to 40 mg [66]. All of these women had menstrual disturbances associated with glucocorticoid treatment, and the investigators found that prednisolone reduced the peak luteinizing hormone response to intravenous gonadotropin-releasing hormone by about 60%. This suggests an inhibitory effect of glucocorticoids on the pituitary gonadotroph. Glucocorticoids also inhibit estradiol-stimulated uterine growth [67], possibly by reducing intracellular estrogen receptor concentrations. However, other molecular mechanisms have been hypothesized: glucocorticoid receptor-mediated inhibition of the c-fos/c-jun transcription factor by protein-protein interaction is primarily responsible for this inhibition [68]; this factor is used in the signal transduction pathways of many growth factors and is directly or indirectly stimulated by estrogen.

Estrogen can induce hyperresponsiveness of the hypothalamic-pituitary-adrenal axis to stimuli, via a stimulation of CRH neurons (which innervate and stimulate central noradrenergic neurons) and direct effects on the production or metabolism of norepinephrine [69]. Estrogen stimulation of the hypothalamic-pituitary-adrenal axis may be exerted through interaction of the ligand-activated estrogen receptor with specific DNA sequences, the estrogen-responsive elements, in the promoter of the human CRH gene [70]. Estrogen may exert some of its physiologic negative feedback effect on the reproductive axis through a subpopulation of CRH and proopiomelanocortin neurons that inhibit gonadotropin-releasing hormone and, hence, follicle-stimulating hormone and luteinizing hormone secretion. Evidence from studies in nonhuman primates suggests that in the period immediately before ovulation, a decrease in estradiol levels leads to reduced hypothalamic CRH secretion. This effectively disinhibits the gonadotropin-releasing hormone (GnRH) neuron and possibly participates in the generation of the ovulatory luteinizing hormone surge [71]. This takes place simultaneously with a delayed estrogen-induced central noradrenergic surge that has an additional positive effect on the gonadotropin-releasing hormone neuron [69]. Estradiol also downregulates glucocorticoid receptor binding in the anterior pituitary, the hypothalamus, and the hippocampus; this tends to increase hypothalamic-pituitary-adrenal axis activity by interfering with glucocorticoid negative feedback, whereas progesterone opposes these effects [72].

Again leptin can have a role: it suppresses the hypothalamic-pituitary-adrenal axis by inhibiting hypothalamic CRH and adrenocortical cortisol secretion, other the stimulating actions on HPO axis. Low leptin levels may be involved in the adaptive activation of the hypothalamic-pituitary-adrenal axis and the inhibition of gonadal function that takes place in starvation and anorexia nervosa [73]. Some of the effects of leptin on the central nervous system are mediated by the inhibition of the potent orexogen neuropeptide Y, which normally stimulates the CRH neuron and inhibits the locus ceruleus-norepinephrine system [51].

The marked changes that take place in a woman's reproductive system during her life are bound to affect the functioning of the stress system. The first of these changes takes place at puberty, when gonadarche is slowly established with increasing ovarian follicle growth and circulating estradiol levels first and then the establishment of ovulatory menstrual cycles within the next two to three years. During this time, the stress system receives increasing intermittent positive input from estradiol. Puberty is a period of increasing vulnerability to disorders or states characterized by disturbances or changes in hypothalamic CRH secretion [59], such as melancholic and atypical depression, eating disorders, chronic active alcoholism or other addictions, and chronic active athleticism, as well as seasonal affective disorder, the chronic fatigue and fibromyalgia syndromes, and several autoimmune disorders. Once established, the monthly fluctuations of estradiol that accompany menstrual cycles are expected to influence the secretion of central nervous system CRH and catecholamines until menopause. Decreased secretion of CRH in the late luteal and menstruation phases would be expected and might help explain the presence of luteal dysphoric mood disorder (the premenstrual tension syndrome) and the increased incidence of suicides and enhanced vulnerability to autoimmune and allergic inflammatory phenomena seen during these phases [62,74]. Finally, during the perimenopausal period and early menopause, there is a progressive, intermittent decrease in estradiol levels that would be expected to be associated with decreased activity of the CRH and locus ceruleus-norepinephrine systems and that might help explain the characteristic “hot flashes” and so-called climacteric depression.

CRH and its receptors are also present in rat and human ovaries. Ovarian CRH is primarily found in the theca and stroma and also in the cytoplasm of the ovum itself [75]. Corticotropin-releasing hormone receptors, which are type 1 (similar to those of the anterior pituitary), are also found primarily in the stroma and theca and in the cumulus oophorus, whereas the follicular fluid contains CRH. as well. The findings suggest that CRH may participate in the communication between the ovum and the cumulus oophorus and may influence ovarian steroid biosynthesis. Incubation of granulosa-lutein cells with CRH suppresses estradiol and progesterone secretion in a dose-dependent, interleukin-1-mediated manner [76]. In this sense, ovarian CRH has antireproductive actions that might be related to the earlier menopausal failure of ovaries in women exposed to high psychosocial stress. We believe that a major physiologic function of ovarian CRH is its participation in the "aseptic" inflammatory phenomena of the ovary, including ovulation and luteolysis.

The human endometrium also contains CRH [77]; finally "reproductive," CRH has been identified in various reproductive tissues and can, accordingly, be ovarian, testicular, endometrial, or placental. It is a form of "tissue" corticotropin-releasing factor (CRH found in peripheral tissues) and is analogous to the "immune" CRH found in immune organs and inflammatory sites. It plays a role as proinflammatory hormone.

In conclusion, CRH, in addition to coordinating the behavioral, neuroendocrine, metabolic, and immune components of the stress response, seems to have direct reproductive regulatory roles at the hypothalamus, influencing gonadotropin-releasing hormone secretion, and at the periphery, promoting inflammatory phenomena, such as ovulation and implantation [59].

5. Complications of Menstrual Dysfunction

Menstrual dysfunction in adolescents with eating disorders can have effects even at long distance and exert a negative influence on growth and pubertal development, peak bone mass acquisition, and cognitive function. These complications may not be completely reversible, as recently reviewed [1].

Growth and Pubertal Development

Eating disorders often present with the onset of puberty, when normal changes in body composition may combine with the developmental challenges of adolescence to produce body image disturbance. Pubertal delay or arrest may be associated to malnutrition [78]. Pubertal delay is a common finding in adolescents who develop AN prior to the completion of puberty. Seventeen percent of adolescents with AN of the restricting type have sexual maturity ratings that were two standard deviations below the mean for age [78]. Of particular concern is the effect of eating disorders on achievement of menarche. Misra et al. [79] found that of the female adolescents who had AN and had not attained menarche, 94% were above the mean age at menarche (12.8 years) for white girls in the United States, and 35% were delayed more than two standard deviations (>15.3 years). Of the AN girls who had attained menarche, 32%, manifested it at an age greater than the mean age of normal population. Others have also found the age of menarche to be delayed in females with early-onset AN compared to healthy adolescent females. Impairment of linear growth and permanent short stature occur in some adolescents with eating disorders. During normal puberty, estrogen levels increase simultaneously with increases in GH and IGF-I. Both estrogen and IGF-I are bone-trophic hormones that stimulate longitudinal bone growth. Regulation of longitudinal bone growth is likely due to a complex interplay between estrogen, other hormones, and the GH-IGF axis

[80]. Levels of estrogen and IGF-I are low in adolescents with AN, which may contribute to alterations in linear growth [81].

Peak Bone Mass

Peak bone mass acquisition occurs during adolescence. The development of an eating disorder during adolescence can result both in failure to acquire peak bone mass and in low bone mineral density with a potential increased risk for fractures [81]. Failure to acquire peak bone mass is related to the menstrual disturbances that occur in eating disorders (see Chapter 4 for a more detailed discussion).

Cognitive Function

Brain development involves increases in total white and occipital gray-matter volumes from ages 4 to 20 years in healthy children and adolescents, while temporal gray-matter volumes increases in childhood and adolescence, reaching a maximum at age 16.7 years and then declines [82]. Research on brain changes in AN suggests that the development of an eating disorder during this critical developmental period may cause structural and functional changes that may or may not be reversible [83,84]. MRI studies [83] have demonstrated increased cerebrospinal fluid (CSF) volumes associated with decreased total gray- and total white-matter volumes in adolescent females with AN compared to healthy controls. In a cross-sectional and longitudinal follow-up study [85], patients who had recovered from AN showed persistent increases in CSF volume and deficits in gray matter compared to healthy controls; however, these values were both improved when compared to values in low-weight patients with AN. In a long-term follow-up study of brain structure and cognitive function, women with adolescent-onset AN had larger lateral and third ventricles and showed cognitive deficits over a broad range of neuropsychological domains. Both weight recovery and cortisol were important modifiers of the structural brain changes. However, the women who remained amenorrheic had deficits in cognitive function across a variety of domains, including recall, verbal memory, working memory, visual reproduction, reading, math, and oral language [86]. Low circulating levels of estrogen have been shown to have an adverse impact on cognition in postmenopausal women, surgically menopausal women, and women with premature ovarian failure and Turner syndrome [87,88]. The relationship between amenorrhea and cognition in AN has yet to be fully elucidated.

6. Conclusions

Menstrual dysfunction is a common feature of all types of eating disorders. The etiology of menstrual dysfunction in adolescents with eating disorders is multifactorial and the result of a complex interplay of many factors including body weight, body fat, eating attitudes and behaviors, exercise, and psychological stressors, leptin and other hormones. This is further complicated by the fact that eating disorders are common among adolescent girls, a time of profound physical and mental growth and development. The significance of menstrual dysfunction in adolescents with eating disorders is particularly important when considering its impact on linear growth, pubertal development, bone mineral accretion, and cognitive functioning [89]. Research on menstrual dysfunction in eating disorders has produced a base of knowledge, albeit one with major gaps. Most of the research on menstrual function and eating disorders has focused on adults, and the findings may not apply to younger individuals. Thus, the research agenda for menstrual function and eating disorders among adolescents is vast. Further study of the many factors that influence menarche and menstruation is needed. The identification of clinically useful biological markers to predict menarche and return of menstrual function is critical in the treatment and prevention of significant morbidity in this population. Menstrual dysfunction in adolescents with eating disorders has far-reaching effects. Future research in patients with AN will help us appreciate the impact of estrogen on cognition, and this may have important implications for understanding the treatment and prognosis of AN. Finally, research on the causes of menstrual dysfunction in adolescents with eating disorders will provide researchers and clinicians with a clearer understanding of the physical and psychological implications that these disorders can have on the adolescent's overall health.

REFERENCES

[1] Vyer, E; Steinegger, C; Katzman, DK. Eating Disorders and Menstrual Dysfunction in Adolescents. *Ann N Y Acad Sci,* 2008, 1135, 253–264.

[2] Bulụn, SE; Adashi, EY. The physiology and pathology of the female reproductive axis. In: Larsen, PR; Kronenberg, HM; Melmed, S; Polonsky, KS; Editors. Williams *Textbook of Endocrinology.* 10th Ed. Philadelphia: WB Saunders; 2003; 617-618.

[3] Marshall, J & Kelch, R. Low dose pulsatile gonadotropin-releasing hormone in anorexia nervosa: a model of human pubertal development. *J Clin Endocrinol Metab,* 1979, 49, 712–718.

[4] Apter D. Development of the hypothalamic-pituitary-ovarian axis. *Ann N Y Acad Sci,* 1997, 816, 9–21.

[5] Boyar, RM; Rosenfeld, RS; Kapen, S; Finkelstein, JW; Roffwarg, HP; Weitzman, ED; Hellman, L. Human puberty: simultaneous augmented secretion ofluteinizing hormone and testosterone during sleep. *J Clin Invest,* 1974, 54, 609–618.

[6] Marshall WA & Tanner JM. Variations in pattern of pubertal changes in girls. *Arch Dis Child,* 1969, 44, 291-303.

[7] Boyar, RM; Katz, J; Finkelstein, JW; Kapen, S; Weiner, H; Weitzman, ED; Hellman, L. Anorexia nervosa: immaturity of the 24-hour luteinizing hormone secretory pattern. *N Engl J Med,* 1974, 291, 861–865.

[8] Golden, NH; Jacobson, MS; Schebendach, J; Solanto, MV; Hertz, SM; Shenker, IR. Resumption of menses in anorexia nervosa. *Arch Pediatr Adol Med,* 1997, 151, 16–21.

[9] Swenne, I. Weight requirements for return of menstruations in teenage girls with eating disorders, weight loss and secondary amenorrhoea. *Acta Paediatr,* 2004, 93, 1449–1455.

[10] Swenne I. Changes in body weight and body mass index (BMI) in teenage girls prior to onset of an eating disorder. *Acta Paediatr,* 2001, 90, 677–681.

[11] Mason, HD; Key, A; Allan, R; Lask, B. Pelvic ultrasonography in anorexia nervosa: what the clinician should ask the radiologist and how to use the information provided. *Eur Eat Disord Rev,* 2007, 15, 35–41.

[12] Treasure, J.L. The ultrasonographic features in anorexia nervosa and bulimia nervosa: a simplified method of monitoring hormonal states during weight gain. *J Psychosom Res,* 1988, 32, 623–634.

[13] Key, A; Mason, H; Allan, R; Lask, B. Restoration of ovarian and uterine maturity in adolescents with anorexia nervosa. *Int J Eat Disord,* 2002, 32, 319–325.

[14] Frisch, R.E. & Mc Arthur, JW. Menstrual cycles: fatness as a determinant of minimum weight for height necessary for their maintenance or onset. *Science,* 1974, 185, 949–951.

[15] Frisch, RE. The right weight: body fat, menarche and ovulation. *Baill Clin Obstet Gynaecol,* 1990, 4, 419-39.

[16] Misra, M; Prabhakaran, R; Miller, KK; Tsai, P; Lin, A; Lee, N; Herzog, DB; Klibanski, A. Role of cortisol in menstrual recovery in adolescent girls with anorexia nervosa. *Pediatr Res,* 2006, 59, 598–603.

[17] Miller, KK; Grinspoon, S; Gleysteen, S; Grieco, KA; Ciampa, J; Breu, J; Herzog DB; Klibanski, A. Preservation of neuroendocrine control of reproductive function despite severe undernutrition. *J Clin Endocrinol Metab* 2004, 89, 4434–4438.

[18] Hurd, HP; Palumbo, PJ; Gharib, H. Hypothalamic-endocrine dysfunction in anorexia nervosa. *Mayo Clin Proc* 1977, 52, 711–716.

[19] Loucks AB; Verdun, M; Heath, EM. Low energy availability, not stress of exercise, alters LH pulsatility in exercising women. *J Appl Physiol,* 1988, 84, 37–46.

[20] Warren, MP & Perlroth, NE. The effects of intense exercise on the female reproductive system. *J Endocrinol* 2001, 170, 3–11.

[21] Marcus, M.D; Loucks, TL; Berga, SL. Psychological correlates of functional hypothalamic amenorrhea. *Fertil Steril* 2001, 76: 310–316.

[22] Schneider, LF & Warren, MP. Functional hypothalamic amenorrhea is associated with elevated ghrelin and disordered eating. *Fertil Steril* 2006, 86, 1744–1749.

[23] Davis, C; Katzman, DK; Kaptein, S; Kirsh, C; Brewer, H; Kalmbach, K; Olmsted, MP; Woodside, DB; Kaplan, AS. The prevalence of high-level exercise in the eating disorders: etiological implications. *Compr. Psychiatry* 1997, 38, 321–326.

[24] Warren, M.P. Health issues for women athletes: exercise-induced amenorrhea. *J Clin Endocrinol Metab,* 1999, 84, 1892–1896.

[25] Litt, IF & Glader, L. Anorexia nervosa, athletics, and amenorrhea. *J Pediatr,* 1986, 109, 150–153.

[26] Golden, NH. A review of the female athlete triad (amenorrhea, osteoporosis and disordered eating). *Int J Adolesc Med Health,* 2002, 14, 9-17.

[27] Falk, JR & Halmi, KA. Amenorrhea in anorexia nervosa: examination of the critical body weight hypothesis. *Biol Psychiatry* 1982, 17, 799–806.

[28] Herzog, DB; Keller, MB; Sacks, NR; Yeh, CJ; Lavori, PW. Psychiatric comorbidity in treatment-seeking anorexics and bulimics. *J Am Acad Child Adolesc Psychiatry,* 1992, 31, 810–818.

[29] Young, EA & Korszun, A. The hypothalamic-pituitary-gonadal axis in mood disorders. *Endocrinol Metab Clin North Am,* 2002, 31, 63–78.

[30] Hull, KL & Harvey, S. Growth hormone: roles in female reproduction. *J Endocrinol,* 2001, 168, 1–23.

[31] Izadyar, F; Hage, WJ; Colenbrander, B; Bevers, MM. The promontory effect of growth hormone on the developmental competence of in vitro matured bovine oocytes is due to improved cytoplasmic maturation. *Mol Reprod Develop,* 1998, 49, 444–453

[32] Bartke, A. Role of growth hormone and prolactin in the control of reproduction: what are we learning from transgenic and knockout animals? *Steroids,* 1999, 64, 598–604.

[33] Danilovich, N; Bartke, A; Winters, TA. Ovarian follicle apoptosis in bovine growth hormone transgenic mice. *Biol Reprod,* 2000, 62, 103–107.

[34] de Boer, JA; Schoemaker, J; van der Veen, EA. Impaired reproductive function in women treated for growth hormone deficiency during childhood. *Clin Endocrinol,* 1997, 46 681–689.

[35] Homburg, R & Farhi, J. Growth hormone and reproduction. *Curr Opin Obstet Gynecol,* 1995, 7, 220–223

[36] Shoham, Z; Homburg, R; Owen, EJ; Conway, SS; Ostergaard, H; Jacobs, HS. The role of treatment with growth hormone in infertile patients. *Baillieres Clin Obstet Gynecol,* 1992, 6, 267-281.

[37] Shaker, AG; Yates, RWS; Fleming, R; Coutts, JRT; Jamieson, ME. Absence of effect of adjuvant growth hormone therapy on follicular responses to exogenous gonadotropins in women – normal and poor responders. *Fertil Steril* 1992, 58, 919–923.

[38] Dor, J; Ben-Shlomo, I; Lunenfeld, B. Insulin-like growth factor-I (IGF-I) may not be essential for ovarian follicular development: evidence from IGF-I deficiency. *J Clin Endocrinol Metab* 1992, 74, 539–542.

[39] Untergasser, G; Kranewitter, W; Schwarzler, P; Madersbacher, S; Dirhnofer, S; Berger, P. Organ-specific pattern of the human growth hormone/placental lactogen gene cluster in the testis. *Mol Cell Endocrinol,* 1997, 130, 53–60.

[40] Bagnato, A; Moretti, C; Ohno, Y; Frajese, G; Catt, KJ.Expression of the growth hormone-releasing hormone gene and its peptide product in the rat ovary. *Endocrinology,* 1992, 130, 1097–1102.

[41] Pekary, AE; Yameda, T; Sharp, B; Basin, S; Swerdloff, RS; Hershman, J. Somatostatin-14 and -28 in the male rat reproductive system *Life Sci,*1984, 34, 939–945.

[42] Harvey, S & Hull, K. Growth hormone: a paracrine growth factor? *Endocrine,* 1997, 7, 267–279.

[43] Mantzoros, CS. Role of leptin in reproduction. *Ann N Y Acad Sci,* 2000, 900: 174-183.

[44] Chehab, FF; Lim, ME; Lu, R. Correction of the sterility defect in homozygous obese female mice by treatment with the human recombinant leptin. *Nat Genet,* 1996, 12, 318–320.

[45] Rogol, AD. Leptin and puberty. *J Clin Endocrinol Metab,* 1998, 83, 1089–1090.

[46] Mantzoros, CS; Flier, JS; Rogol, AD. A longitudinal assessment of hormonal and physical alterations during normal puberty in boys. V: rising leptin levels may signal the onset of puberty. *J Clin Endocrinol Metab,* 1997, 82, 1066–1070.

[47] Clement, K ; Vaisse, C ; Lahlou, N; Cabrol, S; Pelloux, V ; Cassuto, D ; Gourmelen, M; Dina, C; Chambaz, J; Lacorte, JM; Basdevant, A; Bougnères, P; Lebouc, Y;

Froguel, P; Guy-Grand, B. A mutation in the human leptin receptor gene causes obesity and pituitary dysfunction. *Nature,* 1998, 392, 398–401.

[48] Yu, WH; Kimura, M; Walczewska, A; Karanth, S; McCann, SM. Role of leptin in hypothalamic-pituitary function. *Proc Natl Acad Sci USA,1*997, 94, 1023–1028.

[49] Licinio, J; Negrao, AB; Mantzoros, C; Kaklamani, V; Wrong, ML; Bongiorno, PB; Mulla, A; Cearnal, L; Veldhuis, JD; Flier, JS; McCann, SM; Gold, PW. Synchronicity of frequently sampled, 24 hour concentrations of circulating leptin, luteinizing hormone and estradiol in healthy women. *Proc Natl Acad Sci,* 1998, 95, 2541–2546.

[50] Ahima, R; Prabakaran, D; Mantzoros, C; Qu, D; Lowell, B; Maratos-Flier, E; Flier, JS. Role of leptin in the neuroendocrine response to fasting. *Nature,* 1996, 382, 250–252.

[51] Sivan, E; Whittaker, PG; Sinha, D; Homko, CJ; Lin, M; Reece, EA; Boden G.. Leptin in human pregnancy: the relationship with gestational hormones. *Am J Obstet Gynecol,* 1998, 179, 1128–1132.

[52] Ballauff, A; Ziegler, A; Emons, G; Sturm, G; Blum, WF; Remschmidt, H; Hebebrand, J. Serum leptin and gonadotropin levels in patients with anorexia nervosa during weight gain. *Mol. Psychiatry,* 1999, 4: 71–75.

[53] Hebebrand, J; Muller, TD; Holtkamp, K; Herpertz-Dahlmann, B. The role of leptin in anorexia nervosa: clinical implications. *Mol. Psychiatry,* 2007, 12, 23–35.

[54] Kopp, W; Blum, WF; Von Prittwitz, S; Ziegler, A; Lubbert, H; Emons, G; Herzog, W; Herpertz, S; Deter, HC; Remschmidt, H; Hebebrand, J. Low leptin levels predict amenorrhea in underweight and eating disordered females. *Mol Psychiatry,* 1997, 2, 335–340.

[55.] Welt, CK; Chan, JL; Bullen, J; Murphy, R; Smith, P; DePaoli, AM; Karalis, A; Mantzoros CS. Recombinant human leptin in women with hypothalamic amenorrhea. *N Engl J Med,* 2004, 351: 987–997.

[56] Audi, L; Mantzoros, CS; Vidal-Puig, A; Vargas, D; Gussinye, M; Carrascosa, M. Leptin in relation to resumption of menses in women with anorexia nervosa. *Mol Psychiatry,* 1998, 3, 544–547.

[57] Khamsi, F; Roberge, S; Yavas, Y; Lacanna, IC; Zhu, X; Wong, J. Recent discoveries in physiology of insulin-like growth factor-1 and its interaction with gonadotropins in folliculogenesis. *Endocrine,* 2001, 16, 151-165.

[58] Woods, SC & D'Alessio, DA. Central control of body weight and appetite. *J Clin Endocrinol Metab,* 2008, 93 (11 Suppl 1), S37-50.

[59] Chrousos, GP; Torpy, DJ; Gold, PW. Interactions between the hypothalamic-pituitary-adrenal axis and the female reproductive system: clinical implications. *Ann Intern Med,* 1998, 129, 229-40.

[60] Chrousos, GP & Gold, PW. The concepts of stress and stress system disorders. Overview of physical and behavioral homeostasis. *JAMA,* 1992, 267, 1244-1252.

[61] Berga, S. Functional hypothalamic chronic anovulation. In: Adashi, EY; Rock, JA; Rosenwaks, Z, eds. *Reproductive Endocrinology, Surgery, and Technology.* Vol. 1. Philadelphia: Lippincott-Raven; 1996; 1061-1075.

[62] Collins, A; Eneroth, P; Landgren, BM. Psychoneuroendocrine stress responses and mood as related to the menstrual cycle. *Psychosom Med,* 1985, 47, 512-27.

[63] Rivest, S & Rivier, C. The role of corticotropin-releasing factor and interleukin-1 in the regulation of neurons controlling reproductive functions. *Endocr Rev,* 1995, 16, 177-199.

[64] Chen, MD; O'Byrne, KT; Chiappini, SE; Hotchkiss, J; Knobil, E. Hypoglycemic 'stress' and gonadotropin-releasing hormone pulse generator activity in the rhesus monkey: role of the ovary. *Neuroendocrinology,* 1992, 56, 666-673.

[65] Plant, TM. Gonadal regulation of hypothalamic gonadotropin-releasing hormone release in primates. *Endocr Rev,* 1986, 7, 75-88.

[66] Sakakura, N; Takebe, K; Nakagawa, S. Inhibition of luteinizing hormone secretion induced by synthetic LRH by long-term treatment with glucocorticoids in human subjects. *J Clin Endocrinol Metab,* 1975, 40, 774-779.

[67] Rabin, DS; Johnson, EO; Brandon, DD; Liapi, C; Chrousos, GP. Glucocorticoids inhibit estradiol-mediated uterine growth: possible role of the uterine estradiol receptor. *Biol Reprod,* 1990, 42, 74-80.

[68] Bamberger, CM; Schulte, HM; Chrousos GP. Molecular determinants of glucocorticoid receptor function and tissue sensitivity to glucocorticoids. *Endocr Rev,* 1996, 17, 221-244.

[69] Zukowska-Grojec, Z; Shen, GH; Capraro, PA; Vaz, CA. Cardiovascular, neuropeptide Y, and adrenergic responses in stress are sexually differentiated. *Physiol Behav,* 1991, 49, 771-777.

[70] Vamvakopoulos, NC & Chrousos, GP. Evidence of direct estrogenic regulation of human corticotropin-releasing hormone gene expression. Potential implications for the sexual dimorphism of the stress response and immune/inflammatory reaction. *J Clin Invest,* 1993, 92, 1896-1902.

[71] Kerdelhué, B; Jones, GS; Gordon, K; Seltman, H; Lenoir, V; Melik Parsadaniantz, S; Williams, RF; Hodgen, GD. Activation of the hypothalamo-anterior pituitary corticotropin-releasing hormone, adrenocorticotropin hormone and ß-endorphin systems during the estradiol 17 ß-induced plasma LH surge in the ovariectomized monkey. *J Neurosci Res,* 1995, 42, 228-235.

[72] Peiffer, A; Lapointe, B; Barden, N. Hormonal regulation of type II glucocorticoid receptor messenger ribonucleic acid in rat brain. *Endocrinology,* 1991, 129, 2166-2174.

[73] Heiman, ML; Ahima, RS; Craft, LS; Schoner, B; Stephens, TW; Flier, JS. Leptin inhibition of the hypothalamic-pituitary-adrenal axis in response to stress. *Endocrinology,* 1997, 138, 3859-3863.

[74] Hayward, C; Killen, JD; Wilson, DM; Hammer, LD; Litt, IF; Kraemer, HC; Haydel, F; Varady, A; Taylor, CB. Psychiatric risk associated with early puberty in adolescent girls. *J Am Acad Child Adolesc Psychiatry,* 1997, 36, 255-262.

[75] Mastorakos, G; Scopa, CD; Vryonidou, A; Friedman, TC; Kattis, D; Phenekos, C; Merino, MJ; Chrousos, GP. Presence of immunoreactive corticotropin-releasing hormone in normal and polycystic human ovaries. *J Clin Endocrinol Metab,* 1994, 79, 934-939.

[76] Ghizzoni, L; Mastorakos, G; Vottero, A; Barreca, A; Furbini, M; Cesarone, A; Ferrari, B; Chrousos, GP; Bernasconi, S. Corticotropin-releasing hormone (CRH) inhibits steroid biosynthesis by cultured human granulosa-lutein cells in a CRH and interleukin-1 receptor-mediated fashion. *Endocrinology,* 1997, 138, 4806-4811.

[77] Mastorakos, G; Scopa, CD; Kao, LC; Vryonidou, A; Friedman, TC; Kattis, D; Phenekos, C; Rabin, D; Chrousos, GP. Presence of immunoreactive corticotropin-releasing hormone in human endometrium. *J Clin Endocrinol Metab,* 1996, 81, 1046-1050.

[78] Palla, B. & Litt, IF. Medical complications of eating disorders in adolescents. *Pediatrics,* 1988, 81, 613–623.

[79] Misra, M; Aggarwal, A; Miller, KK; Almazan, C; Worley, M; Soyka, LA; Herzog, DB; Klibanski, A. Effects of anorexia nervosa on clinical, hematologic, biochemical, and bone density parameters in community dwelling adolescent girls. *Pediatrics,* 2004, 114, 1574–1583.

[80] Juul, A. The effects of oestrogens on linear bone growth. *Hum. Reprod Update,* 2001, 7: 303–313.

[81] Misra, M. & Klibanski, A. Anorexia nervosa and osteoporosis. *Rev Endocr Metab Disord* 2006, 7: 91–99.

[82] Giedd, JN; Blumenthal, J; Jeffries, NO; Castellanos, FX, Liu, H; Zijdenbos, A; Paus, T; Evans, AC; Rapoport, JL. Brain development during childhood and adolescence: a longitudinal MRI study. *Nat Neurosci,* 1999, 2, 861–863.

[83] Katzman D.K., E.K. Lambe, D.J. Mikulis, Ridgley, JN, Goldbloom, DS; Zipursky, RB. Cerebral gray matter and white matter volume deficits in adolescent girls with anorexia nervosa. *J. Pediatr,* 1996, 129, 794–803.

[84] Lambe, EK; Katzman, KK; Mikulis, DJ; Kennedy, SH; Zipursky, RB. Cerebral gray matter volume deficits after weight recovery from anorexia nervosa. *Arch Gen Psychiatry,* 1997, 54 537-542.

[85] Katzman, DK; Zipursky, RB; Lambe, EK; Mikulis, DJ. A longitudinal magnetic resonance imaging study of brain changes in adolescents with anorexia nervosa. *Arch Pediatr Adolesc Med,* 1997, 151, 793–797.

[86] Chui, HT; Christensen, B; Zipursky, RB; Katzman, DK. Effects of menstrual function and weight restoration on cognitive function in females with adolescent-onset anorexia nervosa. *J Adolesc Health,* 2006, 40, S12–S12.

[87] Miller, KJ; Conney, JC; Rasgon, NL; Fairbanks, LA; Small, GW. Mood symptoms and cognitive performance in women estrogen users and nonusers and men. *J Am Geriatr Soc,* 2002, 50, 1826–1830.

[88] Ross, JL; Stefanatos, GA; Kushner, H; Bondy, C; Nelson, L; Zinn, A; Roeltgen, D. The effect of genetic differences and ovarian failure: Intact cognitive function in adult women with premature ovarian failure versus Turner syndrome. *J Clin Endocrinol Metab,* 2004, 89, 1817–1822.

[89] Katzman, DK. Medical complications in adolescents with anorexia nervosa: a review of the literature. *Int J Eat Disord,* 2005, 37, S52–S59.

In: Anorexia Nervosa: A Multi-Disciplinary Approach
Editors: A. Mancini, S. Daini, L. Caruana, pp. 75-85
ISBN: 978-1-60876-200-2

Chapter 4

ANOREXIA NERVOSA: MEDICAL COMPLICATIONS

A. Bianchi, F. Veltri, L. Tartaglione, L. Tilaro, L. De Marinis
Division of Endocrinology, Catholic University of the Sacred Heart, Rome, Italy

ABSTRACT

Anorexia nervosa is a debilitating psychiatric disorder with serious biological, psychological and social consequences. This condition can cause significant medical complications. Cardiovascular alterations include bradycardia, arrhythmias, hypotension, mitral valve prolapse, reduced left ventricular mass and impaired myocardial performance; sudden death has been reported. Biochemical abnormalities range from fluid and electrolyte depletion, hypoglicemia, and liver enzymes alteration, to severe dehydration with renal damage, hypoproteinemia, edema, cardiovascular collapse and renal infarcts. Gastrointestinal complications include gastric dilatation, liver impairment, pancreatitis and malabsorption. Laboratory tests often reveal hematologic alteration: anemia and leucopenia are frequent, as well as morphologic alterations of red blood cells and thrombocitopenia. Bone marrow atrophy is reported in almost 50% of the patients. Finally, anorexia nervosa is associated with failure to obtain normal peak bone mass, markedly reduced bone density, increased long-term risk of fractures. Re-feeding syndrome is related to high incidence of confusion, convulsions, coma and death. Although many of these medical complications improve with nutritional rehabilitation and recovery from the disorder, some are potentially irreversible.

1. INTRODUCTION

Anorexia Nervosa is a debilitating psychiatric disorder with serious biological, psychological, and social consequences. Anorexia nervosa is still a serious cause of morbidity and mortality that may result in premature death or life-long medical and psychosocial morbidity. This condition causes significant and often life-threatening medical complications, including cardiovascular dysfunction, electrolyte disorder and gastrointestinal involvement

[1,2]. Although many of these medical complications improve with nutritional rehabilitation and recovery from the disorder, some are potentially irreversible.

Immediate management of medical complication and correction of nutritional deficits are necessary before patients can benefit from psychotherapy [3].

Medical Complications of Anorexia Nervosa
Cardiovascular
Bradycardia and hypotension
Heart failure
Peripheral edema
Sudden death
Mitral valve prolapse
Re-feeding syndrome
Biochemical abnormalities
Gastrointestinal
Gastric dilatation
Constipation
Pancreatitis
Malabsorption
Hematologic
Anemia
Leukocytopenia
Thrombocytopenia
Bone marrow atrophy and transformation
Bone
Osteoporosis

2. Physical Examination

Patients with anorexia nervosa usually have few physical disturbances.

Hypothermia is characteristic and may present with cold intolerance and an inability to compensate for changes in temperature. The hands and feet may be discoloured due to cyanosis *(acrocyanosis)* and cold, with a thready pulse (unless the patients vomit regularly, in which case they may be sweating). Sometimes there can be present thin and soft hair (*lanugo*), especially on the back. An enlargement of salivary glands, due to fasting and compulsive hyperalimentation followed by vomiting, can be found. Some patients who eat large amounts of vegetables rich in vitamin A have a yellowish colouring of the skin (*carotenodermia*) that is noticeable especially on the palms of the hands [4].

3. Cardiovascular Complications

A variety of cardiovascular complications are described in anorexia nervosa [5]. These include bradycardia and hypotension, lengthening of the QT interval and other electrocardiographic abnormalities, reduced left ventricular mass and impaired myocardial performance, mitral valve prolapse and sudden death. Endocarditis is also reported. Almost 80% of patients have cardiovascular abnormalities, mainly bradycardia, hypotension, arrhythmias and repolarization disorders; sudden death has been reported in 10% of the patients.

Bradycardia and Hypotension

The most common cardiovascular complications are electrocardiographic abnormalities, such as sinus bradycardia, decreased voltage and prolonged QT and orthostatic hypotension. Electrocardiographic abnormalities are very common, and sinus bradycardia is reported in up to 95% of adolescents with anorexia [6-8]. Rare cases of patients with second-degree heart block were reported [9]. A reduced noradrenergic activity in the central and peripheral nervous system of patients, an increased vagal tone and decreased metabolic rate are the physiopathologic mechanisms involved. The clinical consequences of these changes are hypotension, hypothermia and depression. Evidence is presented that the reduced activity of the sympathetic nervous system is caused by starvation. These patients have low cardiac output and demonstrate increased peripheral vascular resistance, despite the presence of hypotension [1-5]. Increased clinical disease severity seems correlated with increased bradycardias and decreased left ventricular forces. It is important to remember that in anorexia nervosa, there may be other potential causes of electrocardiographic changes such as metabolic and electrolyte disturbances (e.g., hypokaliemia) or drug effects.

Heart Failure

Congestive heart failure may appear in anorexia nervosa. Patients with anorexia have been reported to have systolic and diastolic ventricular dysfunction, low cardiac output and demonstrated increased peripheral vascular resistance, despite the presence of hypotension. The heart is atrophic, pericardial effusions were reported and regional wall motion abnormalities on echocardiography or radionuclide ventriculography were present, often in absence of shortness of breath, palpitations or chest pain. In one study, the majority of adolescents with AN had decreased left ventricular mass and cardiac output at the basal state, indicating early structural and functional heart involvement [7]. Cardiomyopathy may be also related to both prolonged elevated sympathetic activity and hypoglycaemia. Ohwada et al. [10] reported evidence of ampulla cardiomyopathy, which is characterized by extensive akinesis of the apical region with hypercontraction of the basal segment of the ventricle, in three young women with anorexia nervosa, all of whom had experienced a hypoglycemic coma.

Deficiencies of magnesium, phosphorus, thiamine and selenium can also weaken cardiac muscular contraction. Ingestion of ipecac syrup can result in weakening of the cardiac muscle [11,12].

After re-feeding in anorexia nervosa, we observe a consistent increase in cardiac dimensions, wall thickness, ventricular mass, and cardiac output, reflecting reversibility of these abnormalities.

Peripheral Edema

Some patients develop peripheral edema, especially during weight restoration or on cessation of laxative and diuretic abuse.

Sudden Death

As mentioned earlier, QT interval is usually normal in patients with anorexia, but QT prolongation and ventricular arrhythmia may develop in the setting of severe hypokalemia, exposing patients to a high risk of a sudden cardiac event [5].

Abnormalities of the autonomic nervous system might be a cause of cardiac dysfunction. Recent studies suggest that patients with anorexia nervosa have reduced cardiovascular sympathetic nervous responsiveness, increased parasympathetic nervous responsiveness, and increased complexity of the interbeat interval time series compared with healthy controls [13]. Isner et al. proposed that sudden cardiac death in anorexia nervosa patients may result from ventricular tachyarrhthmias related to prolonged QT intervals [6].

Mitral Valve Prolapse

One of the commonest cardiovascular complications of AN is mitral valve prolapse (MVP). MVP has been reported in 33% to 37% of adolescents with AN examined by echocardiography. The association can be explained by the valvular-ventricular disproportion theory of MVP, which proposes that MVP results from either too much valve tissue or too small a ventricular cavity. Left ventricular cavity size is reduced in AN. Some authors suggest that MVP might have an associated arrhythmogenic propensity that poses an additional risk to these adolescents. Although it is not yet clear, MVP may resolve with weight restoration [2]. The fact that MVP disappeared in patients with AN after they had received therapy and regained weight but recurred during follow-up in those patients who lost weight again supports this theory.

One of mitral valve prolapse complications is sudden death; still mitral valve prolapse may also play a role in sudden death in some patients with anorexia nervosa [14-17].

4. Re-feeding Syndrome

Re-feeding syndrome is a syndrome consisting of metabolic disturbances that occur as a result of reinstitution of nutrition to patients who are starved or severely undernourished. Re-feeding syndrome is of particular concern in severely malnourished adolescents with AN. It is defined as severe shifts in fluid and electrolyte levels, in particular phosphate levels, from extracellular to intracellular spaces in severely malnourished patients who have total body phosphorus depletion and are undergoing re-feeding, whether orally, enterally, or parenterally [18]. On re-feeding, the absorbed glucose leads to increased blood glucose levels, which increase insulin and decrease glucagon secretion. The net result of these changes is the synthesis of glycogen, fat and protein. This anabolic state requires minerals such as phosphate and magnesium and cofactors such as thiamine. Insulin stimulates the absorption of potassium into the cells (via the Na-K ATPase symporter), with both magnesium and phosphate also taken up. Water is drawn in to the intracellular compartment by osmosis. This decreases serum levels of phosphate, potassium and magnesium further, and results in the clinical features of re-feeding syndrome. The clinical picture consists of cardiovascular, neurological and hematological complications and can be associated with significant morbidity and mortality. Patients can develop fluid and electrolyte disorders, especially hypophosphatemia, along with neurologic, pulmonary, cardiac, neuromuscular, and hematologic complications. Most effects result from a sudden shift from fat to carbohydrate metabolism and a sudden increase in insulin levels after re-feeding, which leads to increased cellular uptake of phosphate. Re-feeding increases the basal metabolic rate. Intracellular movement of electrolytes occurs along with a fall in the serum electrolytes including phosphate, potassium, magnesium, glucose, and thiamine [19]. Significant risks arising from re-feeding syndrome include confusion, coma, convulsions, and death. This syndrome can occur at the beginning of treatment for anorexia nervosa when patients are reintroduced to a healthy diet, and cardiac sequelae occur early in the cascade of events that arise during re-feeding. The shifting of electrolytes and fluid balance increases cardiac workload and heart rate. This can lead to acute heart failure. Oxygen consumption is also increased, which strains the respiratory system and can make weaning from ventilation more difficult. Treatment recommendations include early administration of supplemental phosphorous, gradual increase in prescribed nutrition, and close monitoring of electrolyte levels and cardiac status [2, 20-22].

5. Biochemical Abnormalities

Nutritional abnormalities are common, including sodium depletion and hypovolemia, hypophosphatemia and hypomagnesemia [1,3].

With severe vomiting, major fluid and electrolyte abnormalities arise. Hypokalaemia and hypochloraemic alcalosis occur, blood urea and creatinine may be elevated due to dehydration, liver enzymes can be increased, blood glucose is often low, and seric cholesterol is usually moderately high; severe laxative abuse can lead to severe dehydration and electrolyte depletion [4]. Persistent electrolyte abnormalities resulting from continued vomiting or purgative abuse may lead to permanent renal damage (mesangial hyalinisation and sclerosis and interstitial renal fibrosis) [4]. Hyponatraemia is frequently found and can be derived from excessive fluids incomes and abnormalities in secretion of ADH. Hyponatraemia further compounds the potassium loss as a reduction in the plasma sodium releases renin angiotensin and aldosterone [4]. Aldosterone then promoves further potassium loss from the kidneys. Peripheral edema is commonly encountered during re-feeding; it is usually mild and resolves with diuresis, but a more severe form is found in association with hypoproteinaemia. The resultant fluid shifts can precipitate shock, cardiovascular collapse and renal infarcts [4].

6. Gastrointestinal Complications

Disturbances in the functioning of the gastrointestinal tract have been described in both anorexia nervosa and bulimia nervosa [23]. Gastrointestinal complications can be serious, including gastric dilatation and severe liver dysfunction [1]. Patients with anorexia nervosa experience substantial delays in gastric emptying, as well as constipation [23]. These problems may give rise to significant medical complications and may contribute to increased difficulties with re-feeding and weight restoration.

Gastric Dilatation

Gastritis, delayed gastric emptying, gastric motor dysfunction, delayed small bowel transit time and gastric dilation typically occur after binge-eating and become manifest in spontaneous vomiting and upper abdominal pain [1]. Conservative treatment is usually sufficient; in rare cases, however, circulation disorders of the gastric wall occur, leading to necrosis and gastric perforation. An impairment of esophageal motility and gastric emptying is a typical consequence of malnutrition but has also been found variably in patients with bulimia nervosa. After an increase of food intake and stabilisation of weight, this disturbance seems to be fully reversible [24].

Megaduodenum and duodenal immobility are also secondary complications and are reversible..

Constipation

Constipation is frequent and, in most cases, is a result of poor nutrition and hypokalemia due to purging behaviour such as laxative abuse.

The possibility of constipation due to antidepressant medication, particularly tricyclic antidepressants, should be considered [23,24].

Pancreatitis

An increase in serum amylase levels is found in about 50% of anorexia nervosa patients. In most cases, it is due to vomiting and is not a result of pancreatitis. Correspondingly, the increase is caused by the iso-amylase of the parotid gland. However, both acute and chronic pancreatitis are associated with eating disorders, also as result of re-feeding or binge eating [24]. Recent studies show that either chronic malnutrition, or re-feeding after periods of malnutrition, may precipitate acute pancreatitis through several pathogenetic mechanisms. In anorexia, protein energy malnutrition is associated with increased levels of proinflammatory cytokines (IL-1, IL-6, TNF-α) and depleted antioxidant status. High tripsinogen levels, reflecting acinar cell damage and ductal disruption, have also been demonstrated in protein energy malnutrition. At the cellular level, pancreatitis is believed to ultimately depend on activation of trypsinogen to trypsin within the pancreas, leading to the subsequent activation of other proteases. Together, these enzymes cause cell damage and trigger further inflammatory processes [25,26].

Malabsorption

Anorexic patients have metabolic and nutritional characteristics that differ from those present in other gastrointestinal disorders that are always associated with weight loss. In anorexia nervosa, there is frequently found a decrease in energy expenditure or a decrease in the amount of fat body mass and lean body mass. Decrease of lean body mass is related with an increased turnover and with an increased protein catabolism, with increased urinary loss of nitrose [27]. Lean body mass consists essentially of muscle and bone mass and is considered the body compartment that is metabolically active, so energetic metabolism in anorexic patients can be reduced. Moreover, in these patients, there is an increased turnover of free fatty acids, low secretion of insulin and reduced glucose-induced thermogenesis [27].

In literature, there are also described several cases of patients with both celiac disease and eating disorders. There are complex ways in which celiac disease and eating disorders interact with important clinical implications for the diagnosis and treatment of both illnesses [27].

Nutritional factors also play an important role in loss of bone density in patients with anorexia nervosa.

7. Osteoporosis

Anorexia nervosa is associated with failure to obtain normal peak bone mass, markedly reduced bone density and an increased long-term risk of fractures. Low-weight patients are at high risk for osteopenia/osteoporosis, and anorexia nervosa is associated with markedly reduced bone density, especially at the lumbar spine, but also at the proximal femur and dista, with bone fractures in 44% of them [28]. In patients who have had the disorder for an average of 5.8 years, the risk of fractures occurring is seven times higher than in healthy women of the same age [29]. Normally, optimizing bone growth and achieving peak bone mass occurs during adolescence. Therefore, it is not surprising that anorexia nervosa, with its attendant failure to attain normal peak bone mass, is associated with a markedly increased long-term risk of nontraumatic fractures. The mechanism underlying bone loss in anorexia nervosa is still unclear, but it seems complex and multifaceted. Osteoporosis may develop as a consequence of a lack of estrogens, low calcium or vitamin D intake, hypercortisolemia or the duration of the illness [30].

Anorexia nervosa appears to be a low turnover state, characterized by increased bone resorption without concomitant increased bone formation. This imbalance contributes to the significant bone loss that characterizes anorexia nervosa. Markers of bone resorption, such as N-teleopeptide and deoxypyrydoline, are higher in patients with anorexia nervosa, and markers of bone formation, such as osteocalcin, are not concomitantly elevated.

The mechanisms underlying the phenomenon of bone loss observed in anorexia nervosa patients are still unclear. Amenorrhea is a diagnostic criterion for anorexia nervosa, and estrogen deficits have been reported as a major etiological factor for bone loss in this population. However, hypoestrogenia alone cannot account for the loss in bone mass observed in anorexia nervosa patients. Other factors are involved in this bone loss, and nutritional factors in particular, seem to play an important role. The role of the latter has been confirmed by several authors who have found good correlations between bone mineral density in anorexia nervosa patients and nutritional indices such as body mass index, lean body mass, fat mass, insulin-like growth factor I (IGF-I), and leptin. Finally, in a recent study involving 45 anorexic, osteoporotic patients, the authors showed that two years of hormone replacement therapy (HRT) (consisting in one or two percutaneous doses of 0.5 mg 17βestradiol from day 1 to day 21, and 10 mg of dydrogesterone 1 cp from day 11 to day 21) do not prevent the bone loss. The increase in weight is the most important predictor of gain in bone mass at the spine and the hip, and physiological menstrual cycle recovery seems to be an important factor in the recovery of bone mass [31].

8. Hematologic Complications

Changes of the peripheral blood cell count in patients with anorexia nervosa are frequent. Anemia and leukopenia are observed in one-third of these patients [32].

Routinely performed laboratory tests often reveal mild alterations of the total blood cell count. However, dramatic changes can occur, mimicking a severe hematological disease such as acute leukaemia or idiopathic thrombocytopenia.

Anemia

Anemia, defined as reproducibly low hemoglobin level less than 14 g/dl in men or 12 g/dl in women, is a common observation in patients with malnutrition. The incidence rate of anemia in patients with anorexia nervosa varies from 21% to 39%. Characteristically, the mean corpuscular hemoglobin (MCH) and the mean corpuscular volume (MCV) are normal. Anemia with elevated MCV or MHC without a lack of folic acid or vitamin B12 is rare. The most frequent morphologic alterations of red blood cells in peripheral blood in patients with anorexia nervosa are anisocytosis, poikilocytosis, and, occasionally, acanthocytosis. The pathophysiological reasons of an anemia in AN are not clarified. Most authors agree upon the theory that the lack in the red cell production corresponds to morphological changes in the bone marrow, but there are several cases of anemia without any morphological impairment of the bone marrow.

An acquired hemolytic syndrome was reported in a patient suffering from anorexia nervosa and hypophosphatemia. Hypophosphatemia accompanying anorexia nervosa is a potentially life-threatening complication during the re-feeding process. Iron deficiency is not a typical finding of anorexia nervosa, and 33% of patients demonstrated an elevated level of serum ferritin [32].

Leukocytopenia

Although leukocytopenia can be observed in 29% to 36% of the patients with anorexia nervosa, severe cytopenias with a granolucyte count below 0.5/nl are rather uncommon. Leukocytopenia is more frequent in anorexia nervosa patients who are strict dieters than in those who vomit or purge.

Analysis of the differential blood cell counts reveals a significant lymphocytopenia in patients with anorexia nervosa.

Thrombocytopenia

The incidence of thrombocytopenia in patients with AN ranges between 5% and 11%. Platelet counts below this value are rather uncommon, but in contrast to other diseases with severe thrombocytopenia (e.g., aplastic anemia or idiopathic thrombocytopenia), the hemorrhagic tendency in patients with AN appears more frequently. It is supposed that other factors, such as increased fragility of blood vessels, may be superimposed.

Bone Marrow Atrophy and Transformation

Examination of the bone marrow reveals signs of bone marrow atrophy in almost 50% of the patients with anorexia nervosa, and they can additionally suffer from a gelatinous bone marrow transformation.

Morphologic changes in the bone marrow, combining an atrophy of fat cells and a loss of hematopoietic cells with the deposition of an amorphous gelatinous material, has been described as ''gelatinous transformation'' (GMT) or ''serous atrophy.'' For diagnosis, bone marrow aspirate is feasible, but bone marrow biopsy remains as the gold standard. The pathophysiologic mechanism of this feature of bone marrow atrophy is unknown. Morphological studies revealed an increase in the fat fraction and a relative increase in the size and number of adipocytes in the bone marrow in AN patients leading to a partial reduction of normal hematopoietic tissue.

Bone marrow atrophy and gelatinous transformation are more likely associated with body fat mass index than with duration of the illness. It has been suggested that anorexia nervosa leads to an atrophy of the bone marrow in half of the patients. In fact, peripheral blood cell count cannot predict the severity of bone marrow atrophy, but interestingly, 50% of patients with hematological changes in the peripheral blood count display morphological signs of a gelatinous transformation in the bone marrow aspirate. It is important to mention that all hematological and morphological alterations disappear completely and rapidly after sufficient re-feeding [32].

References

[1] Mitchell, JE & Crow, S. Medical complications of anorexia nervosa and bulimia nervosa. *Curr Opin Psychiatry,* 2006, 19, 438-443.

[2] Katzman, DK. Medical complications in adolescents with anorexia nervosa: a review of the literature. *Int J Eat Disord,* 2005, 37 (Suppl), s52-59.

[3] Comerci, GD. Medical complications of anorexia nervosa and bulimia nervosa. *Med Clin North Am,* 1990, 74, 1293-1310.

[4] Hamilton Crisp, A & McClelland, L. *Anorexia Nervosa: Guidelines for Assessment and Treatment in Primary and Secondary Care.* London: Psychology Press, 1996.

[5] Vázquez, M; Olivares, JL; Fleta, J; Lacambra, I; González M. Cardiac disorders in young women with anorexia nervosa. *Rev Esp Cardiol,* 2003, 56, 669-673.

[6] Isner, JM; Roberts, WC; Heymsfield, SB; Yager, J. Anorexia nervosa and sudden death. *Ann Intern Med,* 1985, 102, 49-52.

[7] Mont, L; Castro, J; Herreros, B; Paré, C; Azqueta, M; Magriña, J; Puig, J; Toro, J; Brugada, J. Reversibility of cardiac abnormalities in adolescents with anorexia nervosa after weight recovery. *J Am Acad Child Adolesc Psychiatry,* 2003, 42, 808-813.

[8] Nahshoni, E; Weizman, A; Yaroslavsky, A; Toledano, A; Sulkes, J; Stein, D. Alterations in QT dispersion in the surface electrocardiogram of female adolescents diagnosed with restricting-type anorexia nervosa. *J Psychosom Res,* 2007, 62, 469-472.

[9] Bravender, T; Kanter, R; Zucker, N. Anorexia nervosa and second-degree atrioventricular block (Type I). *Int J Eat Disord,* 2006, 39, 612-615.

[10] Ohwada, R; Hotta, M; Kimura, H; Takagi, S; Matsuda, N; Nomura, K; Takano, K. Ampulla cardiomyopathy after hypoglycemia in three young female patients with anorexia nervosa. *Intern Med*, 2005, 44, 228-233.

[11] Casiero, D & Frishman, WH. Cardiovascular complications of eating disorders. *Cardiol Rev,* 2006, 14, 227-231.

[12] Birmingham, CL & Gritzner, S. Heart failure in anorexia nervosa: case report and review of the literature. *Eat Weight Disord,* 2007, 12:e7-10.

[13] Ishizawa, T; Yoshiuchi, K; Takimoto, Y; Yamamoto, Y; Akabayashi, A. Heart rate and blood pressure variability and baroreflex sensitivity in patients with anorexia nervosa. *Psychosom Med,* 2008, 70, 695-700.

[14] Cheng, TO. Anorexia nervosa and mitral valve prolapse. *Postgrad Med,* 1987, 82, 32-35.

[15] Meyers, DG; Starke, H; Pearson, PH; Wiken, MK. Mitral valve prolapse in anorexia nervosa. *Ann Intern Med,* 1986, 105, 384-385.

[16] Cheng, TO. Mitral valve prolapse: an overview. *J Cardiol*, 1989, 19 (suppl 21), 3-20.

[17] Cheng TO. Mitral valve prolapse. *Disease-a-month,* 1987, 33: 481-534.

[18] Crook, MA; Hally, V; Panteli, JV. The importance of the re-feeding syndrome. *Nutrition,* 2001, 17, 632-637.

[19] Mehanna, HM; Moledina, J; Travis, J. Re-feeding syndrome: what it is and how to prevent and treat it. *Br Med J,* 2008, 336 (7659), 1495-1498.

[20] Hearing, S. Re-feeding syndrome. *Br Med J,* 2004, 328 (7445), 908–909.

[21] Tresley, J & Sheean, PM. Re-feeding syndrome: recognition is the key to prevention and management. *J Am Diet Assoc,* 2008, 108, 2105-2108.

[22] Kraft, M; Btaiche, I; Sacks, G. Review of the re-feeding syndrome. *Nutr Clin Pract,* 2005, 20, 625–33.

[23] Hadley, SJ & Walsh, BT. Gastrointestinal disturbances in anorexia nervosa and bulimia nervosa. *Curr Drug Targets CNS Neurol Disord,* 2003, 2, 1-9.

[24] Zipfel, S; Sammet, I; Rapps, N; Herzog, W; Herpertz, S; Martens, U. Gastrointestinal disturbances in eating disorders: clinical and neurobiological aspects. *Auton Neurosci,* 2006, 129, 99-106.

[25] Morris, LG; Stephenson, KE; Herring, S; Marti, JL. Recurrent acute pancreatitis in anorexia and bulimia. *JOP,* 2004, 5, 231-234.

[26] Wesson, RN; Sparaco, A; Smith, MD. Chronic pancreatitis in a patient with malnutrition due to anorexia nervosa. *JOP,* 2008, 9, 327-331.

[27] Gasbarrini, G; Mingrone, G; Capristo, E; Greco, AV. (eds): *Proceedings of Meeting "Problemi nutrizionali in gastroenterologia: Malassorbimento e alterazioni metaboliche: quale ruolo per la nutrizione."* Cenesthesis, Bologna, 1997.

[28] Mehler, PS & Mackenzie, TD. Treatment of osteopenia and osteoporosis in anorexia nervosa: A systematic review of the literature. *Int J Eat Disord,* 2009, 42, 195-201.

[29] Zipfel, S; Seibel, MJ; Löwe, B; Beumont, PJ; Kasperk, C; Herzog, W. Osteoporosis in eating disorders: a follow-up study of patients with anorexia and bulimia nervosa. *J Clin Endocrinol Metab,* 2001, 86, 5227-5233.

[30] Legroux-Gérot, I; Vignau, J; D'Herbomez, M; Collier, F; Marchandise, X; Duquesnoy, B; Cortet, B. Evaluation of bone loss and its mechanisms in anorexia nervosa. *Calcif Tissue Int,* 2007, 81, 174-82.

[31] Legroux-Gérot, I; Vignau, J; Collier, F; Cortet, B. Factors influencing changes in bone mineral density in patients with anorexia nervosa-related osteoporosis: the effect of hormone replacement therapy. *Calcif Tissue Int,* 2008, 83, 315-323.

[32] Hütter, G; Ganepola, S; Hofmann, WK. The hematology of anorexia nervosa. *Int J Eat Disord,* 2009, 42, 293-300.

In: Anorexia Nervosa: A Multi-Disciplinary Approach ISBN: 978-1-60876-200-2
Editors: A. Mancini, S. Daini, L. Caruana, pp. 87-95

Chapter 5

NUTRITION IN ANOREXIA NERVOSA

Meniconi Paola[2], Giraldi Alessandra[2], Magini Marinella[2], Meucci Elisabetta[1] and Martorana Giuseppe Ettore[1,2]

Institute of Biochemistry and Clinical Biochemistry, School of Medicine, Catholic University of the Sacred Heart, Rome, Italy.

Dietetics Service, Dept. of Laboratory Medicine, Policlinico Universitario "A. Gemelli," Rome, Italy.

ABSTRACT

Nutritional intervention and counseling, together with all the proper medical and psychological measures, are essential tasks in the management of patients with anorexia nervosa. The approach to each patient by the dietician or nutrition professional or specialist should be tailored to fit the personal needs and cultural and religious beliefs of the patient. A personalized re-feeding program should be, therefore, agreed upon with the patient, with the aim of achieving nutritional rehabilitation, weight restoration, and reversal of the metabolic, medical and psychological complications. These efforts should always be seconded by a constant nutritional education aimed at changing the eating behavior of patients with anorexia nervosa and by steady dietetic counseling supporting the patients in the ups and downs of chronic illness. In order to help patients to meet their nutritional needs and achieve their targets, diets with high-energy density and a great variety of foods are recommended. Enteral feeding by nasogastric tube and parenteral nutrition are to be limited to patients with the most severe restrictive forms of anorexia nervosa and low body mass index hospitalized in specialized units under strict medical indication and supervision. Special attention should also be paid to avoid the re-feeding syndrome and to correct the medical complications. Finally, a set of motivations could also be useful in keeping the patient on the proposed dietary program, thus lowering the incidence of relapse.

1. Introduction

Good nutritional management of patients with anorexia nervosa requires attention to a number of areas. As with any other eating disorder, during assessment and throughout treatment, attention to the complexities of anorexia nervosa, such as influencing factors, comorbid illness, medical and psychological complications, is critical for its effective treatment. Nutrition intervention, including dietetic counseling, by a dietician or a nutrition expert is an essential component of the team treatment of patients with anorexia nervosa [1].

When a restricted diet appears to be a permanent feature of the patient's lifestyle, education in achieving good nutrition should form part of the treatment. The aim is to ensure that the patient knows how to meet nutritional needs. Particular attention should be given to energy, protein, and mineral and vitamin supplementation. As with other aspects of the management of anorexia nervosa, a complex negotiation with the patient may be needed and issues of motivation are paramount.

Ultimately, the objective of treatment must be the return of body composition to normal; this requires a competent metabolic machinery [2]. Therefore, the first step must be to repair the machinery, with tissue repletion being a secondary consideration during the early phase of treatment.

For some patients with a long history of anorexia nervosa, the best option may be to maintain a weight safe enough to allow some quality of life and prevent hospital admission. This normally requires a BMI of at least 15Kg / m2. Maintaining a low body weight requires a low energy intake, but the requirement for most essential nutrients is at least as high as that recommended for healthy people. Achieving an adequate dietary intake of all nutrients, therefore, requires a diet with a high nutrient density overall. This can be planned in discussion with the patient, using foods that the individual feels able to tolerate and that are acceptable within the context of cultural and religious practices. Planning the diet should include particular attention to the following [1]:

- regular, stable intake of carbohydrate, to prevent erratic weight changes;
- adequate intake of protein, especially for vegetarians, those who avoid dairy products and those with increased protein requirements (e.g., in infection or in puberty)
- adequate intake of essential fatty acids;
- adequate intake of nutrients necessary for bone mineral density (calcium, vitamin D, magnesium);
- iron and zinc for those who do not eat red meat;
- fat-soluble vitamins;
- the need for long-term, well-balanced vitamin and mineral supplementation;
- the need for supplementation with specific nutrients that are difficult to provide in adequate amounts from the diet, especially when there are increased requirements.

A number of approaches may help the patient to manage meals and snacks, including adequate amounts of starchy carbohydrate and, if possible, some fat in the diet, and constructing meals with the largest possible variety of foods.

2. Nutritional Rehabilitation

Although re-feeding a malnourished patient may look easy, nutritional rehabilitation in patients with anorexia nervosa who are resistant to weight gain can be extremely challenging and, a few times, unrewarding.

Nutritional rehabilitation can be defined as the restoration of normal eating habits, body weight and functions and, more specifically, involves: a) metabolic recovery; b) weight restoration; c) improvement in eating behavior; and d) reversal of the medical complications.

a. Metabolic Recovery

In states of malnutrition, as in anorexia nervosa, basal metabolic rate slows down as an adaptive response to starvation. Resting energy expenditure decreases and may be as low as 50% to 70% of predicted values. Consequently, in the malnourished state, initial caloric requirements are low. With nutritional rehabilitation and metabolic recovery, caloric requirements increase dramatically [3,4].

While there is wide variability in individual cases and in different studies, approximately 7,500 kcals of energy are required on average for one kg of weight gain.

b. Weight Restoration

Weight gain should be achieved in inpatient, partial hospitalization, and outpatient settings.

Rate of weight gain should be 0.9-1.4 kg per week for inpatient programs, 0.5 to 0.9 kg per week for partial hospitalization programs (when such programs are step-down programs from inpatient units) and 0.2 to 0.5 kg per week for outpatient management [5].

For most inpatient units, a behavioral contract is the backbone of the program. Weight gain is rewarded by an increase in privileges and weight loss is accompanied by a loss of privileges; similar deals should be agreed upon with outpatients, too.

Such programs work without necessarily needing to resort to nasogastric feeding or to total parenteral nutrition [6]. What is clear, however, is that during the first five to seven days of nutritional rehabilitation, there is often no weight gain. In fact, initially there can be even some weight loss to below admission weight. These five to seven days, termed the "phase of stabilization," is the time during which the body changes from a state of catabolism to a state of anabolism. Weight gain cannot be expected to occur during this time.

Gradual increases in caloric prescription can be made every 24 to 48 hours, as tolerated. The advantages of eating regular meals is that it teaches the patient to eat normally. This method, however, requires a greater need for nutritional or dietary input to ensure that the meals provide the correct amount of calories. Liquid supplements alone provide the necessary calories in a balanced formula but, in this way, normal eating behavior is not necessarily reinforced. On the other hand, voluntary nasogastric feeding, accompanied by oral feeding, does increase the rate of weight gain but does not impact on psychological recovery [7]. Total parenteral nutrition should rarely be necessary for nutritional rehabilitation in anorexia nervosa and should be used for the shortest amount of time.

Independent of the type of nutritional rehabilitation, the content should provide a balanced diet containing 45% to 65% of intake from carbohydrates, 10% to 35% from protein and 20% to 35% from fat [8]. An adequate calcium intake, which for an adolescent is 1,200 to 1,500 mg a day, should be ensured. A multivitamin containing 100% of the RDA should be prescribed to provide adequate intakes of vitamin D, other fat-soluble vitamins and trace elements in order to compensate for the increased requirements during metabolic recovery.

c. Improvement in Eating Behaviour

With nutritional rehabilitation, eating disorder symptoms, such as food hoarding and abnormal eating behaviors, lessen. Food choices improve, and the obsession about food decreases in frequency and intensity (5). In this regard, continuous nutritional education and dietetic counseling is of paramount importance.

d. Reversal of Medical Complications

Although medical complications are mainly under the care and responsibility of the medical and psychiatric staff, a proper nutritional program should be also undertaken and associated to the medical and psychological therapy.

Among the most common complications in this respect are the electrolyte disturbances of hypokalemia and hyponatremia. The former occurs in those who are vomiting and/or abusing laxative or diuretics, while the latter is more likely to occur in those who drink excessive amounts of water, and both can be corrected using standard formulae.

Serum phosphorus levels may be normal on presentation but can drop precipitously on re-feeding [9]. Over three quarters of the patients reach their phosphorus lowest point within the first week of hospitalization [10]. Hypophosphatemia is thought to be one of the more important etiologic factors in the development of the re-feeding syndrome [11].

Other laboratory findings suggest a sort of metabolic derangement, especially with regard to cholesterol metabolism [12,13].

Cardiological complications in anorexia nervosa include reduction of heart size and exercise capacity [14,15], but cardiac output and left ventricular function are usually preserved [14]. The cardiac structural and functional abnormalities are reversible after re-feeding [15]. Bradycardia and orthostatic blood pressure changes are frequent findings in anorexia nervosa and are often the reason for medical hospitalization [16]. With nutritional rehabilitation, orthostatic blood pressure changes (defined as a drop in systolic blood pressure of more than 20 mm Hg and/or a drop in diastolic blood pressure of >10 mm Hg) usually resolve within a day or two, but orthostatic pulse changes (defined as an increase in pulse rate of more than 20 beats per minute on standing) take longer to resolve and usually occur when patients reach a weight approximately 80% of expected body weight [17].

Amenorrhea is one of the cardinal features of anorexia nervosa and is associated with suppression of the hypothalamic-pituitary-ovarian axis [18]; weight restoration is accompanied by restoration of hormonal levels and resumption of menses. A weight approximately 90% of ideal body weight is the average weight at which menses return, and 86% of patients with anorexia nervosa who reach this weight will resume menses within six months [19].

Several computed tomography and magnetic resonance studies of patients with anorexia nervosa imply loss of brain substance or cerebral atrophy [20-26]. Cognitive impairment is also well documented in anorexia nervosa, but it is not clear whether the cognitive deficits are directly related to the structural brain changes [27]. More recent studies, however, with a longer follow-up period, have shown that the ventricular enlargement and white matter changes are reversible with nutritional rehabilitation [21,28], but that gray matter volume deficits and regional blood flow disturbances can persist despite weight restoration [28,29].

Osteopenia occurs in over 90% of adolescents and young adults with anorexia nervosa and is associated with increased fracture risk [30,31], and it may not be entirely reversible, despite medical and nutritional intervention [32].

Malnutrition is associated with depressed mood, cognitive impairment and preoccupation with food, weight and shape. Both Kingston et al. [27] and Jones et al. [33] found that patients with anorexia nervosa had impaired focusing, verbal memory and visuo-spatial reasoning. With nutritional rehabilitation, there is improvement in mood and cognitive function, although it is difficult to correlate the subtle neuropsychological changes with objective measures of nutritional status [34] or brain magnetic resonance imaging findings [27].

3. Conclusions

Energy intake during re-feeding must achieve a compromise between the need to restore normal nutrition as quickly as possible and the patient's limited physical and psychological ability to tolerate eating.

An individualised approach may, therefore, be best for those not being treated in a specialised eating-disorder unit [35]. In specialised units, a standardised program can instead be used, with appropriate flexibility for individual needs.

A weekly weight gain of 0.5-1.0 kg is generally regarded as optimum. There is some preliminary research evidence that a minimum weight gain of 0.5 kg per week results in greater weight gain at discharge than use of a higher minimum [36].

It is common practice in many units to set a target weight at the beginning of treatment. This gives definition to the treatment program and may help to soften and delay the patient's anxiety about being allowed to gain weight and being overweight. There is no clear consensus as to how the target weight should be determined. A reasonably common practice is to base it on a low normal body weight, such as a BMI of about 19 Kg/m2.

In chronic starvation, the energy requirement is depressed because body cell mass is depleted and there is a conservative metabolic response to starvation. It is, therefore, possible to promote weight gain with a relatively low energy intake at first and to increase it gradually; this allows the patient some time to adapt to an increasing intake [37]. The rate of increase in intake depends on the patient's motivations, and the level of support and supervision that can be provided.

Enteral feeding has a limited role in the treatment of anorexia nervosa; however, there are some situations in which it may be required. If enteral feeding is considered necessary, the nasogastric route is normally preferred because it reinforces the view that enteral feeding is a short-term measure, and there is less medical risk involved than with other procedures. Occasionally, patients find an artificial means of feeding preferable as it takes away one's sense of responsibility for eating [38]. In critically ill patients, enteral feeding may allow a greater degree of control over the patient's nutritional intake. There is a risk of hypophosphataemia and acute thiamine deficiency at the outset of enteral feeding. It is, therefore, recommended that such patients are given phosphate supplements before feeding starts [39], and additional mineral supplement ation and intravenous B and C vitamins may also be required.

Many of the principles of inpatient re-feeding can also be applied to outpatients. However, outpatients are a heterogeneous group, and an individualised approach to re-feeding is mandatory. In view of the risk of complications if weight gain is too rapid, weight gain of more than 0.5 Kg per week is probably unwise. In patients who are gaining significant amounts of weight (0.3 Kg per week or more), regular monitoring of serum electrolytes is recommended, together with prescription of a complete micronutrient supplement. The patient should be also monitored clinically for evidence of edema and other complications of re-feeding.

Recently, a paper by Mehler et al. [40] reviewed the criteria for the use of total parenteral nutrition re-feeding in patients with severe anorexia nervosa, i.e., abnormal vital signs (very low heart rate, symptomatic hypotension, <70%-75% of ideal body weight, rapid and severe weight loss unresponsive to outpatient treatment, cardiac arrhythmias), where the traditional modes (re-feeding through oral or nasogastric routes) have previously failed. The use of parenteral nutrition has also started a debate on its applications to patients with anorexia nervosa. The controversy is about the correct clinical indications, relative efficacies and risks of parenteral vs. enteral feeding in AN patients [41,42]. More recently [43], Thiels considered the clinical, ethical and legal approaches to "forced treatment" of patients with anorexia nervosa with a BMI ~ 13 Kg/m2 or below. The author's final recommendations are listed in the paper and include: "Coercion should not be used instead of psychotherapy; use coercion carefully and for the shortest time; patients should be motivated to eat with increasing independence; the aim is not a particular weight but the continuation of treatment without coercion." For further details, the reader is invited to refer to this review [43] and to the literature quoted therein.

Not everything is problematic: a recent paper by Schebendach et al. [44] reported that patients with higher scores of diet energy density and diet variety in hospitalized, weight-restored AN patients predict a better outcome, suggesting that the intake of energy-dense foods and a greater variety of foods are essential for relapse prevention. Another issue that comes in handy for instilling more motivations in patients with anorexia nervosa is represented by the alterations of laboratory hematochemical parameters [12,13]. Although the molecular mechanisms are not yet clear, high cholesterol levels are frequently found in sera of AN patients, who seem to need longer periods of treatment with further weight gain to fully normalize [45]. This unexpected metabolic alteration could be used as an additional motivation for informed AN patients, always at odds with "fats" in their very restrictive diets, in order to adhere more willingly and for a longer time to the proposed nutritional therapy.

REFERENCES

[1] Council Report CR130 July 2005. Royal College of Psychiatrists, London. *Guidelines for the nutritional management of anorexia nervosa.* Approved by Council: October 2004. Due for review: 2008.

[2] Neville, H; Golden, MD; Meyer, W. Nutritional rehabilitation of anorexia nervosa. Goals and dangers. *Int J Adolesc Med Health,* 2004, 16, 131-144.

[3] Schebendach, JE; Golden, NH; Jacobson, MS; Hertz, S; Shenker, IR. The metabolic responses of starvation and re-feeding in adolescents with anorexia nervosa. *Ann N Y Acad Sci,* 1997, 817, 110-119.

[4] Vaisman, N; Rossi, MF; Corey, M; Clarke, R; Goldberg, E; Pencharz, P B. Effect of re-feeding on the energy metabolism of adolescent girls who have anorexia nervosa. *Eur J Clin Nutr,* 1991, 45, 527-537.

[5] Yager, J; Anderson, A; Devlin, M. American Psychiatric Association Practice Guideline for the Treatment of Patients with Eating Disorder. *Am. J Psychiatry,* 2000, 157(suppl):1-39.

[6] Solanto, MV; Jacobson, MS; Heller, L; Golden, NH; Hertz, S. Rate of weight gain of inpatients with anorexia nervosa under two behavioural contracts. *Pediatrics,* 1994, 93, 989-991.

[7] Zuercher, JN; Cumella, EJ; Woods, BK; Eberly, M; Carr, JK. Efficacy of voluntary nasogastric tube feeding in female inpatients with anorexia nervosa. *JPEN J Parenter Enteral Nutr,* 2003, 27, 268-276.

[8] Trumbo, P; Schlicker, S; Yates, AA; Poos, M. Dietary reference intakes for energy, carbohydrate, fiber, fat, fatty acid, cholesterol, protein and amino acids. *J Am Diet Ass,* 2002, 102, 1621-30.

[9] Kohn, MR; Golden, NH; Shenker, IR. Cardiac arrest and delirium: presentations of the re-feeding syndrome in severely malnourished adolescents with anorexia nervosa. *J Adolesc Health,* 1998, 22, 239-243.

[10] Ornstein, RM; Golden, NH; Jacobson, MS; Shenker, JR. Hypophosphatemia during nutritional rehabilitation in anorexia nervosa: implications for re-feeding and monitoring. *J Adolesc Health,* 2003, 32, 83-88.

[11] Solomon, SM & Kirby, DF. The re-feeding syndrome: a review. *JPEN J. Parenter Enteral Nutr,* 1990, 14, 90-97.

[12] Weinbrener, T; Zuger, M; Jacoby, GE; Herpertz, S; Liedtke, R; Sudhop, T; Gouni-Berthold, I; Axelson, M; Berthold HK. Lipoprotein metabolism in patients with anorexia nervosa: a case-control study investigating the mechanisms leading to hypercholesterolaemia. *Br J Nutr,* 2004, 91, 959-969.

[13] Zak, A; Vecka, M; Tvrzicka, E; Hruby, M; Novak, F; Papezova, H; Lubanda, H; Vesela, L; Stankova, B. Composition of Plasma Fatty Acids and Non-Cholesterol Sterols in Anorexia Nervosa. *Physiol Res,* 2005, 54, 443-451.

[14] Moodie, DS & Salcedo, E. Cardiac function in adolescents and young adults with anorexia nervosa. *J. Adolesc Health Care,* 1983, 4, 9-14.

[15] Mont, L; Castro, J; Herreros, B; Pare, C; Azqueta, M; Magrina, J; Puig, J; Toro, J; Brugada, J. Reversibility of cardiac abnormalities in adolescents with anorexia nervosa after weight recovery. *J Am Acad Child Adolesc Psychiatry,* 2003, 42, 808-813.

[16] Fischer, M; Golden, NH; Katzman, DK; Kreipe, RE; Rees, J; Schebendach, J; Sigman, G; Ammerman, S; Hoberman, HM. Eating disorders in adolescents: a background paper. *J Adolesc Health,* 1995, 16, 420-437.

[17] Shamin, T; Golden, NH; Arden, M; Filiberto, L; Shenker, JR. Resolution of vital sign instability: an objective measure of medical stability in anorexia nervosa. *J Adolesc Health,* 2003, 32, 73-77.

[18] Golden, NH & Shenker, IR. Amenorrhea in Anorexia Nervosa: Etiology and Implications. In: Nussbaum, MP; Dwyer, JT, eds. Adolescent Nutrition and Eating Disorders 3 edition. *Philadelphia: Hanley & Belfus,* 1992, 503-518.

[19] Golden, NH; Jacobson, MS; Schebendach, J; Solanto, MV; Hertz, SM; Shenker, JR. Resumption of menses in anorexia nervosa. *Arch Pediatr Adolesc Med,* 1997, 151, 16-21.

[20] Enzmann, DR & Lane, B. Cranial computed tomography findings in anorexia nervosa. *J Comput Assist Tomogr,* 1997, 1, 410-414.

[21] Golden, NH; Ashtari, M; Kohn, MR; Patel, M; Jacobson, MS; Fletcher, A; Shenker IR. Reversibility of cerebral ventricular enlargement in anorexia nervosa, demonstrated by quantitative magnetic resonance imaging. *J Pediatr,* 1996, 128, 296-301.

[22] Katzman, DK; Lambe, EK; Mikulis, D; Ridgley, JN; Goldbloom, DS; Zipursky, RB. Cerebral gray matter and white matter volume deficits in adolescent girls with anorexia nervosa. *J Pediatr,* 1996, 129, 794-803.

[23] Nussbaum, M; Shenker, JR; Marc, J; Klein, M. Cerebral atrophy in anorexia nervosa. *J Pediatr,* 1980, 96, 867-869.

[24] Krieg, JC; Pirke, KM; Lauer, C; Backmund, H. Endocrine, metabolic, and cranial computed tomographic findings in anorexia nervosa. *Biol Psychiatry,* 1988, 23, 377-87.

[25] Dolan, RJ; Mitchell, J; Wakeling, A. Structural brain changes in patients with anorexia nervosa. *Psychol Med,* 1998, 18, 349-953.

[26] Artmann, H; Grau, H; Adelmann, M; Schleiffer, R. Reversible and non-reversible enlargement of cerebrospinal fluid spaces in anorexia nervosa. *Neuroradiology,* 1985, 27, 304-312.

[27] Kingston, K; Szmukler, G; Andrewes, D; Tress, B; Desmond P. Neuropsychological and structural brain changes in anorexia nervosa before and after re-feeding. *Psychol Med,* 1996, 26, 15-28.

[28] Katzman, DK; Zipursky, RB; Lambe, EK; Mikulis, DJ. A longitudinal magnetic resonance imaging study of brain changes in adolescents with anorexia nervosa. *Arch Pediatr Adolesc Med,* 1997, 151, 793-797.

[29] Gordon, I; Lask, B; Bryant-Waugh, R; Christie, D; Timimi, S. Childhood-onset anorexia nervosa: identifying a biological substrate. *Int J Eat Disord,* 1997, 22, 159-165.

[30] Golden, NH; Lanzkowsky, L; Schebendach, J; Palestro, CJ; Jacobson, MS; Shenker IR. The effect of estrogen-progestin treatment on bone mineral density in anorexia nervosa. *J Pediatr Adolesc Gynecol,* 2002, 15, 135-143.

[31] Grinspoon, S; Thomas, E; Pitts, S; Gross, E; Mick, D; Miller, K; Herzog, D; Klibanski, A. Prevalence and predictive factors for regional osteopenia in women with anorexia nervosa. *Ann Intern Med,* 2000, 133, 790-794.

[32] Bachrach, LK; Katzman, DK; Litt, IF; Guido, D; Marcus, R. Recovery from osteopenia in adolescent girls with anorexia nervosa. *J Clin Endocrinol Metab,* 1991, 72, 602-606.

[33] Jones, BP; Duncan, CC; Brouwers, P; Mirsky, AF. Cognition in eating disorders. *J Clin Exp Neuropsychol,* 1991, 13, 711-728.

[34] Green, MW; Elliman, NA; Wakeling, A; Rogers, PJ. Cognitive functioning, weight change and therapy in anorexia nervosa. *J Psychiatr Res,* 1996, 30, 401-410.

[35] Salisbury, JJ; Levine, AS; Crow, SJ; Mitchall, JE. Re-feeding, metabolic rate and weight gain in anorexia nervosa: a review. *Int J Eat Disord,* 1995, 17, 337-345.

[36] Herzog, T; Zeeck, A; Hartmann, A. Lower targets for weekly weight gain lead to better results in in-patient treatment of anorexia nervosa. *Eur Eat Disord Rev,* 2004, 12, 164-168.

[37] Strober, M; Freeman, R; Morrell, W. The long-term course of severe anorexia nervosa in adolescents: survival analysis of recovery, relapse, and outcome predictors over 10 to 15 years in a prospective study. *Int J Eat Disord,* 1997, 22, 339-360.

[38] Neiderman, M; Zarody, M; Tattersall, M; Lask, B. Enteral feeding in severe adolescent anorexia nervosa: a report of four cases. *Int J Eat Disord,* 2000, 28, 471-475.

[39] Birmingham, CL; Alothman, AF; Goldner, EM. Anorexia nervosa: re-feeding and hypophosphataemia. *Int J Eat Disord,* 1996, 20, 211-213.

[40] Mehler, PS; Kolpak, S; Padilla, R. Anorexia Nervosa and the Use of Total Parenteral Nutrition Re-feeding. *Current Nutrition,* 2005, 1, 97-104.

[41] Diamanti, A; Basso, MS; Castro, M; Bianco, GX; Ciacco, E; Calce, A; Caramadre, AM; Noto, C; Gambarara, M. Clinical efficacy and safety of parenteral nutrition in adolescent girls with anorexia nervosa. *J Adolesc Health,* 2008, 42, 11-18.

[42] Melchior, JC & Corcos, M. Parenteral Nutrition and anorexia nervosa: is it useful, is it ethical? *J Adolesc Health,* 2009, 44, 410-411.

[43] Thiels C. Forced treatment of patients with anorexia. *Forensic psychiatry,* 2008, 21, 495-498.

[44] Schebendach, JE; Mayer, LES; Devlin, MJ; Attia, E; Contento, IR; Wolf, RL; Walsh, BT. Dietary energy density and diet variety as predictors of outcome in anorexia nervosa. *Am J Clin Nutr,* 2008, 87, 810-816.

[45] Nova, E; Lopez-Vidriero, I; Varela, P; Casas, J; Marcos, A. Evolution of serum biochemical indicators in anorexia nervosa patients. *J Hum Nutr Diet,* 2008, 21, 23-30.

SECTION II: PSYCHOLOGICAL ASPECTS

In: Anorexia Nervosa: A Multi-Disciplinary Approach ISBN: 978-1-60876-200-2
Editors: A. Mancini, S. Daini, L. Caruana, pp. 99-113

Chapter 6

INFANTILE ANOREXIA

S. Daini, L. Petrongolo and L. Bernardini
Institute of Psychiatry, Catholic University of the Sacred Heart, Rome, Italy.

ABSTRACT

Anorexia has extremely deep roots reaching back to the first few moments of life. Some complications experienced by the newborn during birth and immediately after can play a role in the aetiopathogenesis of eating disorders that the child may show over the course of his/her life. The newborn immediately establishes a significant and poignant relationship with his/her mother; he/she learns from her how to express his/her own personality through the feeding behavior. Therefore, observing the dynamics of this relationship represents a particularly interesting analysis for further, in-depth study of the anorexic disorder. Different types of treatment can be applied following direct observation of the relationship among father, mother and child; this can be behaviorist when the therapist, with play therapies and lunch-sessions, works on the communication exchange between parents and children, observing the complementary and symmetrical exchanges and the cooperation skills in the management of the feeding relationship with the child.

1. INTRODUCTION

"Infantile eating disorders" include a variety of specific problems with different etiologies and outcomes, whose long list of symptoms reflects its heterogeneous nature. Some of these symptoms refer directly to the eating skills and behaviors: oro-motor, oro-sensorial and oro-pharyngeal developmental disabilities, selective refusal of food, vomiting, rumination, swallowing of non-nourishing substances, food-related panic. Other symptoms are vague and not specific: colic during the first three months of life. Transitory eating problems are also common during early childhood, in particular in some critical developmental phases, and they do not necessarily underlie a disorder. Between the seventh and the ninth month of life, during weaning and when anxiety for the unknown may develop, or between the second and third year of life, when the child starts eating autonomously, food refusal behavior is a common phase of the maturation process when the child's biological, cognitive and affective skills are reorganized into a more complex developmental level. Such phases require a negotiation between the child the and caregiver in order to reach a new interactive set of rules and adjustments that take into account the growing sense of individual autonomy that the child is acquiring. Moreover, from birth, children show clear, individual differences in hunger and satiety cycles; some newborns request food as soon as they wake up, others passively accept being nourished or communicate discontinuous signs of hunger. Some children are hypersensitive in the oral and oro-pharyngeal area; they have difficulty in accepting contact with the food on their lips, in their mouths or in swallowing it. These children may be particularly sensitive to food texture and its temperature. Hyposensitivity to food, to its taste and texture is rarer. When this happens, newborns can keep milk in their mouths for several minutes without swallowing it, and children may keep solid food in their mouths without swallowing it for a long time. With children who show non-organic failure to thrive, caregivers can address these changes in several ways that often reflect their developmental experience during the separation-individuation process; some will encourage the child's autonomy, others feel uncomfortable and become hyperprotective.

The diagnostic expression "Feeding Skills Disorder," was suggested by Ramsay & co. [1] to define clinical case histories with developmental disabilities in the feeding patterns. When assessing a clinical status, it is fundamental to take into account that feeding represents an essential aspect of the children's caretaking. Feeding is of particular importance to parents as a source of satisfaction and reassurance, or to the contrary, as a source of intense worry, should a disorder manifest. As a result, bad care giving behaviors may be started, thus complicating the child's eating difficulties. Hence, there is the need to determine when a problem becomes a disorder.

2. Early Anorexia

Childhood psychopathology defines early anorexia as a syndrome characterized by inadequate and troublesome feeding associated with failure to thrive or with growth stunting, when no organic causes can explain the child's disorder.

From birth, the newborn has a very well-developed neuro-physiologic system at suction behavior level: the reflex of cardinal points, accompanied by the head rotation; the reflex of escape; the reflex of suction and swallowing, accompanied by attempts of finger grasping; all represent an immediately functional motor unit. However, children with eating disorders do not behave as above when it comes to feeding. If we analyse the rhythm of suction and the frequency of the interruptions, we can find infants who suck with a fast rhythm, almost without a pause, and others whose rhythm of suction is slower and often interrupted. Other variables accompany such behaviors. Some children cry and toss and turn when confronted with what is for them an intolerable tension; others seem to wait for feeding more serenely. Some suck with their eyes open, others with closed eyes. Regardless of these individual differences, suction seems to be a need in itself for the baby; when he/she eats too quickly, the baby tries to extend the suction time with its fingers or with another object; but the feeding in babies cannot be limited to a mere satisfaction of the physiological hunger. It represents the prototype of human relations. Freud distinguished between the satisfaction of the feeding need itself (hunger) and the pleasant reward (suction) that baby gets; the ontogenetic trace of this pleasure will continue, schematically, in his/her appetite. Currently, the handling of the child [2]—like body contact, maternal words, glances, rocking and his/her need for bonding [3] —are also considered important. However, the suction remains the strongest element of this exchange, and it represents the privileged way through which the baby will begin to explore the world outside; this is proved by that phase when the baby will systematically bring everything to his/her mouth (from the fourth to fifth month to the tenth to twelfth month). This does not mean that there is no aggressiveness in this exchange; we have only underlined the libidinal dimension so far. Swallowing, making disappear, eliminating are aggressive movements. While we welcome with due caution the hypothesis of precocious aggressiveness against the mother's breast [4], we must recognise that feeding a newborn means making disappear the tension, the previous desire. If the feeding exchange is not satisfactory, the infant may feel the disappearance of this need like a loss, a threat or a danger of annulment.

Thmother's approach depends on her child's behavior and on his/her feelings about oral skills, but also on the baby's ability to learn and adapt to new situations. At the beginning, it is not easy for the mother to hold her baby in her arms, to handle him, to calm him/her down and to satisfy his/her needs immediately. More often, around the fourth day, mutual adaptation develops; first time mother become conscious of he baby, and she expresses the feeling of being able to take her of him/her. This mutual adaptation develops much more quickly after second delivery.

Besides this process of mutual harmonization, mothers can react differently according to how the baby behaves: some seem scared of the child's voracity, others are proud of it. On the contrary, some mothers are concerned that a slow and irregular suction may be an indication of future feeding disorders. These different feelings that the babies provoke in the mothers are clearly conscious or preconscious "ghosts;" if called back, such ghosts may lead to a pathogenic mother-baby relationship.

Between the fifth and eighth month of life, the infant may develop feeding-skills disorders, progressively rather than suddenly. This sometimes happens during the weaning (hence "weaning anorexia"), and it may be accompanied by constipation. A significant desire for liquids often compensates anorexia for solid food. Moreover, anorexia may happen to concern only the relationship with the mother, while the baby will eat normally with any other person (nanny, child-nurse, grandmother). Usually, the child, with an early development, is lively, toned, dynamic and shows curiosity for the surrounding world. Such refusal for the food, more or less total, causes anxiety in the mother; this leads the mother to adopt a number of strategies aimed at forcing the child to eat. She tries to distract her child, to play with him/her, to seduce the baby; she may wait until he/she feels sleepy or tries to hold his/her hands firmly or even to keep his/her mouth open. Unavoidably, the baby wins, and the mother is defeated and exhausted. Relatives' and friends' advice and opinions will only increase the mother's anxiety. She sees the child's behavior as a refusal towards her; she is distressed, becomes annoyed as the mealtime approaches, and she starts losing the necessary willingness. Under these conditions, the meal does not represent for the baby the nourishing moment anymore, but instead represents the time to absorb his/her mother's anxiety. This phase is often temporary and isolated, while the baby keeps on growing and his/her weight increases.

This is a rare case of acute anorexia. In the baby's evolutionary process, we can distinguish between a simple form of anorexia and a serious mental anorexia [5]; the two are similar at their onset. The anorexic behavior persists, both because the baby's anorexic reaction is deeply rooted in his/her body, and because the mother's behavior does not change. Other changes may occur, such as sleeping difficulties, intense anger, hiccups. The baby shows total lack of interest for food and strong opposition to it. In the latter case, meals turn into a true fight between the mother trying to use all sorts of tricks to introduce food into her baby's mouth (amusement, blackmail, threat, coercion) and the baby floundering, spitting, misbehaving, overturning the dish. Such anorexic behavior may alternate with periods when the baby eats more normally, while throwing tantrums: he only eats sweet food, diary products, and legumes. Vomit is frequent and usually follows the meals. In these conditions, the baby becomes pale and skinny, however, he does not develop a real disease. For a long time, parents try to find an organic origin to this behavior, which is instead very rare (heart condition, digestive problems, infections, encephalopathy or brain tumour).

3. Diagnosing Anorexia in Infants

During the last few years, in the field of Infant research and Developmental psychopathology, we have witnessed that complex structuring of the mental functioning, as well as processes of activation and modulation of the base motivational systems occur during the first years of one's life; among these are the physiological regulation and the attachment process.

The diagnostic systems for children and adolescents provided by DSM-IV and ICD-10 are not appropriate. In the past, Kanner and Chess [6] have proposed specific systems, collected in the appendix of the diagnostic handbook edited by the Group for the Advancement of Psychiatry and published in 1966. In the psychoanalytic field, many authors have criticized the use of adults' diagnostic criteria, deeming them not suitable for adolescents. Anna Freud, in particular [7], thought that criteria connected with individual distress and dysfunctions relevant for adults could not be applied to children, because they do not experience such distress and the functional levels often fluctuate. Anna Freud believed that only a stop to the evolutionary process may represent a disorder, and, for this reason, she proposed a meta-psychological diagnostic profile. With this tool, a physician with a psychoanalytic background may describe the current functioning of a baby using various evolutionary parameters that would allow establishing a rich diagnostic profile, though of an idiographic type.

To this end, the diagnostic Classification 0-3, proposed by the National Centre for Clinical Infant Programs [8] of Washington, seems to introduce an interesting perspective. The task group who created this Classification was formed by psychoanalysts and researchers who significantly contributed to the development of the Infant Research in these last twenty years. Among them were Robert Emde, Stanley Greenspan, Joe Osofsky and Alicia Lieberman. As stated in the introduction to this work, "taking into consideration all the relevant areas of the child's functioning, using all available knowledge in every field, is a specific responsibility of those in charge to make an accurate diagnosis and to formulate an appropriate plan of action." When carrying out a diagnosis on a child, it is necessary to consider the symptoms and the evident behaviors, the developmental process, the family system functioning, the parents' individual characteristics, the features of the adult-child relationship and the interaction patterns, the specific body-build and developmental characteristics of the baby, the recurrent aspects in the affectivity, the language, the cognitive, motor and sensorial activities of the baby.

As the DSM the diagnostic Classification 0-3, as well, proposes a multi-axial classification system: Axis I, the primary classification reflecting the most significant characteristic of the disorder; Axis II, the classification of the relationship; Axis III, physical, neurological, evolutionary and mental conditions and disorders; Axis IV, stressful agents of psychosocial nature; Axis V, developmental level of emotional functioning.

The true innovation is represented by Axis II, which specifically defines the quality of the parent-child relationship; this not only contributes to the baby's personality development and to the structuring of his/her psychological defences, but it also contributes to the representations that the child creates in relation with the others. The disorder shown by the baby is rooted in the parent-child relationship. Diagnosing the relationship disorder should consider not only the observed behavior, but also how the parent describes her/his own subjective experience. The intensity, the frequency and the duration of the relation disorder must be taken in account.

Within this scenario, the following cases must be distinguished:

- Hyper-involvement: the parent tends to interfere with the child's purposes and intentions, over controlling him/her, making inappropriate requests; hence, the child may appear confused, unfocused, submitted, and his/her developmental level may be inadequate. The parent may be anxious, depressed or angry, and the child may react passively or with anger and stubbornness. On the psychological involvement level, the parent perceives the child as part of her/himself and tries to induce or manipulate him/her to satisfy her/his own needs.
- Hypo-involvement: in this case, the parent is little involved and his/her communication is scarce; he/she is insensitive or not sympathetic with the child's signs. For this reason, the parent is unable or refuses to satisfy the child's requests for support, or he/she does not protect his/her son adequately from potential dangers. Within this context, the child may appear neglected on a physical or psychological level. The parent's own history may be characterized by affective deficiencies or negligence.
- Anxious/tense relationship: in this case, the interactions are nervous and poor, and they do not guarantee a mutually satisfactory level. The parent appears very sensitive to his/her baby's signs, but he interacts with him/her in a clumsy way; he/she is anxious and tense on the affective level, hence, he/she can easily fail to understand her/his child's behavior or emotional state.
- Hostile/angry relation: in this case, interactions are negative and abrupt; anger and hostility have a prominent position. The parent is anxious; he/she can handle the child with tension and can at times scoff and mock him/her, perceiving the child's dependency as a burden or an excessive request.
- Mixed relational disorder: the above-described cases are overlapped.

- Abuse: it may be verbal, physical and/or sexual. In the verbal abuse, the boundaries between parent and child are not clear and often the parent exerts hyper-control. When physical, the parent resorts to aggressive physical behaviors with high levels of irritability, anger and hostility. In the case of sexual abuse, there is a lack of attention towards the child's physical boundaries with extreme and erotic intrusive behaviors.

In literature, other classifications exist and more clinical cases are defined.

4. The Observation

The direct and systematic observation of the child and of his/her relationships during development, together with the reports provided by his/her parents, represent a clinical evaluation methodology capable of providing thorough knowledge of both the child's self-organizational, affective, cognitive and social characteristics and of the "child-caregiver" interactive system, regulated by specific relational patterns and mental models [9-13].

Through observation, two types of data can be highlighted: the "objective" data, the behavior indicating the child's developmental and mental state; and the "subjective" data, the causes, the meaning and the attributions on the child, emerging from the parents' reports [12,13].

In line with this theorist-clinical perspective, during the last fifteen years, the Infant research has highlighted how the caregiver's subjective experience and his internal ideas about nurturance relation, studied in a systematic way in the narrative patterns, have a predictive value on child's future relations, development and adaptation [14-16].

In his/her first three years of life, the child interacts with and is involved actively in the relationship with caregivers. For this purpose, we have examined the Feeding Scales (Observational Scales for Mother-Infant Interaction during Feeding), in an overview of instruments and evaluation procedures that allows the clinician to have an integrated vision of the child's evolutionary skills and of the child-caregiver relationship in the developmental context. This is an evaluation scale of the mother-child interactive dynamics in feeding, based on the developmental classification of early infancy eating disorders, by Irene Chatoor [17]. Chatoor's developmental classification of early eating disorders identifies three main developmental areas of food patterns in early infancy: homeostasis, attachment and separation, where it is possible to identify both child's and caregiver's adaptive or ill-adaptive behaviors. The purpose of this scale is to identify child's and mother's adaptive and dysfunctional behaviors, in the mutual interaction during meals, from the first month to three years. It is composed of 46 behavioral items: 26 observed in the mother and 20 in the child. The original scale can distinguish three fundamental types of early feeding pathologies in early infancy: eating disorder of the homeostasis, of the attachment and of the separation (infant anorexia) [18]. The Feeding Scales are applied to video-recorded observations of about twenty minutes of mother-child interaction during feeding. Observation may be carried out at home or in an ad-hoc laboratory.

The American version of this scale gave positive results with regards to its predictive, discriminating and meaning value, as well as to inter-observers and test-retest reliability.

Factor analysis related to the meaning value gave solution to five factors that constitute the five sub-scales of the overall evaluation scale. Identified factors: dyadic reciprocity, dyadic conflict, use of dialogue and elements of distraction during meals, fight for control and maternal non contingency.

Table 1 reports some examples about the dyadic reciprocities, dyadic conflict and maternal non-contingency sub-scale, as per the overall Feeding Scale.

Table 1. Assessment scale of the mother-child interactive behaviors during feeding

Dyadic Reciprocity

Mother	*Never*	*Rarely*	*Often*	*Very often*	*Score*
She positions her child for mutual exchange					
She speaks with her child					
She makes positive comments on her child					
Child					
He/she looks at the mother					
He/her smiles at the mother					
He/she looks happy					

Dyadic conflict

Mother	***Never***	***Rarely***	***Often***	***Very often***	***Score***
She makes negative comments on the way her child takes food					
She feels uncomfortable					
She expresses anger					
Child					
He/she refuses food					
He/she cries when food is offered to him/her					
He/she moves or throws food away					

Maternal non-contingency

Mother	***Never***	***Rarely***	***Often***	***Very often***	***Score***
She manipulates her child excessively					
She does not notice her child's signs					
She interrupts the meal, causing discomfort in the child					
Child					
He/she cries when food or the feeding-bottle is moved away					
He/she vomits or ruminates					

For every item, the observer writes the frequency and/or the intensity with which mother and child follow the listed behaviors. Each item is assigned a score. Each sub-scale gives us three scores: one related to the mother, one to the child and one to the couple. The latter is compared with the standard values of the tool, hence determining the deviation degree from the standard.

The homeostasis eating disorder, arising between the birth and the third month of life, is characterized by a non-regular state of the child during meals. He/she is irritable, gets easily tired and sleepy. The mother-child couple receives a lower score in the sub-scales measuring the dyadic reciprocity and the maternal non-contingency; anxiety, depression, psychiatric disorders or stress-psychosocial factors may lead the mother to be unable to understand her baby's signs and prevent her from facilitating a stable and regular feeding pattern.

In the attachment eating disorder, arising between the third and eighth month of life, we can observe that mother and child are not mutually involved and cannot find pleasure in their relationship during this phase when social exchanges should consolidate the attachment bond. The mother-child couple shows low scores in the dyadic reciprocity and higher scores in the maternal non-contingency. Mother's acute or chronic depression, personality disorders, drug or alcohol abuse and/or high psychosocial stress lie at the base of a dysfunctional pattern in the relationship between child and caregiver.

Finally, in the separation eating disorder, or infant anorexia, arising between the sixth month and third year of life, the mother-child couple show higher scores than in the previous cases in the dyadic conflict sub-scale. This shows an intense conflict in the relationship with regards to the dependency, the control and the autonomy. Interactive exchanges show the emotional fight for control, where the child clearly opposes accepting food from his/her mother, and the caregiver is unable to mediate the negative and hostile aspects arising during the feeding interaction. The caregiver's relational history, the child's behavior characteristics, the problems in appropriately recognizing the hunger/satiety signs, may be at the base root of the difficulties in establishing autonomy and regularity in the feeding pattern [17,18].

As in the first years of life, the regulation between caregiver and child develops above all within the caretaking; the analysis of the feeding interactive dynamics through a codified system of behaviors, can be extremely useful. It can contribute to the diagnostic assessment process, incrementing data obtained from the anamnesis and the parents' reports on the relationship with their children and helping to early identify specific dysfunctional patterns in the couple relationship models.

The study of the child-caregiver relationship during the early eating regulation disorder allows observers to recognize interactive dysfunctional patterns in the organization of the emotional-affective regulation and attachment systems during the early developmental phases (homeostasis and attachment eating disorders); later in the years, we can identify developmental conflicts related to the child's separation-individuation and autonomy processes (separation-individuation eating disorder or infant anorexia) [17-19].

In these last few decades, infantile psychoanalysis has given great consideration to a psychodynamic and developmental model, where mother-child interactions and communication are assumed great value. Particularly the attachment theory, proposed by Bowlby [3], allowed researchers to draw attention on the primary relation as a psychobiological *primum movens* aimed at finding protection and reassurance. According to Bowlby, when the child is hungry, tired, cold, sick or suffers for any reason, the attachment behavior is initiated, as a primary cause, with the aim of obtaining the mother's reassuring closeness and getting in physical contact with her to re-establish an affective balance. Therefore, the eating behavior is a fundamental part in developing the attachment behavior, consolidated by two meaningful variables: the caregiver's sensitivity in responding to the child's signs and the nature of the interaction between the caregiver and the child [20]. Inner functioning models develop during the first years of life; they are inner representations of the experienced attachment relations. If the mother has an insecure attachment history, the attachment behavior to her child is likely to be hostile, and she may transfer over to her child insecure attachment patterns, which may show in the specific feeding context.

5. Aetiopathology

At first, the attention was focused on anorexic mothers. Though they are often described as authoritarian, manipulative and invasive, they do not show a precise psychopathologic profile. On the contrary, for all of them, the feeding relation seems to be the main interaction axis, hiding behind the need to feed, a real distress for not being a good mother, fear of being abandoned or abandonment or fear of death. For newborns, food refusal has been interpreted in several different ways, according to the genetic developmental stages. Anorexia may represent the attempt to avoid the filling phase, considered potentially dangerous. Spitz [21] observed that moving the head away from the feeding-bottle or from the breast to signal satiety, represented the prototype of the semantic sign "no," and that, from this perspective, anorexia was a firm refusal behavior in the mother-child relationship that, later on, may prevent access to a more mental symbolization. In the same scenario, the anorexic infants seem to frequently show excessive familiarity towards strangers, in a phase when normally the anxiety for the unknown is most present. Such familiarity would show the inability to identify the mother's face, while focusing the anxiety on strangers' face. Theories on infant anorexia psychopathology are various and have changed during the course of time. Traditionally, a child's feeding dynamics were analysed according to the psychoanalytic framework of the "drive model." According to this theory, personality and behaviors—including feeding—are linked to the impulse intensity and to the appropriateness of the external environment answers [22-24]. Following this theory, oral impulses organize the feeding behaviors during childhood, whether they, as Freud says, are impulses located between the biological and the psychological sphere, or, as Klein says, they are psychic representations of impulses in the form of unconscious fantasies. Potential conflicts at the oral level may develop obsessions and regressions triggered by satisfaction impulse models. Greed, repeatedly unsatisfied requests, resentment, envy, or dependency may play a key role in the development of infantile neurosis, whose consequences with regards to feeding are unusual hunger senses, inhibitions in eating, and refusal to bite, to chew or to swallow food [24]. The above "drive model" has been gradually replaced by the "object relationships model." According to this model, personality and behaviors are structured through the relationship between "me" and the objects of the surrounding environment [25]. The relationship with the objects does not only depend on unavoidable libidinal needs, but also on the "real" adult world and on everyday interactive situations (such as meal time) that significantly influence the precocious developmental stages. The shift from the "impulse" to the "relational" model initiated new theoretical trends in the clinical and developmental field

[3, 25], taking into account the early mother-child relationship during feeding. Starting from the 60s, the mother and child interaction has taken momentum, and studies have been carried out on the basis of direct and systematic observations, rather than only in the light of theoretical models built through analytical history and adult retrospective assessments. This triggered a number of studies called Infant Research, which "has deeply modified the infant and child image during the first years of life." [26].

The attachment theory provided fundamental guidelines for research and treatment. The mother-child attachment relationship has been considered a fundamental experience, especially because the child, participating in repeating relational exchanges, builds mental representations of himself/herself and of the others. The pioneering work lead by Ainsworth and his collaborators [20] identified various attachment models, thanks to the standardized paradigm of the Strange Situation: children are exposed to a lightly stressful situation, in a non-familiar environment, while the mother goes away for a short time. Three main attachment models have been identified in children: confident (B), avoiding (A) and resistant (C) and linked to two main care-giving systems that have been defined as sensitive and insensitive.

A sensitive caregiver is able to answer the child's needs and to communicate adequately with her own son/daughter on an emotional level. The concept of "maternal responsiveness" has therefore been formulated, expressing the emotional availability and the ability to understand and to answer the child's emotional, cognitive and behavioral signs and needs. In synthesis, a "sensitive" parent is the one who establishes a good relationship during feeding (nurturant), is attentive to the child's needs, non-controlling, tolerates a certain degree of crisis and interactive desynchrony that can be renegotiated and recovered with renewed confidence feelings, effectiveness and competence.

On the other hand, an insensitive care-giving situation is when affections and emotions cannot find a common and shared space for the child and the parent; the caregiver is insensitive to her/his child's mental and emotional states. The affective exchange with the child is inconsistent and lacks reciprocity, preventing the baby from understanding his/her own developing emotional state [15]. In this affective interaction, participants are blocked inside negative and non-coordinated relational patterns: the messages sent by the parent and by the child are not read, understood and decoded within the relationship. A scenario of insensitive and unforeseeable caretaking can be disorganizing for the child's mental and affective state. He/she, in turn, may develop inadequate relational strategies and insecure attachment mental models to his/her own caregiver. Further studies have shown how, with a sensitive parent who is able to answer promptly and adequately his/her child's needs and requests, the baby develops a model of secure attachment (B). He/she elaborates a "primary" behavioral strategy that allows to him/her to look for protection and care and to establish closeness and contact when he/she needs them [20]. At the same time, the child develops an inner functioning model according to which the parent is perceived and considered as an available and loving figure, and he/she perceives himself/herself as able to ask for help and care. The child is confident that his/her mother will be available and sensitive when the child is frightened or in danger. An insensitive parent, instead, who shows a refusal attitude, has an unforeseeable and inconsistent behavior in answering the child's needs, and/or triggers an insecure attachment model in her/his own child (avoiding/A or resistant/C). Particularly, children who do not show any discomfort during separations, do not search for contact with the caregivers and move their attention away from them, are defined I nsecure-avoiding; children who show jointly and look for closeness but refuse contact are defined insecure-resistant.

More recently, groups of children with inconsistent and conflicting behaviors of attachment have been identified. Such behaviors are shown in the presence of seriously insensitive mothers. They develop atypical attachment models (disorganized/disoriented/D, avoiding/ambivalent/A/C, unstable/avoiding/U/A) [27]. Their behavior is highly contradictory, badly directed and incomplete, due to a collapse of the adaptation strategies; they are not able to organize and plan consistent behaviors to ask their caretaking figures for protection and care. The atypical attachment models are more often associated with a maternal psychiatric pathology, unresolved losses and/or traumas in the parents' histories, and/or serious familiar stressor in abuse and violence situations [28].

In this perspective, some authors have considered verifying empirically if there is a relation among the child's attachment models, the caregiver and precocious anorexia. Various researches have highlighted that, in the event of infant anorexia, both the mother and the child are classifiable in the following "unsecure" attachment categories: avoiding/A, resistant/C or disorganized-disoriented/D in the children; outdistancing/D or worried-involved/E in the mothers. Moreover, if infant anorexia is developed, unsecure attachment can increase problems and lay the foundations for chronic malnutrition. Particularly, children with a moderate to serious non-organic failure to thrive syndrome tend to have more often atypical attachment models (disorganized-disoriented/D, avoiding-resistant/A-C) in association with various types of psychosocial environmental stress (poverty, maternal psychiatric pathology, ill-treatment and abuse, conflict and unstable familiar contexts) [29].

. Results tell us that in order to understand and study infant eating disorders, it is necessary to examine the complicated interlacement among the child, the mother, their relationship characteristics and the developmental tasks that both must face during the process of separation-identification, autonomy. The most recent theoretical and clinical contributions on precocious anorexia present a "multifactor etiological model" according to which various elements can concur to the rising of this illness: the child's regulation difficulties and specific behavior peculiarities (difficult regulation of the state, scarce appetite, negativism, opposition, dependency), the presence of maternal psychopathology (anxiety, depression, eating disorders), caregiver's unsecure attachment style, psychosocial stress [5, 18, 19, 29].

6. Therapeutic Approach

Traditionally, difficulties in the child's growth, when not due to organic factors and relevant food refusal, are considered results of maternal refusal, abandonment or negligence. However, for many years now, studies and the observation of children tell us we should have a more balanced view and focus our attention on the mother-child couple; on the child's side, the interaction is characterized by his/her skills to adapt and adjust himself/herself to the maternal behaviors; on the mother's side, she must be able to correctly understand her child's behaviors, and anticipate his/her needs.

Table 2. Feeding rules applicable to the infants

Follow regular meal; only one extra is admitted
Meals should not last more than 30 minutes
No extras between meals, except natural water
Food should not be given to the child as a reward or positive reinforcement
Always give solid food before liquids
Encourage as much as possible self-feeding
Portions must be small or not excessive
After 10 to 15 minutes, if the child does not eat, remove the food
During the meal, the situation must be the most neutral possible, without any kind of constrictions and/or forcing

Table edited and adapted: Anne-Claude, Bernard-Bonnin: *Feeding problems of infants and toddlers.* Canadian Family Physician - Le Médecin de famille canadien, Vol 52: October, Octobre 2006.

Many approaches are multidisciplinary and encompass nutrition, education and control, observation of the child-caregiver interaction and a survey of the behavior answers of the two figures [30]. In this study, we have seen how important the family doctor's contribution in identifying the child's early problems and giving practical advice to the parents regarding the feeding rules where necessary. Parents should know basic feeding rules that can be adopted with every child, in order to educate him/her to an inner regulation. This will allow the child to learn how to eat according to his/her own physiological hunger and satiety signs. Moreover, this approach focuses the attention on helping the parents to understand their children's behavior in order to facilitate a more serene and structured interaction.

Another study [31] assessed the impact of a training behavioral program for parents, based on the mother-child interaction during feeding at home. The study showed that trained mothers increased their attention level towards their children and, in turn, children increased their acceptance of food that was usually refused and their ability to eat on their own; this demonstrated the functional impact of a specific home training for the parents. Moreover, this study highlighted the importance of systematically assessing the environment during feeding, and it represents an important step in increasing our understandings and possible improvements in the eating disorder treatments.

Other approaches of a psychodynamic nature are based on a model that takes into account at the same time the direct mother-child observation and the subtended intra-psychical phantasmatic network that organizes and gives meaning to this interaction. This unavoidably includes the feeding, which represents one of the first moments of nourishing and affective exchange between the mother and the child. The observer should take into account that in the mother-child interaction, other "children" come into the picture (the real, phantasmatic, imaginary child) who can facilitate or hinder the adaptation between the mother and the child. The phantasmatic child corresponds to the child in the mother's desire—a result of the mother's libidinal and narcissistic conflicts—this child is linked to the maternal Oedipal conflict. The imaginary child is the desired baby linked to the parents couple, to the mother's and father's phantasmatic life; the real child is the one who interacts with his/her background and tries to resonate with the maternal phantasmatic; the resonance can fulfil desires or, on the other hand, confirm some maternal phantasmatic fears [32]. The child's behaviors will acquire a supposed meaning for the mother, who will answer with precise behaviors that, in turn, will structure the child's behavior.

7. Conclusion

Infant anorexia is not always adequately recognized by the parents or the pediatrician, and cannot be effectively treated from a psychological or psycho-educative point of view, especially when it does not cause any serious developmental retardation.

Its psychodiagnostic profile calls for specific observation that is different from that used in adolescents, and its nosographic characteristics are still being studied. Although this can be the basis of disorders that will develop more clearly in the future, it remains close to its psychological matrix (with more difficulty in adolescent and adult therapy): the emotional and affective relation with the maternal figure, as a source of nourishment, and with the paternal figure, as a regulating and containing element of the primary relation with the mother. Therefore, psycho-educational actions, as well as more psychotherapeutic ones, include the family involvement, where the child is totally placed during his/her infant period.

There are still not many studies about treatment outcomes, but the existing ones indicate the positive impact of the relatives' direct participation to both cognitive-behavioral and psychodynamic treatments.

References

[1] Ramsay, M. Feeding disorder and failure to thrive. *Child Adolesc Psychiatr Clin N Am,* 1995, 4, 605-616.

[2] Winnicott, D. W. L'osservazione dei bambini piccoli in una situazione prefissata. In: Dalla pediatria alla psicoanalisi. Original Title: The observation of infants in a set situation, *Int. J. Psycho-Anal.*, XXII, 1941. It. Transl. Firenze: Martinelli, 1975, pp. 66-87.

[3] Bowlby, J. Attaccamento e perdita. Vol. 1; L'attaccamento alla madre. Original title: *Attachement and loss:* Vol. I Attachement, New York, Basic Books, 1969. It. Transl. Torino: Bollati Boringhieri, 1972.

[4] Klein, M. Sull'osservazione del comportamento dei bambini nel primo anno di vita. In: *Scritti 1921-1958.* Original title: Development in Psychoanalysis, London, Hogarth Press. It. Transl. Torino: Bollati Boringhieri, 1978, pp. 494-525.

[5] Kreisler, L. Conduites alimentaires déviantes du bébé: A. L'anorexie mentale; B. La rumination ou mérycisme; C. Les vomissements psychogénes. In: Lebovici, S; Diatkine, R; Soulé, M; Editors. *Nouveau traitéde psychiatrie de l'enfant et de l'adolescent.* Paris: P.U.F., 1995.

[6] Rutter, M. Classification And Categorization in Child Psychiatry. *J Child Psychol Psychiatry,* 1965, 6, 71-83.

[7] Freud, A. Normalità e patologia nell'età infantile. Original title: *Normality and Pathology in Childhood.* New York, International University Press, 1965. It. Transl. Torino: Bollati Boringhieri, 1979.

[8] Zero to Three, *Diagnostic Classification of Mental Health and Developmental Disorders of Infancy and Early Childhood:* Revised Edition (DC: 0-3 R), Washington, DC: Zero To Three Press, 2005. (Original in University of Michigan, digitalized 08/28/2007).

[9] Ammaniti, M. Maternal representations during pregnancy and early infant-mother interaction. *Infant Mental Health Journal,* 1991, 3, 246-255.

[10] Greenspan, SI & Wieder, S. The assessment and diagnosis of infant disorders: Developmental level, individual differences and relationship-based interaction. In: Osofsky, JD; Fitzgerald, HE; Editors. *WAIMH Handbook of Infant Mental Early Intervention, Evaluation and Assessment.* New York: John Wiley & Sons. 2000, 203-237.

[11] Sameroff, AJ & Emde, RN. I disturbi delle relazioni nella prima infanzia. Original title: *Relationships Disturbances in Early Childhood.* A Developmental Approach, New York, Basic Books, 1989. It. Transl. Torino: Bollati Boringhieri, 1991.

[12] Stern, DN. Il mondo interpersonale del bambino. Original title: *The interpersonal world of the child.* New York, Basic Books, 1985. It. Transl. Torino: Bollati Boringhieri, 1987.

[13] Stern, DN. La costellazione materna. Il trattamento psicoterapeutico della coppia madre bambino. Original title: *The Motherhood Constellation. A unified view of parent-infant psychotherapy,* London, Karnac Books, 1995. It. Transl. Torino: Bollati Boringhieri.

[14] Beetherton, I. Modelli operativi interni e trasmissione intergenerazionale dei modelli di attaccamento. In: Ammaniti, M; Stern, DN (editors). *Attaccamento e psicoanalisi,* Bari: Laterza, 1992, 21-46.

[15] Fonagy, P; Moran, GS; Steele, M; Steele, H. L'integrazione della teoria psicoanalitica e del lavoro sull'attaccamento: la prospettiva intergenerazionale. In: Ammaniti, M; Stern, DN; Editors. *Attaccamento e psicoanalisi,* Bari: Laterza, 1992, 61-84.

[16] Main, M; Kaplan, K; Cassidy, J. La sicurezza nella prima infanzia, nella seconda infanzia e nell'età adulta: il livello rappresentazionale. Original title: Security in Infancy, Childhood and Adulthood: A move to the Level of Representation, in: I. Brettherton E. Waters (Eds.), Growing Points of Attachment Theory and Research, Monographs of the Society for Research in Child Development, 50, 1985, 66-104. It. Transl. Riva Crugnola, C. (Ed.): *Lo sviluppo affettivo del bambino.* Milano: Raffaello Cortina Editore, 1993, 109-152.

[17] Chatoor, I; Loeffler, C; McGee, M; Menvielle, E (Editors). *Observational Scale for Mother-Infant Interaction During Feeding.* Manual, 2nd edition. Washington DC: Children's National Medical Center, 1988.

[18] Chatoor I., Ganiban J., Colin V., Plummer N., Harmony R. J. (1998). Attachment and feeding problems: a reexamination of non-organic failure to thrive and attachment insecurity. *Journal of the American Academy of Child and Adolescent Psychiatry,* 37, [1217-1224].

[19] Chatoor, I. Infantile Anorexia Nervosa: A developmental disorder of separation and individuation. *J Am Acad Psychoanal,* 1989, 17, 43-64.

[20] Ainsworth, M.D.S., Blehar, M.C., Waters E., Wall S. *Patterns of Attachment: A Psychological Study of the Strange Situation.* Hillsdale, N. J.: Lawrence Erlbaum Associates, New York Distributed by Halsted Press Division of Wiley, 1978.

[21] Spitz, RA. Il primo anno di vita del bambino. Original title: *Genese des premieres relations obiectales in Revue Francaise de psychoanalyse,* 4, 1954. It. Transl. Roma: Armando, 1965.

[22] Abraham, K. Ricerche sul primissimo stadio pregenitale della libido. In: Opere, Vol. 1. Original title: Untersuchungen über die frühesten praegenitalen Entwicklungsstufen der Libido, in *Int. Z. Psychoanal.,* 4, 71, 1916. It. Transl. Torino: Bollati Boringhieri, 1975.

[23] Freud, S. Tre saggi sulla teoria sessuale: Opere, Vol. 4. Original title: *Drei Abhandlungen zur Sexualtheorie,* Leipzig-Wien, Franz Deuticke, 1905. It. Transl. Torino: Bollati Boringhieri, 1970.

[24] Klein, M. Invidia e Gratitudine. Original title: *Envy and Gratitude,* London-New York, Tavistock-Basic Books, 1957. It. Transl. Firenze: Martinelli, 1969.

[25] Winnicott, DW. Dalla Pediatria alla Psicoanalisi. Scritti scelti. Original title: Collected Papers (1931-1956). T*hrough Pediatrics to Psycho-Analysis,* New York, Basic Books, 1958. It. Transl. Firenze: Martinelli, 1975.

[26] Ammaniti, M. *Manuale di Psicopatologia dell'infanzia.* Milano: Raffaello Cortina, 2001.

[27] Main, M. *Procedure for identifying infants as disorganized/disoriented during the Ainsworth Strange Situation.* Chicago: University of Chicago Press, 1990.

[28] Lyons-Ruth, K. Attachment relationships among children with aggressive behavior problems: The role of disorganized early attachment patterns. *J Consult Clin Psychol,* 1996, 64, 64-73.

[29] Chatoor, I; Ganiban, J; Hirsh, R; Borman-Spurrell, E; Mrazek, DA. Maternal characteristics and toddler temperament in infantile anorexia. *J Am Acad Child Adolesc Psychiatry,* 2000, 39, 743-751.

[30] Anne-Claude, Bernard-Bonnin. Feeding problems of infants and toddlers. *Canadian Family Physician - Le Médecin de famille canadien,* 2006, 52 (10), 1247-1251.

[31] Werle, MA; Tria, B; Murphy and Karen S. Budd, Treating chronic food refusal in young children: home-based parent training. *J Appl Behav Anal,* 1993, 26 (4), 421-433.

[32] Lebovici, S. Il neonato, la madre e lo psicoanalista. Le interazioni precoci. Original title: *Le nourrisson, la mère et le psychanalyste.* Paris, Le Centurion, 1983. It. Transl. Roma: Borla, 1988.

In: Anorexia Nervosa: A Multi-Disciplinary Approach ISBN: 978-1-60876-200-2
Editors: A. Mancini, S. Daini, L. Caruana, pp. 115-134

Chapter 7

ANOREXIA AND PARENTS

S. Daini and C. Panetta

Institute of Psychiatry, Catholic University of the Sacred Heart, Rome, Italy.

ABSTRACT

Making reference to the numerous studies that demonstrate the importance of family regarding the etiopathogenesis and in the treatment of eating disorders, this chapter deals with, in the first part, a panorama of the psychoeducational treatments focusing on those relevant in helping the family of anorexic patients; while in the second part, it describes the experiences in the Day Hospital of the Psychiatry Institute of Agostino Gemelli Hospital located in Rome, Italy, related to the realization of a psychoeducationl project geared to the family of patients with severe psychological disturbances. The project had two aims: the first being to supply useful information to anticipate and, above all, to effectively manage acute crisis as well as to build a holding environment able to represent a valid emotional support for the families of patients admitted to Day Hospital.

The project consisted of a limited number of meetings involving a precise quantity of family members and took into consideration families of patients with various psychopathologic profiles concurrently undergoing treatment; among which, parents of anorexic patients, allowing a profitable comparison among different situations and stimulating a reasonable separation from the emotional events and, thus, consenting family members to provide more effective help and to contain the regression of the patient.

Encounters with the family members had the following objectives: providing the correct information regarding the genetic transmission of the psychological illness; the correct "management" for moments of crisis: which behaviors to adopt and which not; the importance of family for anorexic patients during moments of psychological crisis; the correct relationship between family members and the treating medical team during patient's hospital stay and return to home; with regards to medication : in which cases the patient can autonomously manage their own pharmacology therapies and in which cases it is not opportune.

From the point of view of psychodynamics, this study shows how psychoeducation, offering information about the psychopathology and simultaneously offering moral support to the family members in situations where the patient takes care of herself, can positively influence the psychological state of the patient.

1. Introduction: Psychiatric Family History and Genetics Studies

When one talks about anorexia, talking about family begins as early on as discussing the role of family history in the pathogenesis of the illness. In previous years, studies on family history of eating disorders have tried to better understand the role of the genetic factors and of the non-genetic family-related factors of anorexia pathogenesis and of bulimia nervosa [1].

The studies on the psychiatric family history are based essentially on two techniques: one focuses on the technique of inquiring about the family history (family history method) and the other regards a direct study of the family (family-study method). Both approaches have advantages and disadvantages. The first method is the simplest and is based on the gathering of family information through a patient interview and, if necessary, an interview of another family member; while the second method entails carrying out an interview directly with the immediate family members in order to evaluate the existence of any other psychological pathologies. Obviously, the last technique results in being more reliable and precise, even if it is more "expensive" [2]. It was shown, in fact, how both of these types of factors linked to the family are of considerable importance [3]. A high number of affective disorders, substance abuse, and eating disorders were observed in the families of patients with eating disorders. An interesting observation is that in patients with eating disorders, it is more commonly seen a co-morbidity for affective disturbances present in a family member with a medical history positive for affective disturbances [4,5]. Subsequent to these observations, scientific literature explored the possibility that anorexia nervosa could represented a "variant" of depressive disorders and that, therefore, anorexia and affective disorders shared a common etiology [6]. Other studies analyzed the differences within the various subgroups pertaining to eating disorders. Strober [7] observed, for example, a greater frequency of obesity, affective disturbances and substance abuse within the family circle of patients with anorexia nervosa binge/purging type with respect to the families of restrictive anorexia patients. Similar results were verified when comparing patients with bulimia nervosa and patients with restrictive anorexia [8], while Laessle & Coll. [9] pointed out that the patients that have a higher psychiatric percentage within their families are those with anorexia binge/purging type as compared with patients affected by restrictive type anorexia or by bulimia nervosa. Other studies, nevertheless, did not find differences amongst the various subgroups. [10,11]. The genetic studies do not seem to indicate the presence of a common diathesis between eating disorders and affective disturbances [3,12], nor between eating disorders and substance abuse [3,13]. Lilenfeld & Coll. [14], in a study using the family-study method, evaluated the aggregation of psychiatric disturbances in families with anorexic bulimic patients and in healthy families, as controls. In the families of patients with eating disorders, an increased risk for eating disorders was seen under threshold levels and greater depressive and obsessive-compulsive disturbances with respect to the families of the control group. The authors conclude affirming that it is possible that there is a common vulnerability for anorexia nervosa and bulimia nervosa.

These studies seem to indicate an important family component regarding the onset of anorexia nervosa. Few studies, nevertheless, have tried to understand how much this family component is of an environmental or genetic origin. Holland & Coll. [15], in one of the first studies carried out on twins, had verified a significantly greater number monozygotic twins concordant of diagnosis with respect to dizygotes, with an estimate of heritability of approximately 80%. However, this study is limited by the fact it was carried out on subjects who had requested treatment. Since a family case history positive for anorexia nervosa results more likely in a request for help, the data of this study could overestimate the familial aggregation of this pathology.

In a recent study carried out on twins in Sweden [16], heritability of anorexia (additive genetic effects) was estimated at approximately 0.56, with a residual variance attributable to environmental factors. In the same study, the neuroticism (prospectively assessed neuroticism) was associated with the successive development of anorexia, which, therefore, is a predictive factor.

An analogous study made in Norway [17] on monozygotic twins and dizygotic twins, estimated an inferior contribution of heritability for anorexic syndrome (overall, heritability 0.22), while different symptoms of the disturbance have had a different heritability; they are greater for the symptoms correlated to weight loss and less correlated to the worry for bodily weight.

In any case, a genetic component constitutes a risk factor for the development of this eating disorder.

2. The Role of the Family in the Genesis of Anorexia Nevosa

Scientific literature has been interested in various aspects concerning the families of patients with anorexia nervosa: what is the family's role in the etiopathogenesis of the disorder, what demographic characteristics can influence the onset of this disorder, and finally which variables linked to family can influence the prognosis and the response to the treatment of the disorder in question. Many studies have highlighted the familial factors that intervene in the etiopathogenesis of anorexia nervosa, underlining the role of the family in the development of this pathology (Gull, [18]).

Authors having different theoretical viewpoints have described the possible role of family members [19-23], however, the studies of family characteristics of patients with anorexia nervosa is not easy to compare because of the different methodologies used and of the large variability of the social-cultural and demographic feature of the subjects studied. The evaluation of the patient and of his/her families, at the moment of their request for help, is strongly influenced from the "crisis" situation, secondary to the illness, that brought the patient and his/her family to ask for treatment, as well as from how close the patient is to his/her family. Dependency problems, the drive towards autonomy, to gain a stable and secure identity, constitute important elements that rotate around individuation-separation and can weigh heavily on the course of the illness. For these motives, the patient's attitude and that of his/her family towards the evaluation of the problems, can vary according to the phase of the treatment: generally, in the acute phase, anorexic patients tend to deny any problem. The desire to be liked and for approval of the family manifests throughout the course of the treatment, with an attitude of hypercompliance towards the therapists, which makes it more difficult to have an authentic understanding of the familial problems. Conflicting families or negative familial atmospheres, instead, are often described in anorexic –bulimic patients and in bulimic patients [23].

Minuchin & Coll. [21] identified some characteristics of familial interaction that seem specific of the families in which there are people affected from anorexia nervosa; for example, being overprotective, instability of individual boundaries, and the rigidity and the insufficient ability to resolve conflicts. In Italy, Mara Palazzoli-Selvini [22] widespread the systemic model and fundamentally sustains that the anorexic patient constitutes the "homeostasis" and stability factor of the familial system. Beyond the theories and family therapies, for most of the therapists, it is often evident that anorexia nervosa represents the patient's difficulty to reach his/her own autonomy, independence and individuality. These themes are very common during adolescence, which, in fact, constitutes the moment of greatest individual and familial vulnerability.

The demographic characteristics of the families in which an anorexia nervosa cases are present were objects of interest for many scholars and include different aspects like social class, order of geniture, age of the parents at patient's birth, and parental integrity. Many psychiatric disturbances show a greater predominance in the lower socioeconomic classes, but it is difficult to understand how much this is secondary to a "social" selection process or if it is, instead, caused by social factors.

A factor that, instead, seems significantly associated with a greater predominance of eating disorders is the degree of urbanization of the patient's residence. It seems, in fact, that in greater urbanized areas, there is a greater predominance of eating disorders and in particular, of bulimia nervosa [21,25]. The controlled studies of order of geniture, parents' ages and integrity of the familial unit of patients with anorexia nervosa are very few and often contradictory. Beginning from Hilde Bruch [19], some authors observed a more advanced age in the parents of patients with anorexia nervosa, but controlled studies denied this observation. Bruch later reported that patients with anorexia nervosa were more often first-born or last-born children, but this fact was also later denied from observations on larger sample sizes [26]. Finally, regarding the integrity of the familial unit, the few studies present in literature seem to point out similar or lower percentages, with respect to data on the general population, of families not integrated because of separation or death of the parents.

3. Family Factors that Influence the Prognosis and the Response to Treatment

A common data of observation that is extracted from the epidemiological studies on the general population and from those on clinical populations is that anorexic patients arrive at medical observation in a percentage much lower with respect to the severity of the disorder; and as is clearly evidenced by its manifestation, when these cases seek medical attention, the duration of illness is rather long. This fact can also depend upon the great difficulty that the parents encounter to convince their child of the necessity of a medical examination and treatment. In this perspective, the familial factors may be determining to anticipate or to delay the onset of treatment and influence, also in this way, the long-term result. In fact, it was noted that an early beginning of treatment reduces the risks of chronicization and facilitates the therapeutic approach. The possible negative influences of the family on the evolution of the disorder are at the base of a practice already very widespread in the first clinical descriptions of anorexia: that to separate the patient from his/her family, for therapeutic purposes, above all by hospitalization. Vandereycken and Pierloot [27], evaluating the response to treatment of an anorexic group of patients, observed that the rigid use of the rule of "parentectomy," that is to say, the total distancing of the patient from their family until the entire weight recovery, was able to have some advantages in the short-term, but had also numerous and serious collateral effects. One of the most important collateral effects was the drop-out, that is, the abandonment of treatment by the patient. This is one of the main reasons that the treatment proposed by Vandereycken then transformed into a therapy that involves the family and that takes into account the needs of the family as well [23]. Indication of an involvement of the family in the treatment comes also from some studies that have observed a worsening of the familial symptoms in parallel to the improvement of the anorexic patient's physical state. Crisp & Coll. [28], for example, had observed a significant increase of the psychoneurotic symptomathology in fathers as in mothers during the weight recovery of their child.

This increase concerned anxiety and phobic symptoms, in particular. It is interesting to note that the changes were more net as the relationship between spouses was poor, thus underlining what effect the illness of the child can have on the familial balance. The same study had then observed a significant connection between the result of the treatment and the initial symptomathology of the parents. Morgan and Russell [29], in their follow-up study, reported that the sole familiar factor that seemed to influence the prognosis was the problematic relationship between the patient and other family members before the onset of the eating disorder. Other factors, like the rivalry between sisters, the presence of psychiatric disturbances amongst family members, and/or the social class or anomalies of the familial structure did not seem to have any impact. In a study of North & Coll. [30], it was verified that a good result of two years from the beginning of treatment, in a sample of adolescent patients, anorexia nervosa is associated with a good initial family functioning. Moreover, the perception of the familial functioning provided by the patients corresponded substantially to the evaluation carried out by interviews of the families. In a long-term follow-up study carried out on adolescent patients with anorexia nervosa, Strober [7], investigating different family aspects—for example, the presence of familial psychiatric disturbances, familial relationships, social adaptation, encouragement towards autonomy, areas of conflict—verified that the familial variables were able to be considered predictive of long-term results. Particularly, the presence of hostile attitudes towards the family seemed to increase the slowness of remission and the risk of onset bulimia. The passage from anorexia to bulimia, factors that hinder or slow down the process of full recovery, also were significantly associated with a scarcity of empathy or parental affection towards their child.

Other methods already tested with other psychiatric pathologies and later on used also for the evaluation of familial problems in anorexia nervosa are the evaluation of emotional expression and the evaluation of the familial burden. The concept of expressed emotions was derived from research carried out on schizophrenia [31] that had observed how family attitudes and behaviors could significantly influence the rate of readmission (understood as the necessity of rehospitalization) of the schizophrenic patients. The measurement of expressed emotions, carried out in a specific interview—the Camberwell Family Interview (CFI)—includes five main scales: criticism (that is, the presence of critical comments towards the patient), hostility, emotional over-involvement, warm affection and positive comments. The studies carried out on patients with eating disorders, using the concept of expressed emotions, reported rates of criticism inferior with respect to the family members of schizophrenic patients [32,33]. Both of these studies observed significantly higher criticism rates in the families with bulimic patients with respect to those with anorexia nervosa patients. Bulimia is, in fact, often interpreted like scarcity of will and not like a pathological state, thus provoking hostility and criticism from the parents. Expressed emotion in the families with patients affected by anorexia nervosa is, however, significantly greater with respect to families of patients with cystic fibrosis and with families of control groups [34].

As with schizophrenia, some studies have tried to evaluate what role expressed emotion covered in the response to treatment of anorexia nervosa and the course of the illness. Szmukler & Coll. [32] had verified that in adolescent patients who undertook family therapy, the level of drop-out was significantly associated with the level of familial criticism. Familial criticism, on the contrary, seemed not to influence the patient drop-out that randomly continued with an individual treatment. Le Grange & Coll. [33] carried out an interesting study that, other than evaluating predictive effectiveness of expressed emotion variables in the response to the treatment of a group of adolescent patients (age <18 years) with anorexia nervosa, also evaluated the effect on expressed emotion of the parents of two different types of treatment: the family therapy or the psychoeducational approach (involvement of the parents in the treatment, but the parents are examined and seen by doctors separately). Even if the results are interpreted with some caution for the rather low numbers of the sample size, the study of Le Grange seems to indicate a greater effectiveness of the psychoeducational approach to decrease familial criticism. On the contrary, the family therapy seems to provoke an increase of criticism after 32 weeks of treatment, although the weight and the clinical state of the patients improve in the same manner in both groups. The patient improvement, as well, seems to be significantly correlated to the initial level of familial criticism and, in the group of patients with a scarce response to treatment, the criticism seems more elevated. This fact underlines the possible role of the familial factors in the maintenance of the symptomatology. The commentaries, in fact, can install a greater sense of uselessness and inability of patients who already have very low self-esteem and who turn to the caloric restriction like sole methods of self-realization and reassurance. The difficulty in achieving recovery and the scarcity of results from the therapy can, at times, increase the levels of criticism with the establishment of a dangerous vicious circle that only with a treatment involving parents can it be brought to an end [35].

Another study concerning the influence of expressed emotion in response to the treatment and as the result of a year's time was carried out by Van Furth & Coll [36]. Also, this study solely took into account patients with anorexia nervosa in the age of adolescence. The initial familial criticism of the patients was rather low and tended to improve after the treatment that included also, in all of the cases, some form of family consultation. Nevertheless, the authors verified that the variable best able to predict both the response to the treatment and result in a year's time was the presence of maternal commentaries.

The problems and the difficulty that fall on the family members of the patients affected from a severe pathology constitutes instead what comes defined as a family "burden" [37]. In the psychiatric field, it was defined as the presence of problems, difficulties or negative events that torment the life of one or more significant people for a psychiatric patient [38]. Initially, the study of the family burden was mainly addressed with regard to schizophrenic illness, but then interest spread to other chronic psychiatric and somatic pathologies, like depression, anxiety disorders, dementia, cerebral damage, diabetes and renal failure.

Hoenig and Hamilton [39] introduced a fundamental distinction between objective family burden, which concerns the objective problems consequent to the pathology of the patient (such as economical problems, limitations in the working capacity and in free time, social limitations and the side effect on the health of the family), and the subjective burden, which instead pertains to the subjective perception of the family members of the burden. In schizophrenia, the subjective burden resulted in being inferior to the objective burden, but the two components can manifest themselves and vary in an independent manner. Concerning eating disorders, the only studies that evaluate the family burden are studies conducted in Padua [1,40]. These studies used a self-rating scale, the Questionnaire for Family Problems, which includes two relevant subscales to the objective and subjective burden. The studies emphasized that the familiar load is greater in anorexia nervosa with respect to bulimia nervosa, and is especially high in families with anorexic patients pertaining to binge/purging subgroup. The subjective burden seems greater than the objective burden in both anorexia nervosa and bulimia. The second study compared the burden reported from the families with eating disorders with that reported from families of patients with severe schizophrenia (average duration of illness 10 years). The subjective and objective burden resulted significantly higher in schizophrenia than in those with eating disorders. Nevertheless, the subjective burden reported from the families of binging/purging anorexics is not statistically different from that reported from the families of schizophrenic patients. Another important datum of these studies is the correlation verified in anorexia, but not in bulimia, between severity of the attitudes, food disorder symptoms and the family burden. Finally, evaluating some patients' responses to the outpatient treatment, evidence emerged that the parents of the patients who had not improved differentiated themselves from the parents of the patients who had improved for some variables. Particularly, the mothers of the patients who had not improved reported, in the initial phase of evaluation, a subjective burden significantly greater with respect to the mothers of the patients who had answered positively to the treatment. The fathers of the patients who had not improved, instead did not differentiate themselves for the burden perceived, but for the presence, at the initial evaluation, of greater depressive symptoms and of somatization.

Typically, when one thinks of anorexia nervosa, adolescents come to mind; but it is not infrequent now to have to deal with adult patients because the disturbance has a certain percentage of chronicization and, therefore, continues into adult life and because some cases can have a late onset. Since some of these patients are married or live with their partners, it is logical to ask what would be the role of the disorder in relation to the couple and how the relationship is able to influence the course and the response to treatment of anorexia.

If a significant connection exists between these two aspects, it would be important, therefore, to involve the partner in the treatment. This topic received little attention in scientific literature [41]. Scientific literature agrees that a couple in which there is an affected subject from anorexia nervosa manifests a considerable level of dissatisfaction pertaining to the relationship. However, while the patients themselves consider the eating disorder the cause of their problems, therapists often think that it is the opposite: there was, in fact, often a presence of collusion, lack of intimacy, communication deficiencies and avoidance of conflicts between the two partners. These clinical observations on couples were, in part, confirmed from one controlled study [41] that pointed out a deficiency in the ability to open themselves to each other, a significant scarcity of intimacy and an inability of communication in couples with a partner experiencing eating disorders.

4. THE FAMILY AND THE CRISIS: INTERVENTION MODELS

The territorial services delegated in the care of those with psychological problems cannot ignore the importance of the patient's relationship with his/her family, recognized as a fundamental "resource" in every care project. Independently from the pathogenetic theory that the clinician follows, the experiences that the individual has within his/her family context are extremely important and constitute the base for the course of the illness and for its successive result. Particularly, during crisis periods, family support is sought by the patients, and its presence is conveniently directed to help in the therapeutic activity. On the contrary, the absence and, above all, conflict in the family context during a psychological crisis can lead not only to a radical misunderstanding but also to "anti-therapeutic" choices that can weigh on the patient in a more notable manner than in periods of good health, but also in a contained psychological discomfort.

A psychosomatic crisis in the course of anorexic disturbance, for example, can constitute a decisive moment during the course of psychopathological development, a line of cleavage between defense and constructive energies, being able, therefore, to herald a lot to a successive maturing, as to a further regression of the individual psychological organization.

The plasticity of the psychological organization can be considered, therefore, a characterizing element of crisis periods, as much as the fragmentation of the Ego that constitutes the most unfavorable event in a clinical setting.

The moment of crisis constitutes, however, an intense moment in one's identity and of his/her emotional dependencies. In this sense, the family, where present, is not only a helpful instrument, but also a guardian of the patient's "historical" identity,' as well as an elective speaker with regard to emotional relationships.

The multiplicity of the theoretical-clinical lines of thought in family studies and of the possible therapeutic intervention has given origin, in the last years, to attempts to build supplementary models, in which systemic aspects of the family relationships and that of the interpersonal dynamics are taken into account.

The therapeutic model that makes reference to the "cognitive-behavioral theory" is based on the premise that the specific central unit for eating disorders is characterized by a "dysfunctional evaluation form" based in an exclusive manner or predominating on the control of nutrition, of the bodily weight and form. The main objective of this type of theoretical approach is, therefore, to develop an evaluation of oneself less dependent on weight, bodily shape and on the control of nutrition interrupting the factors of cognitive maintenance (thoughts, convictions) and behavioral (iron diet, low weight, vomiting, laxatives, diuretics) of eating disorders. From the point of view of cognitive-behavior, it has been proposed as an operative concept, for possible support, and as cognitive support to the concept of illness that the patient has, in the moment of less clear and possibly more dysfunctional crisis. Therefore, family intervention is also directed to reduce the emotional resonance in the moment of crisis and to have a more rational conception of the events in course. Family therapy, in this type of approach, is directed to help the patient in meal planning and in mechanical nutrition and to reduce expressed emotions and improve familial communication.

The systemic–relational approach considers the bearer of a psychological disorder as one that undergoes the effects of an ambiguous and contradictory communication. In the family system, it is fundamental for the therapy not to focus on the "designated patient" but to expand the inquiry to the *whole family system*, so as to highlight the social and relational context in which the disorder developed and, therefore, take into consideration the resources originating from their environments.

In systemic family therapy, the individual is not, therefore, taken as an isolated element but is introduced in a context of relationships. The family system is seen as a whole, not as a conglomerate of individuals, and this allows elaboration of a new approach that is able to describe phenomena as interpersonal rather than personal. As for the definition of the family life cycle, it is presumed, in the evolution of the family system, an encounter with some "nodal events" that cross the disorganization-reorganization of the same system implicating to overcome some developmental tasks allowing for the entrance in a successive phase. A person's symptoms, other than expressing in metaphorical manner, the subjective psychological conflict acquire, therefore, a precise internal function of the relational system from which they emerged.

A symptom has, therefore, a double valence: it signals to the family the existence of a disorder, and at the same time, makes its destructive power innocuous, centralizing all the worries of the other family members on it.

The growth of a child or the aging process of a parent are only two examples of how change, during the course of time, can have an affect on family members and their relationships. Also the outside world, with its transformations and changes with respect to, for example, the cultural and religious values, to the political and economical climate, deeply influences the entire family system to any generational level: the family is a "multigenerational emotional system.".

The family, therefore, would have to respect two requirements: on one side, modifications according to the changes occurring in time (morphogenetic processes), and on the other, should preserve the actual sense of integrity and continuance in time (morphostatic processes). These orders of processes are absolutely interchangeable: if a family unit is capable of remaining stable in time, it also succeeds to face the changes of its family members and of the external surrounding reality. When an individual or a relationship shows manifestations of discomfort, it is most likely due to the so called internal "rigidity" of a family, characterized from a dysfunctional interactive and persisting model.

Family therapy intervenes across various work techniques on the families, operating on different levels of observation: three-generational history of the family (grandparents-parents-children); the family relational and communicative organization; the function of the individual's symptoms in the family equilibrium; the life-cycle phase of the family in which the symptom of the individual is presented. The techniques, by the utilization of tasks to be carried out in the therapeutic sessions as well as at home, revolve around problems concerning roles, hierarchy, alliances, and the quality of communication. In moments of crisis, family knowledge of its internal dynamics is fundamental, not only in reference to the pathological aspects, but also to be able to rebuild the processes of communication that have developed over time and that have given rise to the patient's problems. The integration with the family through the understanding and the search for collaboration allows the patient to have continuance course of treatment and continuous informative resources on the patient.

Family therapy based on the object relations theory is currently the most important example of psychodynamic family therapy. In 1960, working with married couples at the Tavistock Clinic, Henry Dicks [42] began to observe that some relatively healthy couples succeeded in their marriage at a primitive level of object relations. He observed that these couples tended to emotionally live with the spouse according to a symbolic unconscious meaning. What Dicks observed was a form of transfer: the spouses placed in action a relationship of the past. In terms of the object relations theory, the partner used this mechanism of split and of projective identification to render external, or conjugal, an internal conflict, in which an internal object representation, often a parent, became split and projected in the spouse. Likewise, different authors [43] spread to the entire family this understanding of couples' conflicts based on the theory of object relations. These authors noted that often the patient is the bearer or the container of the unacceptable parts split from the other family members. In this manner, the family balance is maintained from these divisions and of projective identification. The process of psychotherapy begins, therefore, with an attentive diagnosis of the manner in which the representations of the Ego and of the Object have been distributed in the family by means of the division and by projective identification. When this model becomes clear, the therapist seeks to explain how among the various family members an unconscious collusive system was formed, an act to perpetuate the pathological behavior of the anorexic patient. The primary objective of the family support of an anorexic patient from the psychodynamic point of view is, therefore, that of helping all the family members re-internalize the conflicts that were shown through projective identification.

The problem with individual identity results, nevertheless, in an important dynamic element also when observing the family. The crisis, however, deeply involves the concept of individual identity and patient autonomy with respect to their contexts. The common processes of identification with other family members (for example, the parents, but also the children) dramatically are taken into consideration in the moment of crisis, independently from the fact if it is manifested with a specific symptomatology (for example, depression).

Observation of the critical moment and particularly of the "borderline states," convey the recognition and importance of the family relationships, under the most developed aspects not shown in the crisis and as well those more regressive. In fact, at times the crisis is presented in the moment in which the fusional bonds are modified, for example, that between mother and daughter, before the onset of anorexia or the evolution of the bond is not allowed from primitive units present in the patient and in the closer family members. The risk of the critical situation is that it is maintained in a pathological manner, or restored by a serious limit to the patient's psychological evolution, to this type of bond. Therefore, a separate reflection, that is also an action of identification for the patient and for the patient's family members, appears to be an initial moment, able to allow for some less harmful regressions and to free the patients from the painful appearance of this type of bond. In these circumstances, the recovery of a partial identity, also in the difficulty of the moment, is developed in a "protected environment" from the presence of the therapists who share their thoughts with the patient and with the family members.

In view of psychodynamics, the patient's crisis is also the crisis of its family members, where however the refusal of the patient's designation emphasized from relational psychology should not allow that the anguish related with identification paralyzes the entire family, that arranges rationality and operating resources not available to the patient.

It has been noted that the necessity to offer support to the relatives during these situations, in order to develop knowledge and the ability to confront the situation, to produce, if necessary, changes to harmful lifestyles and to obtain a better quality of life not only for the patient, but for all of the family. Support intervention to family members is presented like a psychoeducational tool, with a limited number of meetings with the family beginning during the first moment of crisis. Support to the family members is aimed at observations and reflections together with the families, but not compelled in a rigid manner, proposing, therefore, a dynamic, cognitive and counseling aim.

To the cognitive-informative dimension, psychodynamics of identification and empathy are predominantly added, which therapist allow to receive and comprehend the patient's regression, without overwhelmed results and without family intervention using too rigid and prescribed encouragement or one that is efficient but excessively detached.

The presence of different situations of crisis represents a cue for a confrontation amongst family members, associated with the presence of a family member in crisis allowing other than support also a comparison between different situations able to stimulate a reasonable separation from the emotional events, allowing the family to give more effective help and to contain the regression of the patient.

The delicate balance between these two lines, identification and separation, seems to be an element of the patient's psychological processes and often of collaborative relationship with the therapist. The objective of family support interventions is to try to go along with an evolutionary change of the family relations from the initial moment in which the psychological difficulty is shown, pointing out that the crisis represents an opportunity and not only an acute expression of discomfort

5. The Psychoeducational Treatments

On the basis of the complex studies carried out by Libermann, Falloon and Coll. [44] regarding theories of familial systems, a familiar program was created, focusing on the changes of inadequate communication of needs, desires and feelings, aimed, from one side, to develop behavioral ability, and on the other, to improve the social ability of the patient. Such familial programs result in being a lot more effective than other programs centered solely on the patient's evolution process of social adaptation.

In more recent times, the research in this field is focalizing on the possibility of incorporating families in the treatment plan to more effectively assist the patients after hospital discharge. The reference theoretical model, named Diathesis-Stress, takes into consideration two elements etiologically responsible for the onset of schizophrenic episodes: the biological vulnerability, meaning the person's predisposition to psychological disorders (dithesis) and the environmental stressogeneous factors capable of generating expectations that the individual is not in a position to satisfy. Simultaneously, the theory is joined with an extremely pragmatic approach to the treatment, focalizing attention on the manner in which the family therapy can influence the treatment of the patient's psychotic symptoms and, above all, on how to activate "resistance phenomenon" to the reoccurrences due to stress.

The encounters with the family were centered on the identification of strategies to problem solving: the families had been assisted to identify the problem, to think about a solution, to evaluate the possible results and to choose what was to be the best strategy, to put it into action and, therefore, to report the results. The therapist, by the proposed model, wanted to make the family take on responsibility with respect to the problem solving, focusing the training on the ability of communication, encouraging an open and clear conversation, actively listening and asking precise questions allowing for a transparent expression of the positive and negative feelings. The objective of the intervention was, therefore, to channel the expression of emotions of all family members using the most constructive method.

The study conducted by Hogarty [45] constitutes an important contribution with regard to the area of research that is occupied in analyzing models of intervention that join family treatment, social skills training and pharmacological therapy that are of fundamental importance for the prevention of schizophrenia reoccurrences.

Some aspects of such programs are worth noting: the interventions of psychoeducation remarkably reduce the costs of management of a psychiatric patient; such programs, in fact, even if require a longer time with respect to traditional psychiatric interventions, decrease the number of hospitalizations by means of reducing reoccurrences. All types of families can find benefits from a psychoeducational intervention, increasing the development of coping strategies. Psychoeducational intervention is successful in concomitance with other interventions, such as pharmacological and psychotherapeutic, catered to the patient. The psychoeducational programs represent one of the rings of a more complete and integrated program of care.

6. The Psychoeducational Treatments in Anorexia

The psychoeducational interventions represent, to date, an approach of "good clinical practice" in the enormous majority of programs aimed at the treatment of severe mental disturbances, among which is anorexia. Since the presence of an eating disorder determines catastrophic effects on the family unit in terms of tension, increase in objective and subjective burden, true psychological suffering in one or more of the spouses involved, communicative and relational dysfunctions and, more in general, *burn-out* and isolation, a psychoeducational approach has shown to be able to guarantee the achievement of some objectives that result in being fundamental also for the patient:

1. to supply precise information on the eating disorders and to improve the level of knowledge of the family on the therapeutic resources available;
2. to learn techniques and abilities to improve *coping* with the disorder: the difficulty of the relational and communicative type that characterize the functioning of the "anorexic family" or of the " bulimic family"—beyond every casual interpretation — they concretely exist and must be confronted on a re-educational basis, as soon as possible;

3. offer reciprocal support in an effectively holding atmosphere and to make efforts to resolve problems;.
4. to facilitate an increase, on a social level, the awareness of the problem and a more effective availability of programs that are easily accessible for this disorder. For preventive functioning, such objectives are fundamental to guarantee an earlier access to diagnostic evaluation and rapid use of the multimodal and integrated programs that are the most valid answer for these disturbances.

Between the psychoeducational experiences conducted in Italy on eating disorders, the project of Favaro and Santonastaso [46] foresees a family approach as an integral part of a teamwork in which the family therapist collaborates and maintains contacts with the patient's therapist and with the other healthcare workers involved in the treatment. In the initial phase of case evaluation, the parents of the patients who coexist with the family should be dedicated at least one encounter separately with a psychiatrist or a psychologist that is specifically occupied with the family's problem. The purpose is to give the parents an occasion to talk about their own difficulties about their child's illness and to supply some information on symptoms and behavior. An in-depth examination of the patient's family history is necessary spanning from the tendency of denial of the symptoms to the underestimation of the problem by a great part of many anorexic patients. At times, the therapists supply information on adolescence problems, their present knowledge in the field of eating disorders and the possible treatments available. In the encounter with the family, it is not infrequent to observe that the parents arrive at the consultation not only in a state of comprehensible apprehension for the health of their child, but also tense and with a sense of guilt. Since the main objective of a psychoeducational approach is to seek for the collaboration of the family, in the first encounter, it is best to avoid discussions on anguishing conflicts, in order to establish a comprehensive and cooperative atmosphere, in which the parents feel they are taking part in the therapeutic program, reassured of the possibility to ask indications, alleviated from the feelings of guilt. Contact with the parents can exhaust itself in one or two encounters if special needs or relevant relationship problems are not individualized; other prospective meetings can be done later on, in relation to the evolution of treatment of the daughter. For families with few conflicts, in which the parents as a couple are integrated, they can participate in either individual or group psychoeducational meetings, where discussing the strategies and the behaviors to adopt in special situations that may be created in a family with an anorexic or bulimic patient [46]. In separated couples or in open conflict, the group meetings are unadvisable; while it can be useful meetings with the individual family unit to avoid, where possible, the involvement of the patient in the parental conflict and to help the parents to facilitate their daughter in becoming autonomous.

There exist other cases in which the approach to parents results in being remarkably difficult although there is an apparent scarcity of conflict: it is in those in which the anorexia, although the illness has achieved a considerable severity, is denied by the parents and likewise denied in the same manner from the patient. Situations of high risk may arrive to the observation of a doctor, after a long duration of illness [23]. The presence of like mechanisms inside a family structure can be considered one of the indications for hospitalization.

When working with a single family unit, with successive meetings, the quantity of general information is reduced and the familial problem is deepened in specifics.

The group of parents, besides supplying a psychological support linked to the fact of sharing like experiences, brings a considerable reinforcement to the proposals of change within a family unit: the successful achievement of implementing a strategy in one of the family units provides a practical example of the manner in which some changes can be truly verified. The meetings, in this model, occur on a monthly basis, and, therefore, do not have the purpose of investigating the causes of the disturbance, nor of discussion of the familial dynamics, nor of analyzing the latent conflicts, with the risk of intensifying them. The objective of the therapy is not the family nor the parental couple, but the illness of the daughter and all that can result difficult in her recovery. The formal procedure of psychoeducational intervention appears, therefore, to be flexible, marked by the concreteness of the problems discussed with the parents, to maintain a solid therapeutic alliance.

7. Our Project

In the rehabilitative point of view in which the intervention is placed, because of its dynamic inspiration, it is less prescriptive than in comparison to the cognitive-behavioral, and less orientated, in the descriptive sense of the pathology, but stimulates some reflections in the family members to motive the greater fluidity verified in the defense and in the untying of thought of the family members during crisis periods.

The premise is that the crisis constitutes for the patient, and indirectly for the family, a therapeutic window privileged to favor the changes in the rigid and extremely pathogenic defenses that are able to increase the risk of relapses and of chronicization of the weakest family members. The family members are also, therefore, in the moment of the crisis, less defensive and more motivated to the comprehension of the familial dysfunctional dynamics. It was not wanted to stop at informative or prescriptive interventions that can restrain the emotional changes rather than to favor it or to place the psychopathological event in a cognitive pre-established frame, whose scientific limits are difficult to comprehend by the family members.

This setting does not constitute for itself a psychotherapeutic intervention; for a short term in a temporal arc in which it is developed; it is able, however, to constitute a premise and provide the family intuitions on the familial dynamics otherwise difficult to attain in a psychological context that is more structured or marked by the repetition of the defensive attitudes.

Between the requirements that have been considered, it was of priority in this type of intervention, that of confronting the crisis in the first place where treatment is sought: the psychiatric service that welcomes the critical patient. In connection to this place and therefore to the spontaneous presentation of the request, the intervention is addressed to familial groups that are not unified from the same psychopathology of the less fortunate family member/patient, but that have in common present existence of a family member in crisis. Uniform groups of pathology, in fact, can find usefulness in non-critical moment, also for obvious organizational motives. The stimuli that were used were, therefore, of general character, not bound to a specific psychiatric pathology, leaving space to the expression of the emerging problems, in the family context, rather than to cover them, from the start, with a cognitive scheme constituted solely from information. The previous is, however, expected in the final moment of the course, other that on request by the family, at the moment of the psychiatrist intervention and subsequently to a diagnosis specification of each patient.

The rehabilitative approach, therefore, pertains to the early phases in which the psychopathology is presented as a crisis proposing to limit the devastating effects on the patient's psychology and on their personal and social functionality. These effects would have been present if the crisis were a moment in which thought is absent in the patient (with limits of the psychological state present) and in the family members. Not only do they confront the moment together with him, but constitute at times a place of thought that to the patient is denied but that is able to be immediately returned to after.

The central moment of the rehabilitation in this viewpoint is to make certain that the patient does not lose his/her personal abilities and features, as it often happens also in the course of correct interventions from the biological and psychosocial point of view, but begins the rehabilitative processes as soon as the symptomatology is presented.

The strategic purpose of intervention is, therefore, to create a moment of psycho-educational encounter—aimed at the family members of the patient in psychiatric crisis.

It is intended to underline the possibility for the relatives to meet and to unite in groups, with the aim to gain greater knowledge and competence relevant to the mental illness and to the manner the psychological crisis of the patient are confronted, with the objective to revaluate individual resources and to promote the creation experiences of comparison and of though and reflection.

It is worth noting and underlining the importance of the role and the socio-emotional functions of the parents and of parental figures, as a resource for overcoming the critical phase.

The main objective that the treatment is established to achieve was to help every single family member and the entire family to define personal and group goals and to plan ways and times to attain them and to supply news and specific data relevant to the most correct behaviors to put in action during the critical moments and to identify representatives (employees or not) in a position to help the whole family to emphasize the resources and potential. As well, it was retained opportune to improve the family members' knowledge about the disorder suffered by the patient and supply updated information on the corresponding pharmacological treatment.

The formative pathway has developed in the context of care in which the psychiatric patient was welcomed in the moment of the crisis and, therefore, also experienced by the family, like a familiar and opportune place.

The meeting places used were of adequate logistics for the management of a small group and were equipped with everything necessary for the instrumentation for the projection of slides.

The slides, useful for the presentation of the topic of discussion, formed of short sentences and exemplifying images, were presented following a logical order that started from the interpretive models of psychiatric pathology to pharmacological treatment.

Such psycho-educational intervention was carried out by a team of healthcare workers composed of a psychologist, a rehabilitation specialist and a medical psychiatrist who constantly supervised course of the meetings also in function of the course of the psychological therapy and of the pharmacological therapy of the patient.

Through the development of a welcoming climate, the healthcare workers develop a role of educators and facilitators of the group, promoting in the participants:

- self-consciousness of their own role of care giver and the lifestyle of the family;
- knowledge and deepening of the features of a psychological crisis;
- reflection on the behaviors that interfere with the patient's good course of illness;
- reflection on the relational styles within familial environment and in the relation with the treating therapists. The healthcare workers, through observation and active listening, build an intervention of support to the family, stimulating also the comparison with respect to the socio-emotional experiences inside of the group and the collective discussion.

The healthcare workers, through the information communication to the group relative to the specific psychiatric pathologies, place themselves, above all as containers, favoring, to the same time, a process of individual and group ability of acquisition.

The changes observed in the family members were evaluated with the administration of two questionnaires: the GHQ of Goldberg (General Health Questionnaire)[47], and the SASS scale (Social Adaptation Self-evaluation Scale [48]), activating also a comparison with a control group, always by the administration of the tests previously cited, upstream to the psychoeducational intervention to which the sample participated.

The features of two groups were comparable as to age and social conditions; the sole difference is that the sample is composed almost entirely of women.

The statistical analysis carried out on the tests compiled showed that the two groups present equivalent scores; the data is explicable considering that the subjects did not participate in interventions for the family members of psychiatric patients.

An enhancement is seen in all the sample groups at the conclusion of the psychoeducational program with positive results for the GHQ and SASS tests, taken in examination (comparison per-post significant for both tests).

The parents who participated in this type of psychoeducational group improved their perception of their own psychological state of well-being, put to the test for assistance given to their anorexic family member. Also, they were in a position to improve their own social relations, clashing the tendency of isolation that strikes also the families, as well as the same patient.

These first results make one reflect that the family members, improving their quality of life through teamwork, are also in a better position to effectively help the anorexic patient.

Naturally, parts of the more structured familial dynamics are not accessible to a rapid change and require therapies for a longer duration: the model of intervention proposed is able to be, nevertheless, the premise of a lasting intervention, because it is not entirely based on information, but open to dynamic reflections.

8. CONCLUSIONS

The controlled studies on the results of the familial treatment, both psychotherapeutic type and psychoeducational, are still not very numerous, although their clinical practice have been in action already for years, and the familial interest is included in the interdisciplinary plans, especially of the youngest patients [49,50].

Various types of family intervention seem to have promising results in adolescents, but not in adults [51], and the therapeutic factors associated with the positive result still do not seem to be clear.

One single study confronted the family therapy with the psychoeducational intervention of group [52], verifying an analogous effectiveness of the two types of interventions, above all, for how much it pertains to the recovery of anorexic patients. Both of the techniques did not favor, nevertheless, psychological changes, at least in temporary observations (four months). This study makes one think that, in part, there is a positive effect nonspecific to the interest of the family members in the therapy of anorexic crisis—a sort of bonding reconstruction of the patient to the family, and vice versa, and in the other part, a difficulty to change psychological models to the functioning of the family—that have influenced the psychopathologic aspects of the patient.

These positive results, together with the clinical observations carried out at numerous centers that provide therapy for eating disorders, make one reflect upon, even if the first changes in the patient's family attitudes are not complete, pertaining to the dysfunctional dynamic, some changes are possible and favor the patient's improvement in the critical phase.

Involving the parents in the patient's care processes means to take on an attitude aimed to individualize the needs and to identify the realistic expectations of improvement, with a positive and collaborative behavior. The family members are incorporated inside of the support system of the suffering individual, orientated to find, together along with the therapists, those alternate strategies of coping, indispensable to effectively confront stress factors.

For the accomplishment of a valid psychoeducational project, it is of fundamental importance, the creation of news and "healthier" interpersonal relations between the members of the family and the patient, improving the emotional atmosphere within the whole family unit. To facilitate the clarity and the transparency of the feelings within a family unit, significantly reducing the number of intrusive actions and critics towards the patients, constitutes as the objective to attain an effective psychoeducational program.

All of the psychoeducational programs treated up to now, place in evidence how fundamental it is to treat the family members of the psychiatric patient, in a direct and precise manner, avoiding providing news on the pharmacological treatment and psychotherapeutic in a vague and imprecise manner and avoiding altogether the generation of "fantasized" ideas linked to psychological disturbance. The psychoeducational programs should supply detailed information on the causes of psychiatric illnesses, on its course and on the possible treatments. The encounters organized with the family members must be able to give relief and to build an optimistic climate regarding the improvement of the situation and on overcoming the crisis.

The effectiveness of the new psychoeducational programs aims for the ability to generate, around the patient, a social environment neither hyper-stimulated nor underestimated, capable of protecting the patient from those external agents considered as stressogeneous but, at the same time, being able to avoid social behaviors of withdrawal by the patient.

Concluding, most of the new generation psychoeducational interventions, place at the centre of their attention, the construction of an effective social network in a position to monitor the stimuli that arrive at the patient, and have shown how this constitutes an important predictive factor of possible relapses.

References

[1] Santonastaso, P; Favaro, A; Pollini, B. *Il carico familiare nei disturbi dell'alimentazione: dati preliminari di uno studio controllato*. In: Gentile, MG, editor. Atti giornate di nutrizione clinica. Milano: Franco Angeli., 1997.

[2] Andreasen, NC; Endicott, J; Spitzer, RL; Winokur, G. The family history method using diagnostic criteria. Reliability and validity. *Arch Gen Psychiatry*, 1977, 34, 1229-1235.

[3] Kendler, KS; Walters, E; Neale, M; Kessler, R; Hearth, A; Eaves, L. The structure of the genetic and environmental risk factors for six major psychiatric disorders in women. *Arch Gen Psychiatry*, 1995, 52, 374-383.

[4] Kassett, JA; Gershon, ES; Maxwell, ME; Guroff, JJ; Kazuba, DM; Smith, AL; Brandt, HA; Jimerson, DC. Psychiatric disorders in the first-degree relatives of probands with bulimia nervosa. *Am J Psychiatry*, 1989, 146, 1468-1471.

[5] Walters, EE & Kendler, KS. Anorexia nervosa and anorexic-like syndromes in a population-based female twin sample. *Am J Psychiatry*, 1995, 152, 64-71.

[6] Biederman, J; Rivinus, T; Kemper, K; Hamilton, D; Macfadyen, J; Harmatz, J. Depressive disorders in relatives of anorexia nervosa patients with and without a current episode of nonbipolar major depression. *Am J Psychiatry*, 1985, 142, 1495-1497.

[7] Strober, M; Freeman, R; Morrell, W. The long-term course of severe anorexia nervosa in adolescents: Survival analysis of recovery, relapse, and outcome predictors over 10-15 years in a prospective study. *Int J Eating Disord*, 1997, 22, 339-360.

[8] Piran, N; Kennedy, S; Garfinkel, PE; Owens, M. Affective disturbance in eating disorders. *J Nerv Ment Dis*, 1985, 173, 396-400.

[9] Leassle, RG; Kittl, S; Fichter, MM; Wittchen, HU; Pirke, KM. Major affective disorder in anorexia nervosa and bulimia. *Brit J Psychiatry*, 1987, 151, 785-789.

[10] Gershon ES; Schreiber JL; Hamovit JR; Dibble ED; Kaye WH; Nurnberger JI; Andersen AE; Ebert, M. Clinical findings in patients with anorexia nervosa and affectives illness in their relatives. *Am J Psychiatry*, 1984,141: 1419-1422.

[11] Schmidt, U; Tiller, J; Treasure, J. Setting the scene for eating disorders: childhood care, classification and course of illness. *Psychol Med*, 1993, 23, 663-672.

[12] Strober, M; Lamprt, C; Morrell, W; Burroughs, J; Jacobs, C. A controlled family study of anorexia nervosa. *Int J Eating Disord*, 1990, 9, 239-253.

[13] Kaye, WH; Lilenfeld, LR; Plotnicov, K. Bulimia nervosa and substance dependence. *Alcohol Clin Exp Res*, 1996, 20, 878-888.

[14] Lilenfeld, L; Kaye, WH; Greeno, CG; Merikangas, KR; Plotnicov, K; Pollice, C; Rao, R; Strober, M; Bulik, C; Nagy L. A controlled family study of anorexia nervosa and bulimia nervosa. *Arch Gen Psychiatry*, 1998, 55, 603-610.

[15] Holland, AJ; Hall, A; Murray, R; Russell, GFM; Crisp, AH. Anorexia nervosa: A study of 34 twin pairs and one set of triplets. *Brit J Psychiatry*, 1984, 145, 414-419.

[16] Mitchell, KS; Mazzeo, SE; Aggen, SH; Maes, HH; Kendler, KS; Neale, MC; Bulik, CM. Characteristics of monozygotic male and female twins discordant for overweight: a descriptive study. *Eat Behav*, 2008, 9(3), 366-369.

[17] Mazzeo, SE; Bulik, CM. Environmental and genetic risk factors for eating disorders: what the clinician needs to know. *Child Adolesc Psychiatr Clin N Am,* 2009, 18(1), 67-82.
[18] Gull, WW. Anorexia nervosa. *Transactions of the Clinical Society of London,* 1873, 7, 22-28.
[19] Bruch, H. *Eating disorders: Obesity, anorexia nervosa, and the person within.* New York: Basic Books, 1973.
[20] Dare, C; Eisler, I. Family therapy for anorexia nervosa. In: Garner, DM; Garfinkel, PE, editors. *Handbook of treatment for eating disorders.* New York: Guilford Press, 1997, 34-49.
[21] Minuchin, S; Rosman, BL; Baker, L. *Psychosomatic families: anorexia nervosa in context.* Cambridge, MA: Harvard University Press, 1978.
[22] Selvini Palazzoli, M. *Self-starvation.* New York: Jason Aronson, 1978.
[23] Vandereycken, W; Kog, E; Vanderlinden, J. *The family approach to eating disorders.* New York: PMA Publishing Corp, 1989.
[24] Hoek, HW. Review of the epidemiological studies of eating disorders. *Int Rev Psychiat,* 1993, 5, 61-74.
[25] Santonastaso, P; Ferrara, S; Favaro, A. Disturbi dell'alimentazione nella popolazione generale femminile: Prevalenza e caratteristiche cliniche. In: Scapicchio PL, Vella G. Editors. *Proceedings of XLI National Congress of Italian Society of Psychiatry,* Bari, 25-29 April 1999, 304-306.
[26] Gowers, S; Kadambari, S; Crisp, AH. Family structure and birth of patients with anorexia nervosa. *J Psychiat Res,* 1985, 19, 247-251.
[27] Vandereycken, W & Pierloot, R. Drop-out during in-patient treatment of anorexia nervosa: a clinical study of 133 patients. *Brit J Med Psychol,* 1983, 56, 154-156.
[28] Crisp, AH; Harding, B; McGuinness, B. Anorexia nervosa. Psychoneurotic characteristics of parents: relationship to prognosis. *J Psychosom Res,* 1974, 18, 167-173.
[29] Morgan, HG & Russell, GFM. Value of family background and clinical features as predictors of long-term outcome in anorexia nervosa: four-year follow-up study of 41 patients. *Psychol Med,* 1975, 5, 355-372.
[30] North, C; Gowers, S; Byram, V. Family functioning and life events in the outcome of adolescent anorexia nervosa. *Brit J Psychiatry,* 1997, 171, 545-549.
[31] Vaughn, CE & Leff J. The influence of family and social factors on the course of psychiatric illness: a comparison of schizophrenic and depressed neurotic patients. *Brit J Psychiatry,* 1976, 129, 125-137.
[32] Szmukler, GI; Eisler, I; Russell, GFM; Dare, C. Anorexia nervosa, parental "expressed emotion" and dropping out of treatment. *Brit J Psychiatry,* 1985, 147, 265-271.
[33] Le Grange, D; Eisler, I; Dare, C; Russell, GFM. Evaluation of family treatments in adolescent anorexia nervosa: a pilot study. *Int J Eating Disord,* 1992, 12, 347-357.
[34] Blair, C; Freeman, C; Cull, A. The family of anorexia nervosa and cystic fibrosis patients. *Psychol Med,* 1995, 25, 985-993.
[35] Hodes, M & Le Grange, D. Expressed emotion in the investigation of eating disorders: A review. *Int J Eating Disord,* 1993, 13, 279-288.

[36] Van Furth, EF; Van Strien, DC; Martina, LML; Van Son, MJM; Hendrickx, JJP; Van Engeland, H. Expressed emotion and the prediction of outcome in adolescent eating disorders. *Int J Eating Disord,* 1996, 20, 19-31.

[37] Fadden, G; Kuipers, L; Bebbington, P. The burden of care: the impact of functional psychiatric illness on the patient's family. *Brit J Psychiatry,* 1987, 150, 285-292.

[38] Platt, D. Measuring the burden of psychiatric illness on the family: an evaluation of some rating scales. *Psychol Med,* 1985, 15, 383-393.

[39] Hoenig, J; Hamilton, MW. The schizophrenic patient in the community and his effect on the household. *Int J Psychiatry,* 1966, 12, 165-176.

[40] Santonastaso, P; Zambenedetti, M; Favaro, A; Favaron, C; Pavan, T. Family psychiatric morbidity in eating disorders. *Eur Eating Disord Rev,* 1997, 5, 3-10.

[41] Van den Broucke, S; Vanderycken, W; Vertommen, H. Marital communication in eating disorder patient: a controlled observational study. *Int J Eating Disord,* 1995, 17, 1-22.

[42] Dicks, H.V. *Fifty years of the Tavistock Clinic.* London: Routledge & Kegan Paul, 1970.

[43] Shapiro, D. The training setting in training analysis: a retrospective view of the evaluative and reporting role and other "hampering" factors. *Int J Psychoanal,* 1974, 55(2), 297-309.

[44] Falloon, IRH & Fadden, G. *Integrated Mental Health care. A Comprehensive Community based approach*. Cambridge: Cambridge University Press, 1995.

[45] Hogarty, GE; Anderson, CM; Reiss, DJ; Kornblith, SJ; Greenwald, DP; Javna, CD; Madonia, MJ. Family psychoeducation, social skills training, and maintenance chemotherapy in the aftercare treatment of schizophrenia. I. One-year effects of a controlled study on relapse and expressed emotion. *Arch Gen Psychiatry,* 1986, 43(7), 633-642.

[46] Favaro, A; Santonastaso, P. *Anoressia e bulimia: quello che i genitori (e altri) vogliono sapere.* Verona: Positive Press, Verona, 1996, pp 114.

[47] Goldberg, DP. *The detection of psychiatric illness by questionnaire.* London: Oxford University Press, 1972.

[48] Bosc, M; Dubini, A; Polin, V. Development and validation of a social functioning scale, the Social Adaptation Self-Evaluation Scale. *Eur Neuropsychopharmacol,* 1997, 7 (suppl 1), S57–S70.

[49] Collins, M; Hodas, GR; Liebman, R. Interdisciplinary model for the inpatient treatment of adolescents with anorexia nervosa. *J Adolesc Health Care,* 1983, 4(1), 3-8.

[50] Loeb KL, Walsh BT, Lock J, le Grange D, Jones J, Marcus S, Weaver J, Dobrow Open trial of family-based treatment for full and partial anorexia nervosa in adolescence: evidence of successful dissemination. *J Am Acad Child Adolesc Psychiatry,* 2007, 46(7), 792-800.

[51] Bulik, CM; Brownley, KA; Shapiro, JR Diagnosis and management of binge eating disorder. World Psychiatry, 2007, 6(3), 142-148.

[52] Geist, R; Heinmaa, M; Stephens, D; Davis, R; Katzman, DK. Comparison of family therapy and family group psychoeducation in adolescents with anorexia nervosa.Can J Psychiatry, 2000, 45(2), 173-178.

In: Anorexia Nervosa: A Multi-Disciplinary Approach ISBN: 978-1-60876-200-2
Editors: A. Mancini, S. Daini, L. Caruana, pp. 135-148 © 2010 Nova Science Publishers, Inc.

Chapter 8

TREATING ANOREXIA IN STATE OF EMERGENCY

S. Daini, L. Bernardini and L. Petrongolo
Institute of Psychiatry, Catholic University of the Sacred Heart, Rome, Italy.

ABSTRACT

In anorexic patients, as loss of weight progresses, the fear of losing control and gaining weight grows. With time, this becomes the only law ruling the mind of these girls to the extent that they do not accept any treatment until the crisis becomes uncontrollable. It is more effective to treat anorexia nervosa with hospitalization when the patient is objectively risking her life or when her health conditions are seriously compromised. In this particular treatment context, it is important to carefully consider the relation between the treatment itself and the patient's psychopathological organization; this will now include each member of the medical staff taking care of the patient, just as it had previously involved parents or any other reference model. Indeed, the relationships developed within the hospital, for example, are analyzed not just as simple behaviors but as patterns revealing how the young patient's psyche works, and, at the same time, will indicate the first steps developing a therapeutic relationship.

1. INTRODUCTION

Eating disorders seem to be becoming more frequent. It is a serious problem around which interest has been growing in the last decades. Anorexia and bulimia are typical examples of disorders where individual factors of vulnerability, psychological and biological, are mixed with family and cultural aspects. In both cases, we are looking essentially at a psychological pathology that brings along serious somatic consequences, in turn affecting the psychic state of the patients and contributing to make the disorder chronic and more serious.

In adolescent patients, treatment can be provided in a day-hospital, or hospitalization may be necessary, depending on how serious the somatic and/or psychiatric symptoms are. Nevertheless, while in the case of bulimia, hospitalization is rather rare and its effects do not last long after hospital discharge, in the case of mental anorexia, the importance of the weight loss, and the risks related to the prognosis and the reinforcement of the behavior, call for a well-defined treatment code, more than for bulimia. Often, following hospitalization, patient's collaboration will vary in time. Especially during the initial phase, the patient will try to challenge and show little compliance with the therapy and the doctors. Thoroughly trained staff is,, therefore, necessary to face the problems that will surely arise, especially from a relationship perspective.

Hospitalization of anorexic patients should, therefore, be carefully prepared and supported by a number of rules establishing a real "moral" contract with the patient and her family. Generally, regardless of the operational methods and therapy chosen (psychodynamic, systemic, cognitive behavioral), no particular diet or forced-feeding is prescribed: once the minimum weight is established, we wait until the girl decides to self-feed, without forcing her, so that she can make the decision herself. If forced, and if the weight recovery happens against her will, the patient will feel totally extraneous to it. Once again, she will not feel the responsibly; it will belong to others [1].

On the contrary, voluntary weight recovery allows her to gradually become aware of her wish and her personal involvement; it also helps her to understand the contradictions, the fears and her responsibilities. This delicate period often coincides with a state of depression and is a good time for starting psychotherapy. Resuming feeding is the result of lowering pre-treatment defenses, forcing the patient to consider what is happening in herself and what her real motivations are. In this phase, it is fundamental that the doctor knows how to help her to better understand her conflicts, but without forcing her, since she must consider herself part of this process.

While often, but not always, without a certain weight recovery, the psychotherapeutic treatment of a patient affected by a very serious anorexia can fail; hospitalization and forced feeding can be accepted and tolerated only within a psychological relationship based on openness and trust. This is even more important and difficult as most patients deny their illness or only recognize a few of the symptoms as pathological, for example, they recognize the bulimic crises but not the drive for thinness [2].

2. States of Emergency in Eating Disorders

Often, the clinical picture of anorexia nervosa is associated with other psychiatric imbalances, among which are depression, anxiety, and obsessive-compulsive disorders.

In the most critical situations, significantly underweight people can show depressive symptoms, such as depressed mood, social isolation, irritability, insomnia and decreased sexual drive. Such symptoms may reach the extent of the major depressive episode. Nevertheless, many symptoms of depression can represent an answer to a state of food restriction. It is, therefore, important to analyse the presence of a mood disorder following a partial or total recovery of the body weight.

Anxiety disorder, particularly social phobia, results is often comorbid to AN: the anxiety may be generated by the idea of eating in the presence of other people. However, compulsive eating cannot justify, on its own, diagnosing social phobia.

Compulsive-obsessive disorder is very important and often present in AN. Anorexic patients show many obsessive features: they are obsessed with the idea of the food and their body image; they continually think about the quantity of food, following eating routines such as cutting food into small pieces or meticulously checking the calorific supply. They are perfectionists, meticulous and tidy, keeping rigid control over their body functions, emotions and the environment. Again, obsessive-compulsive disorder can be diagnosed only if food-disorder symptoms are not present.

For personality disorders, there would be a meaningful percentage of their presence, from the 0% to 58%, connected to the AN [3].

Other studies underline how patients with an AN subtype with restrictions and subtype with binge/purging behaviors, more frequently show problems of impulse control, abuse of alcohol and other substances, emotional lability and a higher frequency of suicide attempts. Such symptoms may justify the diagnosis of a borderline personality disorder [4].

The high frequency of psychiatric comorbidity, both in Axis I and Axis II, may lead to difficulties in developing treatment. For this particular reason, it is fundamental to carefully carry out a differential diagnosis between the typical compulsive eating symptoms and psychiatric symptoms [5].

In some cases, AN can be lethal. In many studies, the death-risk rate is estimated to be between 5% and 20% of the treated cases. Such rate is far higher if compared to any other psychiatric disorder, more specifically in patients 15 to 24 years old. [6]. Generally, the most frequent causes of death are linked to the complications resulting from extreme malnutrition, and more specifically, from the cardiovascular and metabolic complications, or suicide. Other authors consider suicide itself as the principal cause of death of anorexic women, in particular for those affected by major depression [7,8,9]. Suicide may be committed when the illness is apparently improving: the patient agrees to eat, but collapses under guilt-feelings and sense of failure [10]. However, in the last years, the death risk has decreased. This is probably due to the possibility of earlier diagnóses, as well as to improvement of the treatments.

Unlike anorexia nervosa, bulimia can develop into a chronic psychopathology. The patient may adapt to it, and the pathology may concentrate in certain moments of the day only, while conducting an apparently standard life in the rest of the day. The clinical course may, therefore, be chronic or intermittent, with remission phases alternating with acute phases. The binge follows rituals for the majority of the cases; these are different for every patient, who chooses her way of feeding herself, according to food or cooking preferences. The weight generally remains within the range, thanks to the adoption of a series of compensation mechanisms like self-induced vomiting, laxative and diuretic abuse and alternation of binge episodes with very restrictive diets. Cases of hypopotassemia are frequent, above all as a consequence of vomiting, of laxative and diuretic abuse, as well as of depressive crisis. However, Sullivan believes that, despite the high risk, death is very unusual for bulimic patients [11].

The therapy for anorexia nervosa would ideally be carried in outpatient treatment. However, this is not always possible, and it is suitable only in those cases where the patients show specific prerequisites: weight loss should be contained (less than 25% of the initial weight), duration of the illness must be shorter than one year, no serious medical complications, good motivation to change and a well-working family environment. If the above favorable conditions are not there, it is worth trying with outpatient treatment for a period of time. However, if within 12 to 16 weeks, no meaningful changes are observed, hospitalization is recommended; extending the outpatient therapy beyond this time can worsen the situation and support chronicisation and the patient's disability.

Moreover, if well organized, the rehabilitation treatment for anorexia nervosa when hospitalized, and the involvement in the rehabilitative program, has a high success rate. In many cases, patients affected by serious forms of anorexia nervosa can be involved in a process of treatment aimed to the recovery; without hospitalization, such serious cases would receive ordinary treatment leading to a high number of extremely negative diagnoses, such as chronicle illness or death.

3. The Hospital Emergency Unit

The Emergency Unit is a hospital operational unit dedicated to emergency cases with scope for short time observation (Emergency Medicine). Here, first medical treatments are given to all urgent and emergency cases, preparatory to urgent hospitalization.

The emergency room is characterized by the presence and the nature of the psychological needs of those needing assistance; emergency patients enter an often new and unknown environment, mostly in bad physical conditions. In case of anorexia, the psychological dynamics have a fundamental significance, even more so as this pathology appears to be "forgotten" by the National Health System, or cannot find adequate support in public health infrastructures across some European countries.[1]

On the contrary, the emergency room and the following hospitalization are possible alternatives, often the only ones, when the patient's life is at risk; a step that may reveal and establish the illness. It is widely acknowledged that, while less serious cases can be treated immediately as outpatients, more serious cases need inward treatment initially, allowing for time to choose the most suitable hospital unit for the ongoing problem: intensive therapy, internal medicine, etc. To this effect, it is extremely important that all involved medical staff are experienced and skilled, and able to go *beyond the Triage and the mere telling of the facts.*

Placing the disorder within the context of a life history or illness often allows a difficult personality, as that of an anorexic, to communicate, to go beyond the physical symptom, and to feel fully cared for, at a human as well as at a medical level. The patient, who has constantly kept herself and others under strict control and indeed challenged the emergency, enters the emergency room and, for the first time, becomes aware her state; this event confirms the illness.

The examination leading to hospitalization, normally carried out by the internist and the psychiatrist, allows for two phases: the diagnostic phase, when each specialist assesses the aspect of his own competence resulting into the definition of the Eating Disorder (type, seriousness, intervention methods and margins), and the therapeutic phase. In the latter, the therapeutic project and the objectives to be reached are agreed upon with the patient.

---

[1] The experience of associations like ABA (Association for the study and the research on Anorexia, Bulimia and eating disorders) tells us that it is not possible to count the number of anorexic and bulimic women who cannot find a place within the National Health Service, even when they reach the Emergency Unit in a state of imminent death. *Cf.* Salute *"Il Servizio sanitario nazionale non dimentichi anoressia e bulimia"* (Roma, 17 Ottobre 2007).

The family and health networks are activated, perhaps for the first time, and the context acts as a meaning matrix, and allows involvement of the patient who has until then not asked for help and has denied and hidden to herself, her partner, relatives and friends, the seriousness of the problem.

Generally, when reaching the emergency room, patients do not ask directly for help as they are in denial, but the relatives will ask as they care about the physical symptoms, or are worried about the clear signs of depression. Emergency room interventions are there to assess the physical condition with the patient and show them the reality and need for hospitalization. This is not easy to achieve in a short time, because of the intensity of the patient's defense state; the staff's empathic and truly sensitive attitude can help the patient. Strictly technical, detached, or too worried and aggressive behaviors may instead lead the patient to continue denying her ill state.

The crisis is accompanied by a significant hypersensitivity to the environmental dynamics and the meta-messages sent by the medical staff. For example, an excessive worry of the emergency unit doctor for the seriousness of the patient's state may significantly increase the patient's anxiety and prevent her from communicating and collaborating. Moreover, unconscious *detachment* mechanisms of the hospital staff (unconsciously understanding the dramatic nature of this kind of patient's psychological state) can lead to an extremely detached behavior or excessive attention to the legal-medical aspects of the decisions to be taken in the emergency room. Such behavior may lead the patient to be more rigid, as she requires an affectionate understanding, given the regression and depression state typical of these moments.

The medical staff of the emergency room may have to deal, themselves, with the issues related to the voluntariness and non-voluntariness of the symptoms. As in the anorexic disorder, the psycho-physical deterioration is mediated by a behavior (control over feeding); unspecialized medical staff can easily unconsciously act as if the patient was voluntarily not eating, and could voluntarily change such behavior. Such misinterpretation can amplify the negative reactions within the family or the social environment around the patient and foster her non-compliance or her refusal to hospitalization.

Because of the fragmentary psychic state of the crisis climax occurring when the patient arrives at the emergency room, relatives need particular attention and reassurance. They unconsciously represent the patient's anxiety; hence, reassuring them is a fundamental element so that this first glimpse of awareness does not turn into a catastrophe.

4. The Inward Treatment

If necessary, an anorexic patient can be hospitalized according to the clinical picture; she may be admitted to an internal medicine or psychiatric unit, or in other specialized infrastructures.[2] In the hospital, anorexia nervosa can be treated in different ways:

Partial or total hospital intervention; these have two general objectives needing different therapeutic protocols, as follows:

[2] Hospitalization in specialized centers may happen in serious cases that do not present life risk; for example, when the clinical picture is chronicized and psychotherapy has not produced results, or with subjects in denial, hostile and reluctant to start any treatment, so as to establish a solid therapeutic relationship.

1. Stabilize the psycho-physical conditions in order to manage the acute complications of the disorder, in patients with low motivation to undertake a treatment aimed at recovery. Ordinary hospitalization is provided within internistic or psychiatric departments, according to the prevailing symptomatology, and it doesn't necessarily ask for the involvement and the commitment of the patient in a therapeutic recovery program.
2. Start or continue a treatment aimed at interrupting factors developing and maintaining the disorder. In many cases, this can lead to full recovery of the patient. This type of intervention calls for direct involvement of the patient in the recovery process, and it must be carried out in intensive rehabilitation hospital infrastructures, or in day-hospital structures.

Admission to Intensive Nutrition Rehabilitation

Unlike ordinary hospitalization, this kind aims at addressing the physical and psychological aspects of the disorder in an integrated manner. It is valid for those serious cases where life is not at risk. There are no universally recognized guidelines for hospital intensive rehabilitation; nevertheless, we use criteria based on clinical experience and broadly accepted by the international scientific community. It has been demonstrated that delaying an intensive rehabilitation hospital treatment can be, in these cases, very dangerous. The mortality of AN patients treated with protocols of intensive nutritional rehabilitation is significantly lower than that of patients treated in medical clinics or in psychiatric hospitals not specialized in DCA [12].

Here are the criteria to be used when choosing an intensive rehabilitation treatment for Anorexia Nervosa:

1. serious or rapid loss of weight connected with medical, psychological and social complications that require hospital treatment;
2. no results to day-hospital or outpatient treatment, with no improvements in body weight or other symptoms of the disorder (binge, self-provoked vomiting, etc.);
3. presence of a related serious psychiatric pathology that hinders day-hospital treatment (major depressive state, severe obsessive-compulsive disorder, borderline personality disorder with impulsive behaviors, abuse or dependence on substances, serious self-harm behaviors); low suicidal risk;
4. presence of severe medical complications (strong hypopotassemia, heart anomalies, presence of diabetes mellitus, etc.);
5. need to separate the patient from her family.

If one or more of these factors are present, hospitalization in a specialist infrastructure is recommended. The essential condition for this type of treatment is, obviously, a suitable level of motivation from the patient as well as her commitment to every phase of the therapeutic treatment. For this reason, hospitalization must always be preceded by a motivational phase (duration varies); this is carried out firstly by the doctor who is recommending the treatment and then mainly by the team who will follow the patient in the hospital rehabilitation treatment.

The specific objectives of the intensive hospital rehabilitation treatment are: to reduce and interrupt the principal physical and psycho-social factors involved in the development and maintenance of the disorder. The treatment should be carried out by a multidisciplinary team, composed of doctors (with internistic and psychiatric skills), psychologist-psychotherapists, nutritionists and specifically trained nursing staff.

Hospitalization in intensive rehabilitation structures has a long duration (between 60 to 120 days, usually); the patient must reach at least 90% of the expected body weight (or a Body Mass Index higher than 18.5), considering an average increase of 1 to 1.5 kg per week.

Compulsory Treatment

In Sullivan's review of 42 studies, the aggregate annual mortality rate from AN averaged 0.56% per year—more than twice that of female psychiatric patients with other diagnoses [11]. However, compulsory hospitalization, in the case of eating disorders is often considered as an essential attempt to save a life.

In Italy, law n. 180/1978, establishes that compulsory health treatments must represent an exceptional case and must last as little as possible. This rather negative interpretation of compulsory treatment has, perhaps, contributed to make its use very rare in cases of anorexia and bulimia, while in the Anglo-Saxon countries, its use is more frequent.[3]

Some have suggested that forced treatment is counterproductive and adversely affects the therapeutic relationship. Hiday found that two hypotheses guide the outcome studies of involuntary commitment [13]. The first is that patients who are hospitalized involuntarily will be angry and negative about their hospitalization and treatment. As a result, they will be less likely to cooperate with inpatient and outpatient treatment and will have to be rehospitalized. The second hypothesis predicts that involuntary patients will become positive toward hospitalization and treatment after their initial anger and negativism subside and after they are treated. Their symptoms will become minimized and functioning maximized, which will help them avoid rehospitalizations.

Actually, compulsory treatment of all mental illnesses represents an ethical and scientific problem: the right to individual freedom and to be different against the need to treat a condition that threatens the life and at the same time jeopardizes free and critical thinking [2]. Ethic positions and scientific matters, i.e., studies and the empirical data, seem to influence each other, if we compare the effects produced by the different choices. However, given the controversy about involuntary treatment in psychiatry and in law, it is surprising that so few empirical studies have addressed involuntary commitment of persons with eating disorders.

A study carried out in London, by the Eating Disorders Unit of the Maudsley Hospital-Bethlehem Royal Hospital, over a period of twelve years (1983-1995), underlined how out of 506 cases of hospitalization for anorexia nervosa, 81 were compulsory.[4] These patients have been compared with similar samples, in dimension and number, in voluntary treatment, both followed for various years. Ramsay, Ward, Treasure, and Russell have reported that

[3] To be precise, with regard to anorexia, English judges have been considering for several years now forced-feeding as an element for treating mental illnesses. This is based on the assumption that refusing to eat is, in these cases, a consequence of the same pathology, and it represents a symptom that must be obligatorily treated, in accordance with the Mental Health Act, 1983.

[4] About 16%, higher if compared to the Italian centers.

involuntary commitment of patients with anorexia nervosa leads to satisfactory short-term results, but found increased morbidity when they followed patients for a mean of 5.7 years after the first admission for treatment. Meaningful differences in mortality have emerged: they are far higher among patients subjected to compulsory health treatment, about 2.17% per year [14]. This result may have a two-fold interpretation post-hoc: the first is that compulsory treatment is counterproductive, and, therefore, leads to worsening; the second is that doctors select the most serious cases for this kind of treatment, already presenting a higher risk of mortality. Only a perspective study could clarify this interpretative doubt.

The mortality rate at follow-up for detained patients was 12.7%, compared to 2.6% for voluntary patients. Undoubtedly, cases requiring compulsory hospitalization are the most chronic and the most resistant to treatment. The low percentage of compulsory hospitalization in Italy leads one to think that, in any case, the majority of the patients are persuaded to voluntary hospitalization, in suitable conditions. This means patients peacefully acquire awareness of the existing problems, and this represents the first step to overcoming the mind-body separation. As it stands, this type of treatment represents both a possibility and a temptation that divides doctors between those who report satisfaction and gratitude from the family and those who prefer to avoid this therapeutic measure.

The resolution of the nuclear conflict autonomy-dependence can be delayed rather than accelerated by forced interventions, and the anxiety can worsen. Risks are even higher if compulsory hospitalization takes place in unsuitable and non-specialized environments. For these reasons, it is always worth experimenting with intelligence and imagination various forms of persuasion and dialogue before resigning to compulsory treatment, calling parents to exercise that forgotten authority and appealing to the fatherly law before turning to the State law [2].

The therapeutic treatment used in all these types of hospital interventions is generally a multidisciplinary treatment and it includes: Multidimensional Diagnostic Evaluation (internistic, psychiatric and nutritional); assistance in eating (nutritional rehabilitation, with the technique of meal planning and mechanical feeding); psycho-educative intervention; psychotherapy (individual and/or group); intervention on the body image disorder; intervention on the family; pharmacological therapy (in some cases).

In many cases, it can be useful to follow hospitalization with outpatient treatment. If so, the patient returns home (if she lives close to the clinic), or she can choose a room or an apartment close to the hospital where she will go for the whole duration of the day-hospital phase. Besides, the patient starts to take control of herself and her body weight: initially, she will only have breakfast outside the hospital, then lunch and finally dinner, while she continues to participate in the therapeutic activities started during the hospitalization and she prepares for the outpatient treatment program [12].

Whatever the type of hospital intervention (total, partial or of intensive rehabilitation) and, despite the fact that there is no universally recognized protocol for assessing eating disorders, everybody agrees that a wide spectrum evaluation is needed, given the heterogeneous and multi-determined nature of these pathologies [15]. The multi-dimensional assessment allows for the analysis of psychological, somatic, socio-environmental and relational aspects [16]. In particular, this method consists of:

- collection of all elements related to the person's history and life (far and near family, personal, physiological and pathological anamnesis);

- evaluation of the psychological functioning model in its cognitive, emotional-affective and behavioral aspects;
- analysis of the personal weight history;
- analysis of the levels of the physical activity;
- evaluation of the feeding behavior;
- study of the health indicators;
- monitoring of the risk factors;
- psychosocial evaluation;
- medical examination;
- laboratory and instrumental tests.

Once information has been collected, the doctor may decide to use some of the numerous psychological tests in order to formulate a complete diagnosis. Certainly, in the initial phase of hospitalization, often during the first meeting, patients appear confused and they refuse medical therapy, even if the physical situation is extremely serious. Nevertheless, during the interview, they often are aware of the real situation, though partially or fragmentarily. The patient is usually worried for her health and hostile towards her parents because of the hospitalization. The interviews touch upon and at times resolve the relationship with the mother, rejected and felt as an anxious and intrusive element; during the meetings, emotions emerge on a deep non-verbal register, due to the impossibility to establish a dialogue or a compromise between mother and daughter. The expression and the physical contact characterize these intense moments, in which a mother can approach her daughter; something that was previously impossible because of the psychological refusal and the physical state. However, despite the difficulties caused by the health state, in some cases patients can quickly establish a therapeutic contact, solicited by the dramatic physical situation they become aware of.

Something to be discussed separately is the treatment within a community: in the last decades, in Italy, the idea of residential community has developed for those patients affected by compulsive eating with a long-lasting pathology or with troubled families who are not able to support their daughters during treatment or rehabilitation. The intervention in community is a social-health intervention with a medium- to long-term duration that needs a multi-disciplinary team, with the following objectives: the change in the dysfunctional behaviors related to the pathology, the development of the personal capacity and resources, the implementation of management capacity and autonomy, aimed at learning how to manage their own everyday life and to plan for medium- to long-term projects [17]. The theoretical approach used is above all the cognitive-behavioral one, whose objective it is to work on the excessive and dysfunctional worry towards one's own weight and body shape, which is typical of this kind of patient. The method includes the application of behavioral exercises and classical techniques of cognitive restructuring [5].

5. The Integrated Treatment and the Experience of the Policlinico Gemelli in Rome

The clinical characteristics of compulsive eating disorders, the complexity and specificity of their nature and, above all, the multiple factors of their causes, make planning a complex, detailed and multi-factor therapy necessary [18]. Besides, in the situations of emergency and refusal of the treatment, the integration of the medical and psychiatric therapies becomes fundamental, even if applying them could be complex [19].

The integrated therapeutic approach of the Policlinico Gemelli in Rome tries to give an answer to the complexity and the multi-factor aspects of compulsive eating disorders, particularly of anorexia. The patient is usually hospitalized in the endocrinology department, where the team is made of different professional figures (psychiatrists, psychologists, internists, endocrinologists, educators and nutritionists) who collaborate and cooperate in order to elaborate an individual and most effective treatment strategy. Involving the above professionals allows for treating in a specialist and qualified manner all affected areas of the patient (organic, psychological, nutritional, and social) leading her, at the same time, to reflect on the various aspects of her own discomfort. The therapeutic course, within an agreed and shared program, is, however, customized and adapted each time to the current situation, the phase of the illness, the actual resources of the patient and her response to the treatment. However, there is a common therapeutic approach to all cases and patients and that is that parents are suggested not to take part to the feeding of their daughter.

In order to make a correct and complete psychiatric and psychological diagnosis, professionals carry out interviews and submit a number of the most used personality tests: Graphic Tests (Human Figure Test; Test Tree Kock ; Family Test); Wartegg Drawing Test; Rorschach; MMPI; ASQ AND CDQ. To these, we add the EDI reactive (Eating Disorder Inventory), a useful self-evaluation questionnaire to identify and measure some psychological traits and groups of symptoms usually associated with eating disorders. The current version of the EDI test [15] includes 64 items from the original version [20] and 27 additional items, for a total of 11 Scales: *Drive for Thinness*; *Bulimia*; *Body dissatisfaction*; *Ineffectiveness*; *Perfectionism*; *Interpersonal distrust*; *Interoceptive awareness*; *Maturity fears*; *Asceticism*; *Impulse regulation*; *Social insecurity*.[5] The psychological assessment also investigates the personality structural aspects of the patients, a fundamental introductory research to all the psychotherapeutic approaches.

Formulating the psychiatric, psychological and medical diagnosis, provide for the most complete picture of such a complex problem, made even more complex by subjective symptoms and confusing objective signs, varying in their clinical expressivity and, therefore,, difficult to categorize. On the contrary, a non-integrated intervention may prove inconsistent, or redundant, and can reinforce the mechanisms of separation while maintaining the status quo. From the doctors' point of view, moreover, working in team can help to face that feeling of impotence and lack of coordination that can occur with extremely complex cases; the single therapist may not know which approach to choose, and that is not due to professional

[5] The EDI results also to be a mean that can be used in the retest, and that, therefore, can easily be used both to establish the necessity of a clinical intervention and as a change indicator of the treatment in progress.

incompetence, but because the situation appears very complex, the family is strongly involved or it is difficult to engage the patient [5].

Unlike other hospital protocols using the cognitive behavioral approach, this therapy does not force or prescribe separation from the family, even during the block of feeding, taking into account the importance of the emotional and affective support the family can give, particularly the mother, in the more seriously regressive states or when life prognosis is uncertain.

The same hospitalization represents a partial but significant separation from the anxious family environment, and it spontaneously creates a number of different reference points (the group of patients, the medical staff) that can develop new identifications. Considered on its own, the isolation from the family is not an effective tool to produce a psychological change, while the first dynamic change seems to affect the unconscious experiences related to the family, with the reconstruction of the feelings of persecution in the hospital environment. The meaning of the psychological separation can instead be attributed to the psychotherapeutic relationship, if this involves a significant investment on the patient side and the progressive acquisition of an autonomous psychic space.

During the first phase of our psychological intervention, the professional experience matured inside the Policlinico Gemelli shows how often patients seem to welcome the diagnostic tests with interest, with a mixture of curiosity and insecurity; they also seem to absorb the diagnostic communication, even when not commented upon. They equally accept psychotherapy, which generally starts with three sessions per week during the hospitalization phase and, after dismissal, it continues at our Psychiatry and Clinical Psychology Day Hospital and is integrated by medical controls.

The psychotherapeutic support function and the move from supportive counselling to the outpatient phase where conflicts are explored, represent a fundamental characteristic of our integrated treatment. Nevertheless, the psycho-dynamic method seems to be more difficult to apply, especially when the psychological, individual and family dynamics take a destructive form. That is maybe why many authors use behavioral techniques in the first phase of treatment. However, a cautious exploration of the current dynamics can help the patient to have some insights into the dynamic causes of the disorder; such intuitions may represent a bridge leading to a more mature awareness, supported by the psychotherapy work that will follow.

6. Starting Point for Debate: The Psychodynamic Perspective

The starting point is in the objective difficulty that young anorexic patients face in starting psychotherapy, especially if the pathological situation includes narcissistic defenses and serious physical conditions.

Also keeping in mind the therapist's initial difficulty in maintaining a stable relationship, it is fundamental that the dialogue begins in the neediest moment, i.e., the crisis time. This is usually the only moment of rational engagement, when the patient lowers her rigid and strong defenses. Besides, crises usually require choices—crisis, in Greek, means choice—and, as the Chinese say, choices are a mixture of dangers and opportunities. That is why it is important to create conditions where people can overcome the emotional ambivalence of a certain situation: falling into depression or reacting? waiting or taking initiative? giving way to the affective or to the practical aspects of the situation? Choosing will allow one to focus all energies in one direction and overcome the crisis.

The human environment and the medical team are, therefore, a reference for projective, adhesive or symbolic identification during the critical period, according to the patient's personality and the crisis' previous development: the coordination and the integration of the interventions are made particularly difficult by the different and quickly varying trends, which are typical of borderline states.

The clinical problem of this pathology calls for an initial concrete commitment; this is particularly important when the death risk is high. First of all, both the doctor and the patient move towards the dimension of the reality, with the risk that the objective of treating the patient's health may cause confusion with regards to the interrelations or cause links that each time can be identified in the different pathologies and in their recovery.

The depth of the medical staff's emotional involvement represents an important element that can be recognized or removed but can alter know-how and the intervention itself. For the medical staff, counter transference in high-risk situations evokes images of patients dying, with the risk that this can happen, and with all related narcissistic consequences of the case.

Empathy is another fundamental element, as a distinctive trait of the psychoanalytic psychotherapy. The self psychology in these particular clinical situations is under intense pressure, given the contemporary presence of the patient's archaic defenses, her somatic objective state and the group resonances.

A common aspect to all those involved in the treatment seems to be the tendency to consider the above-mentioned risky situations, as moments when "thoughts and reflections are potentially zeroed, both in the patient and in the doctors. Such state does obviously not affect the actions aimed at treating the body and its biochemical functions" [21]. The processes of denial, rationalization and isolation, especially when more archaic defenses are raised, lead to attribute to the patient a partial image, as a subject with body and emotional reactions, positive or negative affections, but that hardly embodies a person who can think, with psychic functions of mediation and integration and the interrelation between these two moments. For the patient, the body is or should be at risk of disappearing, while for the doctors, her psyche is running that risk [22].

It is, therefore, difficult to form and maintain an integrated image and identity, as this integration would be more painful and jeopardize, following identification, our own balance. This is why acting (the medical therapy) and addressing the most concrete aspects of the problem and of the relationship with the patient may be one of the consequences.

7. Conclusion

Currently, and in light of the considerations regarding the pathological and serious cases, it is legitimate to wonder if and when the doctor should be directive to the extent of forcing the patient's free will, or to raise her awareness when in denial. The psychiatrist, aware of the psycho-dynamic dimensions (besides questioning the psycho-therapeutic, therapeutic and pharmacological plan like the rest of the medical staff), more than others may doubt how much every decision can represent a therapeutic acting out or an evolutionary occasion. This is because he is above all aware of the risk of relapse, should the body weight be recovered with external interventions, and of the difficulties establishing an alliance with the patient and then a psychotherapeutic contact [23].

On the other hand, the hospital environment, the liaison problems, the need to integrate doctors and psychotherapists do not only represent the actual state, but for the anorexic patients is a group matrix for change.

The psychosomatic crisis underlines how the process of objectification of the death risk and its relevant images are both intra-psychic and interpersonal. Besides, the absence of a cohesive internal organization leads the patient to try to establish fusional relationships with the others and look for cohesion in the hospital environment. The patient moves away from that integration that, instead, would allow her to adapt to real life. In this scenario, psychotherapy represents the first move towards the integration of her own identity, separated from the family and from the surrounding ambience.

From the doctor's point of view, a purely biological intervention involves the risk of losing the patient's thinking dimension; from the psychotherapist's point of view, the exclusive focus on the psyche or its interactions involves the risk of losing the patient's and the environment's real coordinates. In this sense, a convergent attention of both the doctors and the integrated hospital treatment seems to foster a rapid change in the somatisation processes, as well as to help the anorexic patients taking the initial step toward psychic integration.

REFERENCES

[1] Jeammet, P. *Anoressia Bulimia: I paradossi dell'adolescenza interpretati da un grande psichiatra francese.* Milano: Franco Angeli, 2006.

[2] Cuzzolaro, M. *Anoressie e Bulimie.* Bologna: Il Mulino, 2004.

[3] Cassin, SE & Von Ranson, KM. Personality and Eating Disorders : A Decade in Review. *Clin. Psychol. Rev.* 2005, 25 (7), 895-916.

[4] Sansone, S; Levitt, JL: Sansone, LA. The Prevalence of Personality Disorders Among Those with Eating Disorders. *Eating Disorders,* 2005, 13 (1), 7-21.

[5] Caviglia, G & Cecere, F. *I disturbi del comportamento alimentare: L'approccio multidisciplinare per un intervento efficace.* Roma: Carocci Faber, 2007.

[6] Garfinkel, PE *Anorexia Nervosa: A Multidimensional Approach.* New York: Brunner Mazel, 1982.

[7] Patton, G. Mortalità in Eating Disorder. *Psychol. Med.,* 1988, 18, 947-951.

[8] Harris, EC; Barraclough, B. Suicide as an outcome for mental disorders. A meta-analysis. *Br J Psychiatry,* 1997, 170, 205-228.

[9] Pompili, M; Mancinelli, I; Girardi, P; Accorrà, D; Ruberto, A; Tatarelli, R. Suicidio e tentato suicidio nell'anoressia nervosa e nella bulimia nervosa. *Annali dell'Istituto superiore di sanità,* 2003, 39, 275-281.

[10] De Giacomo, P; Renna, C; Santoni Rugiu, A. *Manuale sui disturbi dell'alimentazione: Anoressia, bulimia, disturbo dell'alimentazione incontrollata.* Milano: Franco Angeli, 2005.

[11] Sullivan, PF. Mortality in anorexia nervosa. *Am J Psychiatry,* 1995, 152, 1073-1074.
[12] Piccini, F. Anoressia, Bulimia, *Binge Eating Disorder.* Torino: C.S.E, 2000.
[13] Hiday, VA. Involuntary commitment as a psychiatric technology. *Int J Technol Assess Health Care,* 1996, 12, 585- 603.
[14] Ramsay, R.; Ward, A.; Treasure, J.; Russell, G.F.M. Compulsory treatment in anorexia: short-term benefits and long-term mortality. *Br J Psychiatry,* 1999, 175, 147-153.
[15] Garner, DM. *EDI-2 Eating Disorder Inventory-2. Firenze: Organizzazioni Speciali,* 1995.
[16] Aquilar, F; Del Castello, E; Esposito R; (editors). *Psicoterapia dell'Anoressia e della Bulimia.* Milano: Franco Angeli, 2005.
[17] Brambullo, L; Ferrari, M; Ostuzzi, R; Cuzzolaro, M. La comunità terapeutica residenziale. *Una nuova esperienza di cura per i disturbi del comportamento alimentare.* Psicobiettivo, 2000, 21, 91-98.
[18] Dalle Grave, R. *Anoressia Nervosa: i fatti.* Verona: Positive Press, 1996.
[19] Daini, S.; Barbarino, A.; De Marinis, L. *Fasi critiche dell'anoressia: lineamenti per un intervento d'urgenza. XXXVIII Cong.* Società Italiana di Psichiatria. Salsomaggiore, 20-26 October 1991.
[20] Garner, DM; Olmsted, MP; Bohr, Y; Garfinkel, PE. *Manual for Eating Disorder Inventory (EDI).* Odessa, FL: Psychological Assessment Resources, 1984.
[21] Daini, S. Concretizzazioni. *Minerva Psichiatrica,* 1994, 35, 1-8.
[22] Daini, S & Ferro, FM. *Trasformazioni e silenzi del corpo: Studi sull'anoressia nervosa.* Chieti: Metis, 1995.
[23] Bruch, H. Perils of behavior modification in the treatment of Anorexia Nervosa. *J Am Med Ass,* 1974, 230, 1419-22.

In: Anorexia Nervosa: A Multi-Disciplinary Approach ISBN: 978-1-60876-200-2
Editors: A. Mancini, S. Daini, L. Caruana, pp. 149-157 © 2010 Nova Science Publishers, Inc.

Chapter 9

THE LOGOTHERAPEUTIC APPROACH: AN ANTHROPOGICALLY FOUNDED METHOD

A. Mancini[1], R. Festa[2]
[1]Division of Endocrinology, Catholic University of the Sacred Heart, Rome, Italy
[2]Institute of Clinical Pathology, University "Politecnica delle Marche," Ancona, Italy

ABSTRACT

Among the different psychological interpretations of eating disorders, the logotherapy, based on the anthropologic view known as "existential analysis" by V.E. Frankl, has a special place, since it looks at man as a multidimensional being, with the fundamental characteristic of self-transcendence. He developed a method, born as a reaction against the schools of Freud and Adler, based on the search of meaning (for all human beings, and also applied to many psychological disorders). Interesting considerations can be made, from this point of view, on anorexia nervosa patients, totally fallen back on themselves, on their subjective world, forgetting this opening to the world and other people. This theory tries, therefore, to overcome the restrictive analysis of different psychiatric schools on a man conditioned by his past life.

1. INTRODUCTION

In the field of biomedical research, the study of physiopathology, by finding and linking the significance of the various experimental data, tries to understand the essence of a specific disease. Medical science is featured by a general matter due to the nature of its "object": every etiologic factor interacts within an integrated whole, that is the human being, whose somatic psychic and self-knowledge factors are always present at the same time. This complexity is more evident for psychosomatic diseases, where the nexus between the "psyche" and the "body" is still far to be fully understood [1]. At the top of this topic is anorexia nervosa (AN), a disease at the core of which psychosomatic interrelation just is. In fact, self-imposed fast shows a close connection with own physical image, and this disturbance has much bearing on the patient's relational cultural and social nature. In other words, it is strongly related to the personal oneself. Therefore, if any disease faces these issues, in the case of AN, the peculiarity of the physiopathological study (epistemological aspect) is even clearer: to understand and treat this disease means to investigate the relation psyche-body in a global manner, with the two elements not separable (anthropological aspect).

The question is do psychosomatic medicine and AN particularly put new methodological and epistemological problems? Given the inadequacy of a psychosomatic medicine as conceived by the modern psychiatry, and the danger of a restrictiveness in the attempt to quantify stress, emotions, etc., in an empirical field [2], is it possible to think of man from a more articulate viewpoint?

2. From Psychological to Existential Interpretations

Regarding the various interpretations, the psychoanalytical one, the cognitive-behavioral one, the socio-relational one, etc., some elemental questions arise.

Cognitive psychotherapy and psychoanalysis showed an image of AN patients like subjects at the mercy of their past, totally determined by the events of their childhood [3,4]. According to these viewpoints, the patient is only partially able to decide, so that he is something like a mere victim of the circumstances. Not all authors agree with this interpretation [5]. AN is not simply the effect of the dynamics of childhood and early youth, but an intentionality that marks the clinical symptomatology.

Alfred Adler had noted every psychopathological symptom has got an intentionality and is a way to manipulate the social environment [6]. If it has got an intentionality with an aim, then AN depends on a personal decision, too. Another matter concerns the age of onset of the symptoms. The usual beginning during adolescence, a period in which a person is in search of his/her own personal identity, indicates a crisis involving not only the emotional aspects, but also and above all the dimension of the existential planning.

Finally, a term that is frequent in the characterization of AN patient's world is emptiness [7], which could refer to a personal planning only partially succeeded.

L. Binswanger [8] was the first who interpreted AN under the light of the existentialist anthropology, but another existentialist psychotherapeutical current is the existential analysis and logotherapy by Victor Emil Frankl. Existential analysis is an anthropological conception, that is to say a conception of man and a theory of personality. Logotherapy is a way of interpretation of psychic disturbances and a psychotherapeutic praxis. According to the existential analysis, human being is characterized by a specificity that is the spiritual dimension (not to be mistaken for the religious one). The main features of this dimension are freedom of will, responsibility, self-transcendence, will to meaning, and meaning of life. Logotherapy is a cure rising from the spirit, i.e., as Frankl says "logotherapy is a (psycho)therapy based on the sense. The idea of a cure through the sense is just the contrary of the conventional idea of psychotherapy that might be described as sense through the therapy." Logotherapy accounted for the development and maintenance of psychological and existential disturbances and made up a concrete praxis and some methods for the resolution of neuroses and abnormal behaviors [9].

V. E. Frankl developed the "existential analysis" as reaction to the psychoanalysis, on one side, and the individual psychology, on the other side. It is an anthropological conception, from which a psychotherapeutic praxis results. A human being has got the spiritual dimension as his own specificity characterized by: freedom of will, responsibility, self-transcendence, will of significance and sense of life. Logotherapy is a cure rising from the spirit, i.e., a (psycho)therapy based on the sense [10].

Self-transcendence of the human existence, according to Frankl, brings a new and different perspective with which life and world are perceived. It implies a freedom that is not freedom from every kind of conditioning, but a freedom for something, freedom in order to take up a position regarding the conditionings themselves, freedom in order to decide who one is [11].

3. Victor Emil Frankl

Here is a brief analysis of the main texts by Frankl regarding his theory on the human structure, the role of the science, and the effects of both these issues on the therapeutic method.

In *Logotherapy and Existential Analysis,* [12] Frankl starts from the comparison between the two most important schools (Freud's and Adler's), characterizes their essential nuclei (the function of knowledge and the function of responsibility), and finally highlights the unilateral vision of them both. The aim of Frankl is to recover a unity, though it still remains to be found.

In the appearance of science [13], speaking about traditional medicine, he shows a rigorous methodology is not enough to make an exact science, but the finding of a research must arise from the truth of nature or, dealing with biomedicine, of man. The unity of the various human dimensions, according to Frankl, is made by the category named "existentiality." With respect to the two models by Freud and Adler (which give most importance to the rule of the ego and the recovery of responsibility, respectively), a third category is set, the "existential fulfillment," characterized by a dynamic nature since it is directed to the realization of the values. Spirituality is "singular and unrepeatable," but even the individual refers to a universality.

In the work *At the Beginning Was the Sense*, [14] many elements regarding human structure and the role of science can be found. After confirming the tridimensional structure of man, Frankl states a psychiatric disease has its origin in one of the three dimensions, then it is either a somatogenenic, or a psychogenic, or a noogenic neurosis.

In facing up to reality, it happens like a splitting of the attitude: the pursuit of the truth and the pursuit of the sense. A human faculty is at the basis of both attitudes: the self-transcendence. It is a dynamic vision that moves the three levels of human structure. On the contrary, according to Frankl, a static vision in which man is locked in himself is the mistake of the contemporaneous psychoanalytic theories, based on a "monadological" vision of man.

Frankl criticizes the scientific leaning of his period because it prevalently is a reductionistic one. Frankl does not deny the biological, psychological and sociological conditionings, but he says man always is free to take up a position regarding the conditionings themselves, either submitting to or overcoming them thanks to the "resistance strength of the spirit."

In *Homo Patiens,* [15] we found a strong criticism of the various determinisms. Frankl stresses the spiritual autonomy of man, that is to say the independence of the spiritual dimension from the psychic and physical ones. He highlights the existence of a "psycho-noetical antagonism," which should have as correlate the psychophysical parallelism.

Therefore, man appears to be a dynamic being: not only does he tend to the must-to-be, but also by maturing, he gains the ability to suffer. It is not an innate feature, but the effect of those events in which the attitude values are possible. Suffering is a moral performance. It is not only of ethical dignity, but also of metaphysical significance. Through it, a human being becomes clear in the depth of a metaphysical dimensionality.

In conclusion, the conception of man we deduce is not limited into the immanence, but humanism is overcome by the demonstration of the transcendent nature of human existence. Man is not a measurement of himself. He has to find his creaturality: nostalgia, love and frailty are all ways to a dialogic relationship with the Absolute "You." There are no pretensions to knowledge; man's task is more to ask than to answer, but here may be ways for the knowledge of the truth besides (empirical) science. The value of the right medicine is the consciousness to be open to the transcendence of man [16].

So Frankl proposes a more integrated idea of man, seen as a unity and not a simple composition of the biological, psychological and spiritual dimensions. Therefore, the existential datum and the recovery of self-transcendence are necessary for the therapeutic process. Many elements for the understanding of AN come from Frankl's anthropology [17]. They are possible tracks of thinking and keys to interpretation of the disease. Therefore Frankl's different interpretation needs an in-depth examination.

4. The Logotherapeutic Interpretation

The anthropological conceptions of the various interpretations illustrated above have a more or less strict determinism as common background.

The whole psychic phenomenology seems to refer to unconscious dynamics, learning processes and interpersonal relationships that are altered.

A behaviorist setting [18], though supported by some experimental data, sees a human being as the summation of the learned mechanisms. Cognitive psychology interpretation [4] is perhaps the most consistent, until it deals with the phenomenological investigation. When it tries to give causal explanations, it shows its limits due to the cibernetic model. According to Froggio [5], instead, the world of the patients affected with eating disorders reveals, through a more in-depth examination considering not only the psychological mechanisms, "a refusal of one's freedom of choice, of the inter-subjective dimension, that is to say the ability for self-transcendence that is a human peculiarity realizing in the search and fulfillment of one's own life-planning."

This idea is nothing but the specific application of the "existential analysis" by Viktor Emil Frankl to the field of AN. It is the theoretical basis of his "logotherapy." The first elaboration of this theory was made by Frankl, when he was still a young, in the Vienna of the twenties, the capital of psychiatric culture with the leading personalities of Freud and Adler.

After being a supporter of Freud's theories, Frankl developed his criticism not from the clinical praxis, but the meta-clinical aspects of psychoanalysis and individual psychology [19]. The anthropological systems on which the two theories (by Freud and Adler) are based, are affected with a common defect: the image of a human being presented is reductive and deterministic.[1] For psychoanalysis, man is a being moved by the pursuit of pleasure and is interested in the maintenance of his homeostatic balance. Instead, for individual psychology, a human being is moved only by the pursuit of his own success and will of power. According to both Freud and Adler, man really can not have "true" and uninterested relations, because there are always some unconscious purposes. In these two theories, there is no scope for freedom and self-determination, since a human being is determined by unconscious forces, the instincts of an anarchic and irrational Es or an intolerant and violent aspiration to superiority. Finally, these schools lack a theory of the meanings and values, which are instead conceived as symptoms of disease.

Therefore, at least at the beginning, Existential Analysis developed as a reaction to the reductionistic and deterministic statement of the two psychotherapy Viennese major schools.

According to Frankl, human reality is more complex and neither reducible to unconscious psychic mechanisms, nor understandable only in social or somatic terms. Besides psychological, somatic and social dimensions, there must be something more, something featuring the human being, a spiritual dimension, the dimension of freedom and responsibility, of meanings and values, through which a human being can plan himself, take up an attitude regarding the other dimensions. Frankl defined this dimension noetic (from the Greek *nous* = meaning).

A complex vision of man, with more levels, is well fit for the psychopathological models. AN is a clear example. The disease is psychogenic, at least at the beginning, but the symptoms are organic: a strong loss of weight, amenorrhea, etc. In a second time, the strong physical debilitation, due to the constant fast, affects the psyche: by the means of very complex feedback mechanisms, "secondary psychological alterations" arise. Even social dimension is affected from the disease; an anorexic patient shows a set of social and relational behaviors "altered" with conducts of isolation and warped communication.

Then it is necessary not to favor one to detriment of the other dimensions, but also the problem of their interaction and hierarchy is put. Frankl's answer starts from the studies of two philosophers, Nikolai Hartmann and Max Scheler [22]. Hartmann distinguished three levels in a hierarchical way: the spiritual (different from the religious), the psychic and the somatic one. Scheler, instead, refers to layers, distinguishing the peripheral layers, biological and psychological, from the central layer, the spiritual one. These distinctions, however, might confound the fundamental datum, that is to say, man is the unity of different dimensions. According to Frankl, a hierarchization of the dimensions is not possible, but they have a different position: upper and lower, without any judgment upon the merits and value. Each dimension is in relation with the other two: the totality of the dimensions can be kept

[1] Since from a juvenile manuscript [20], Frankl evidenced that the conscious-being and the responsible-being, respectively underlined by psychoanalysis and individual psychology, in their unilateral and antithetical character, performed effective fulfillment. But, from a philosophical point of view, in the perspective of criticism of knowledge, Frankl asserted that both systems were guilty of a limitation of phenomenic realty, in a material direction (as psychoanalysis is centered on the role of libido) or in a formal one (as individual psychology catches expectations content, but challenges their truthfulness) [21].

and understood only from an upper point of view. Besides, each dimension has its own specificity. If one does not recognize it, he makes a reduction work.

In the case of man, only starting from an upper dimension, the noetic one, we can understand in their whole and right meaning the physical and psychological dimensions. So noetic dimension becomes central, the regulating principle of the other dimensions.

The upper dimension, the spiritual (or noetic) one, besides giving his specificity to a human being, can unify and "regulate" the other dimensions. It represents the central nucleus of a human being around which the other dimensions collect. This dimension is a pure "realty of realization" that can not include and reflect upon itself. It is the proper Ego.

It results in a fundamental characteristic of noetic dimension: self-transcendence [23]. It is not at all closed, but substantially open to the world. In order to explain the characteristic of self-transcendence of human existence, Frankl makes a simile about the eye "Self-transcendence," he writes "stresses the essentially anthropological fact that human self-transcendence is always directed to something or someone beyond himself: a sense to realize or an other human existence to meet. Man is truly a man just when he fully devotes himself to an aim, when he overcomes and forgets himself in serving a cause or loving another person. The same happens for the eye, its function of looking at the world works insofar as the eye does not see itself. In fact, when does the eye see itself? When it is ill: if I am affected with a cataract and I see a "fog," or with a glaucoma and I see the rainbow colors all around my pupil, then my eye perceives something of itself and feels its own illness. But at the same time, my sight makes defective".

Developing this idea, Froggio says "self-transcendence of human existence produces a new and different view to perceive the life and the world. The attention is paid out of oneself, to the questions life asks. Man's duty is to catch and to answer these questions." [5] In this responsibility lies, which, in turn, results in another characteristic, freedom: man is free to decide whether to answer or not the questions life asks.

In short, human freedom is not to be understood as elimination of any conditioning (that is impossible, anyway), but freedom to decide, to take up a position regarding the conditionings themselves and the psychic and somatic mechanisms, which are not eliminable but are not the ultimate nature of man.

Logotherapy, with its specific methods, is being applied successfully to the various fields of psychiatry. Frankl himself used it in curing phobias and obsessions, sexual neuroses, somatopsychic troubles, etc., and later alcohol addiction, neuroses, and even for pedagogical aims.

Born in reaction to the other more unilateral psychiatric schools, logotherapy became later an "existential analysis," a helpful method to anyone for a better consciousness of the spiritual depth of every person.

Man is a being—Frankl says—composed of three dimensions. First of all, the corporeal one, also called somatic or organic, then the psychic one, that is mental in the strictest sense, and finally the spiritual one, that is the dimension proper to man [24].

A psychiatric disease can have one of these three dimensions as base, for example an organic-based depression. Dealing with this issue, Frankl observes that psychotherapists can come to an agreement about the organic basis and the psychopharmacological therapies. He seems in this way to share the idea that only what is organic and measurable can be objectified. More exactly, three types of neuroses can be identified on the basis of the level from which they arise. Then, besides somatogenic and psychogenic neuroses (belonging to the traditional psychiatry), there are the noogenic neuroses. These neuroses are among the most original contributions to psychiatry by Frankl. They are born from ethical conflicts or unresolved problems of existential or religious nature.

So, in facing the facts, a sort of splitting of attitude happens: the pursuit of the truth, on the one hand, and the pursuit of sense, on the other hand.

A human faculty is at the basis of either attitude and drives man beside himself (towards the objective truth or the pursuit of sense): self-transcendence. It is a dynamic vision that puts in movement the three levels of man's structure. So, the three levels contribute to the same purpose that is beside the man himself. It is neither enough to unwind one's own instincts (psychoanalysis) , nor to react to the stimuli (behaviorism), nor to satisfy the needs produced by the consumer society (sociologism). Man wants to make a change in the world, i.e., he wants to do something. Therefore, Frankl recognizes the error of the contemporary psychoanalytical therapies, based on a "monadological" vision of man, just in a static vision that considers man closed in himself.

Self-transcendence means man always stretches out of himself. Frankl does not specify whether self-transcendence is already a conscious and responsible faculty, or if it is just an instinct to go out of oneself —that is to say a need, even if not self-centered, to cover one's own limits and the feeling of dissatisfaction due to one's own limits. Close to the self-transcendence, a second properly human faculty is, the self-distancing ability. Man can grow away from himself, place himself in front of or even against himself [25].

With regard to eating disorders, from that kind of anthropology many elements result, which can be reflection pathways, keys of disease interpretation (or at least elements of the psychopathological picture). They are:

- State of apathy, that means inability to face the truth of oneself (regressive disturbances can result);
- Fear of suffering, that creates a protection preventing a complete solution of problems;
- Illness of the will (or decision). But it seems little to apply to AN, since it follows its own plan strictly particularly in the early fasting period stages;
- An alteration of the self-decision/self-confirmation mechanism. A spiritual growth does not follow the decision, as instead the normal dynamism should.
- Lack of freedom. The subject remains a slave to his instincts, at a level of maturation not leaving him to reach the full expression of the spiritual dimension;
- Stopping at the despair, that is to take to extremes a limited objective;
- Taking to extremes the corporal level, as a means of self-affirmation. Narcissistic behaviors result, with contrasts between aggressive features and insecurities;
- Non-identifying of purposes (that means lack of sense);
- An abnormal scale of values.

By combining these elements, all of which are of the spiritual dimension, we can interpret AN in the way presented by Froggio, like a deficiency, or, to be more exact, a disorder into the scale of values and a non-development of the self-transcendence, leading to fall back on one's own body image. So, the disease is on the level of the values.

5. Conclusions

The world of anorexic patients reveals a refusal of the freedom of choice, of the intersubjective dimension, that is to say, the refusal of the specifically human capacity of self-transcendence that results in the pursuit and the fulfillment of a personal plan. These women, instead, seem to be totally fallen back on themselves, on their own subjective world, without the ability to pay the slightest attention to what is all around.

Frankl's theory seems to find in the man an element able to overcome the restrictive analyses of some psychiatric schools. This analysis is actually fascinating for the ones who believe positivist medicine cannot tell the whole truth of man.

References

[1] Lipowski, ZJ. Psychosomatic medicine in the seventies. *Am J Psychiat,* 1977, 134, 233-244.

[2] Fava, GA & Wise, TN. (Editors.). *Research Paradigms in Psychosomatic Medicine.* Basel: Karger, 1987.

[3] Freud, S. The standard edition of the complete psychological works of Sigmund Freud. London: *The Hogart Press-The Institute of Psychoanalysis,* 1955-1974.

[4] Liotti, G. La terapia cognitivo-comportamentale nei disturbi alimentari psicogeni. In, Pancheri, P, editor. *Trattato di medicina psicosomatica,* vol. II, Firenze, USES, 1984, pp. 1083-1102.

[5] Froggio, G. Mangiare. *Libertà o schiavitù. Cinisello Balsamo* (Milano): Edizioni San Paolo, 1997.

[6] Adler, A. *La psicologia individuale.* Newton Compton: Roma, 1970.

[7] Giordano, S. *Understanding eating disorders.* Clarendon Press: Oxford, 2005.

[8] Biswanger, L. *Il caso Ellen West ed altri saggi.* Milano: Bompiani, 1973.

[9] Fizzotti, E. *La logoterapia di Frankl. Un antidoto alla disumanizzazione psicoanalitica.* Milano: Rizzoli, 1974.

[10] Frankl, VE. Logotherapy and Existential Analysis. A Review. *Am. J. Psychother,* 1996, 20, 252-260.

[11] Frankl, VE. Beyond self-actualization and self-expression. *J. Existent,* 1980, 1, 5-20.

[12] Frankl, VE. *Logoterapia e analisi esistenziale.* Original title: Arztliche Șeelsorge, Wien 1948. It. Transl. by Danilo Cargnello. Brescia: Morcelliana, 1953.

[13] Frankl, VE. Alla ricerca di un significato della vita. Original title*: Das Menschenbild der Seelenheilkunde,* Stuttgart 1952. It. Transl. by Eugenio Fizzotti. Milano: Mursia, 1990.

[14] Frankl, VE & Kreuzer, F. In principio era il senso. Original title: *Im Anfang wan der Sinn.* Von der Psychoanalyse zur Logotherapie, Wien 1982. It. Transl. by Claudia Murara. Brescia: Queriniana, 1995.

[15] Frankl, VE. Homo patiens. Original title: *Homo Patiens: Versuch einer Pathodizee,* Wien 1950. It. Transl. by Eugenio Fizzotti. Varese: O.A.RI., 1972.

[16] Casalone, C. *Medicina, macchine, uomini. Brescia:* Morcelliana, 1999.

[17] Neuringer C & Michael C. (editors). *Behavior modification in clinical psychology.* New York: Appleton-Century-Crofts, 1979.

[18] Frankl, VE. Basic concepts of logotherapy. *J. Existent,* 1962, 3: 111-118.
[19] Frankl, VE. *Le radici della logoterapia. Scritti giovanili 1923-1942,* Fizzotti, E (Editor). Roma: Libreria Ateneo Salesiana, 2000.
[20] Frankl, VE. La problematica spirituale della psicoterapia. Original title: Zur geistingen Problematik der Psychotherapie," 1938, from: Frankl, VE. *Le radici della logoterapia.* It. transl. by Fizzotti, E. Roma: LAS, 2000, pp. 115-126.
[21] Frankl, VE. Filosofia e psicoterapia per la fondazione di una analisi esistenziale. Original title: Philosophie und Psychoterapie. *Zur Grundlegung einer Existenzanalyse,* 1999, from: Frankl, VE, *Le radici della logoterapia.* It. transl. by Fizzotti, E. Roma: LAS, 2000, pp. 42-49.
[22] Frankl, VE. Logoterapia. Medicina dell'anima. Original title: *Logotherapie und Existenzanalyse,* Weinheim 1998. It. Transl. by Eugenio Fizzotti, Paola Florioli, Roberto Tonetti. Milano: Gribaudi Editore, 2001.
[23] Frankl, VE. Dynamics, existence and values. *J Existent,* 1961, 2, 5-16.
[24] Frankl, VE The concept of man in logotherapy. *J Existent,* 1965, 6, 53-58.
[25] Frankl, VE. Psicoterapia nella pratica medica. Original title: *Die Psychotherapie in Der Praxis,* Wien 1947. It. Transl. by Bruno Frick. Firenze: Ed.Universitaria, 1953.

SECTION III: PHILOSOPHICAL ASPECTS

In: Anorexia Nervosa: A Multi-Disciplinary Approach ISBN: 978-1-60876-200-2
Editors: A. Mancini, S. Daini, L. Caruana, pp. 161-171

Chapter 10

ANOREXIA NERVOSA: ETHICAL ISSUES

Maria Luisa Di Pietro, Andrea Virdis, Dino Moltisanti
Institute of Bioethics, Catholic University of the Sacred Heart, Rome, Italy

ABSTRACT

This chapter proposes an ethical reading of the complex reality of anorexia nervosa, analyzing both its anthropological aspects and the clinical problems in its treatment. For this purpose, the first part is devoted to highlight the (fully) human meaning of eating, body construction and relationships, considered as a fundamental key to understanding anorexia nervosa. Eating behaviors are considered in their being carriers of sense, and the food refusal as a moral choice, especially in its meaning of protest and self-affirmation. The action of ingesting is linked to its consequences towards the *bodily aspect* and, for this reason, the relationship between *self* and *body* in the construction of self-identity is taken into account. In particular, the personalistic theory—that conceives the person as a single, unified substance, synthesis of body and soul—is given here as a helpful perspective to understand the moral meaning of refusing one's own body, when it is perceived as something different from the person itself. Finally, relationships, as well, are considered in their moral meaning and in their role in causing pathological behaviors, especially, when inappropriate expectations are exercised on someone, causing suffering. In the second part, the ethical problems that arise from the clinical management of anorexia nervosa are taken into account. In particular, this second part deals with the problem of the conflict between the physician's duty to protect life and the absolute respect of the patient's autonomy. Anorexia nervosa is, in fact, a typical example of treatment refusal clearly asserted by the patient: the authors analyze the argument's pros and cons of compulsory treatment, the problems of the evaluation of competence to refuse treatments in a patient with anorexia nervosa, and they propose an integration of the principle of autonomy with the duty of responsibility towards the objective good of life.

1. Introduction

Teenagers and younger children continue to develop eating disorders at an alarming rate (Rome, 2003): eating disorders and, in particular, anorexia nervosa represent nowadays a challenge not only for physicians (involved at the forefront in the treatment of the pathology), but also for parents, educators, and all those who play an important role in helping people—especially teenagers—to build their self and their body image, through several levels of relationship.

Because of the complex connection among biology, psychology and environment in the development of eating disorders, these disorders must be defined within a biopsychosocial context. In fact, far from being just a "medical" problem, anorexia nervosa suggests many aspects of reflection that can be linked to a socio-cultural, anthropological and ethical point of view. Moreover, clinical management of anorexia nervosa raises particular problems that need a specific ethical analysis. For this reason, ethical considerations regarding this matter can be divided into two main chapters: anthropological (and cultural) aspects concerning the interpretation of all the facts that play a key role in the understanding of anorexic behaviors and in their development, maintenance and prevention (*I part*); and ethical problems that concern more directly physicians, patients and clinical ethicists in the treatment of anorexia (*II part*).

2. Anorexia Nervosa: Anthropological and Cultural Aspects

Since the origins of the clinical research, anorexia nervosa has been noticed for its individuality and originality. Anorexia doesn't deal with a simple symptom, but with a syndrome whose objective elements (the behavior of food restriction, the hyperactivity, the neuroendocrine syndrome) are the apparent elements of a deep modification of the mental functioning and of the whole personality.

Up until now, it is still unclear why people develop such an eating disorder: despite increasing awareness of the major eating disorders, a specific etiology for the pathogenesis of anorexia nervosa remains unclear. Some evidences support a genetic predisposition (Gorwood et al., 1998), some others hormonal factors (Støving et al., 2001), while traditional psychological theory has suggested many factors that might lead to the development of the disorder (enmeshment of mother with daughter, father-daughter distancing, teenagers' disliking their changing bodies, etc.). A combination of these issues, plus cultural values and media messages that dictate "thin is beautiful," "fat is bad," or "buff is tough," create a complex environment that predisposes teenagers to develop anorexia (Sigel, 2009). For this reason, rather than a single-factor causal theory, anorexia nervosa is viewed as a multifactorial disorder with the symptom pattern representing a final common pathway (Garner, 1993).

Well aware of the fact that explanations of the causes of anorexia nervosa given by the different studies on the matter are not conclusive, we propose here a reflection on the moral implication related to some elements that compose the frame in which anorexia develops.

This perspective leads us to understand the "facts" of anorexia in a moral way. In other words, here is proposed a reading of the complex reality of the problem not only from a "medical" point of view, but from an anthropological outlook, where the (fully) human meaning of eating, body construction and relationships are pointed out as a fundamental key to understand (and, in some way, to treat) anorexia nervosa. Therefore, we chose a path going through three main issues closely linked among themselves: eating, self identity and (social and family) relationships.

To point out the "cultural" significance of those elements that characterize eating disorders is necessary to make reference, in first place, to the anthropological meaning of food and eating. The understanding of the anorexic behavior should be included within the frame of those behaviors that occupy a wide space in social and cultural life, such as eating. The meaning of eating has a rich variety that goes from the struggle for survival, to fly from the need, and the internal necessity of nourishment, up to the search of gastronomic refinements and to the luxury that they represent. Eating practice, besides representing an answer to a primary need, is placed in an imaginary and symbolic net, introducing—in this way—really human meanings inside the biological need that binds human being to nature and instinct. The human being—as the only being with symbolic ability—interprets and gives new sense to what just partly unites him/her to the animal world. So much so that, when it comes to food, very often, are the eating habits to determine what is felt as a need: in fact, not always what satisfies corresponds to a real need. Alimentary habits, moreover, change in function of economic development, fashion and advertising, but also in function of the awareness of the value that eating—a certain quality and quantity of food—has regarding person's health and life.

Eating, as well, therefore, for man is not just an "act of man," but a "human act."[1]

The eating behaviors are carriers of sense: they testify moral choices (Coveney, 2006), value adhesion or models and means of differentiation, also becoming attributes of identity of individual and groups.[2] Furthermore, it is important to notice how a meal is generally a collective action, an action in which the individual enters into relations with the community. In this sense, let's think about the educational value that the meal context has in family: it is a kind of mediator of the family relationship parent-child. Especially during childhood and adolescence, a meal becomes a modality through which parents bring children up and, in some way, exercise a certain control over them.

It can be observed how, from a symbolic point of view, the anorexic does not "deprive" of its "biological" meaning so much the food itself as the action of eating, to cloak it with purely representative dimension: food refusal—which becomes often clear just at the table—assumes the meaning of becoming an autonomous person as regards parental action. Food refusal can also have a stronger meaning of protest and rebellion. The anorexic image becomes scandalous, but lends itself to change in a heroic figure when a vocation or a social commitment seems to be at the base of such choice. The hunger strike constitutes the last

[1] "Actus autem humanus dicitur qui non quocumque modo in homine vel per hominem exercetur; cum in quibusdam etiam plantae, bruta et homines conveniant; sed qui hominis proprius est. Inter cetera vero hoc habet homo proprium in suo actu, quod sui actus est dominus. Quilibet igitur actus cuius homo dominus est, est proprie *actus humanus*" (Thomas Aquinas, *De virtutibus*, q. 1 a. 4 co.)

[2] When it comes to the symbolic ability of the man towards food and eating, let's consider—for instance—the fact that in all the civilizations, prohibitions, rules, prescriptions, rituals drive, organize and limit the use of the foods.

means of protest and action that an individual has; it testifies the intensity of his/her motivations and his/her sincerity and it represents a means to make the others feel guilty, especially those who have a part of *moral responsibility* in what happens to the subject.

Moreover, the resolute, methodical restriction, carried out with energy, reveals, after all, a changed meaning of the action of ingesting: eating is lived as an intrusion in the bodily integrity of the subject, not eating is the extreme way to affirm oneself.

So, the implicit intentionality in the anorexic behavior is not focused on the imaginary or the symbolic value of the food, but rather on the action of ingesting and on its consequences towards the *bodily aspect*. This leads us to another core aspect for the comprehension of the facts of anorexia nervosa: the relationship between *self* and *body* in the construction of self-identity. As Rebecca J. Lester (1997) pointed out, the traditional medical model often failed to understand this central point of the question. Myopic medical discourses regarding this matter have produced theoretical dichotomies that preclude the successful theorizing of an embodied self and its particular articulation in anorexia nervosa. The inadequacies of the medical point of view—the medicalization of anorexia as a purely biological dysfunction—are found by Lester in the reification of the Cartesian duality of mind and body, which infuses Western culture, continually produced and socially expressed in its institutions. The body in Western philosophy is the non-self, the base material that grounds the self to the worldly plane of existence. The medical model of anorexia reifies this duality by positing a disembodied self, and then attending to either this ephemeral entity or to the malfunctioning form that houses it (Lester, p. 481). The experience of the self is completely eclipsed. The anorexic body is nothing more than a machine in need of repair, and any subjective perceptions of the self housed in the faulty body are invariably "distortions," products of the incorrect processing of data from an external reality and not to be trusted. But in the anorexic person, the refusal, the "attack" of the body has a deeper meaning. Not wanting the body that one *has*, modifying it at any rate, in fact, has the same value of not wanting to be the one whom a person *is* (Brusset, 1977, p. 15).

This becomes clear from the point of view of personalism, where the human person is conceived as a single, unified substance, a dynamic whole that is the synthesis of body and soul (Sgreccia, 2007). The human person is an incarnate ego, a spiritual being that is unified to the corporeity, which, in turn, is pervaded by the ego and thus spiritualized. The human person is constituted as an "embodied self" or an "acting person" whose body, mind, and soul are integrally connected forming an *individuality* (male or female) and, therefore, wholly affected when it comes to healthcare matters.

In the construction of self, so, all the person is involved (body, mind and soul), and when this construction of self is "affected" in some way, all the aspects of the person are called into question. Furthermore, the construction of self-identity is always a gender (male or female) construction. And with regard to this, it is worth notice that the body the anorexic woman wants to destroy is a *female* body. Many anorexics consider this denial of corporeality as a "male" way of thinking and acting, where the power over the body (exerted through starvation and excessive body training) is seen as the conquering and destroying of their own "weak and detestable" femininity. "Denial of the body is both a philosophical attitude and painful daily practice, which makes them feel stronger, more in control, less vulnerable" (Lester, p. 484).

With regards to this question, from a cultural point of view, it must be noted that the modern interpretation of the relationship self-identity and body, derived from Lacan's,

Derrida's and Focault's post-structuralism, can also contribute to give a certain reading of anorexia. Starting from their idea of the subject viewed just as a product of the discourse, irreducible to any form of identity and able to become other from what it is, the *gender* ideology has affirmed that not only to be man or woman is a "unsettled" reality, but also the body is an entity that can be constructed, as a scientific and aesthetical artifice. And if the gender is just a choice of the subject, also the body—not more "material"—can be deconstructed and built to the point of being useless and, therefore, destructible (Butler, 1990).

Some scholars have observed how the alteration of the relationships of the anorexic adolescent with her own body is the epiphenomenon of a wider conflict: the body itself, perceived as something different from the person, becomes the center of this conflict and the privileged object of both the aggressive attacks and a "narcissistic" claim.

Clinical and sociological studies searching for an explanation of the causes of eating disorders in the relational system (family and society) in which they mainly occur consider relationship as well an important element to be taken into account (Brusset, 1977). There is a certain agreement among them in the consideration that eating disorders are not only the result of a dysfunction *within* the person, or the symptoms of an internal dysfunctional balance, but are significantly linked to the *relationships* that take place in the family and in society. The person who develops anorexia is often overwhelmed by familial and social pressures, and the developing of the syndrome especially would be due to confront these expectations, coping with this type of pressures, and thus to obtain power and control over the surrounding environment as well as over her life. S. Giordano (2003a) proposed recently a re-thinking of relationships in a moral way as a possible explanation of causes of anorexia nervosa, according to the idea that a moral logic, that is a way of thinking of interpersonal relations in moral terms, gives shape to and justifies the clinical condition, and finds consistent expression in abnormal eating behavior. The explanation given by Giordano appears to be original and very interesting from an ethical point of view. She claims that there are deeper reasons that explain why the inappropriate expectations that others have of us should cause us suffering, and these reasons are moral in nature. There are two senses in which we may "suffer" in these cases: one is that we may "feel bad" about being unable to fulfill these expectations, the other is that we see in these expectations a lack of understanding of us ("if they really understood and accepted me, they would not expect this of me"). In both cases, we seem to think that a moral wrong is involved in the disappointment. If we perceive ourselves as the ones who disappoint, we feel guilty. If we perceive ourselves as the ones who are being disappointed ("they should not expect that of us"), then they are the ones who should feel guilty. The person who suffers because "she is disappointing" someone has thus accepted and absorbed a way of thinking, according to which disappointing is something one should feel bad about. But, according to the same logic, those who raise too high expectations also disappoint that person by raising demands that reveal failure to understand and accept the person's inclinations and needs. This way of thinking is called by Giordano moral logic. Within the systems in which interactions are articulated around the dynamics "expectations-disappointments," such as the eating disordered systems, it is inappropriate to talk about persecutors, on the one hand, and victims, on the other, as if they were two groups that confront each other. Both play both roles.

The anorexic, therefore, communicates messages of universal significance: displaying the signs of the consumption, and through the image of the destruction, she solicits the sense of guilt. As an innocent victim, she accuses her executioners with all the strength that the innocent derives from being "punished;" the author of his/her own destruction offers his/her own image weak and strong at the same time. But what is more clearly specific of anorexia nervosa refers to the fact that the destruction is "simply" bodily and appears to the subject as the condition for his/her own personal survival, condition for the maintenance of his/her own value, of the possibility to be loved and of his/her own integrity and identity.

Regarding the issue of body image and expectations, there is an other aspect, typical of our day, that has moral relevance, especially in the prevention of anorexia. In the end of this first part, we also want to mention briefly the problem linked to the role of the media in providing a social context within which eating disorders flourish (and in the etiology of eating disorder symptoms) (Spettigue, 2004) and influence that the media has on body image of children and adolescents (Lawrie, 2006) and on female body satisfaction (Pinhas, 1999).

Although the explanation of the origin of anorexia nervosa in the media messages has been refused as considered too simplistic, there is a certain agreement in considering the ideal of thinness that the media perpetuates as an important element in creating a cultural mentality where there is a negative stigma associated with being overweight, and, therefore, in favoring some condition in which anorexia nervosa can develop.

Body image is an important part of a person's self-concept and body dissatisfaction: not surprisingly, therefore, sociocultural and environmental factors as they relate to ideal body shape are thought to play an important role in the development of eating disorders. Reports of anorexia nervosa are more common in industrialized nations where food is plentiful and where thinness for women is correlated with attractiveness (Rome, 2003). In this regard, the media holds a strong power to influence young women, bombarding them with images of abnormally thin models who seem to represent the ideal. So, when it comes to the role of society in this field, it must be noticed that being aware of the potentially armful impact on conditioning self-perception in people is a first and important step towards a global prevention of those factors that can favor the development of anorexia. A particular attention should be devoted as well to the sly phenomenon of the "pro-ana" community especially developed in the web, where websites espouse anorexia and other eating disorders as a "lifestyle choice" (Atkins, 2002), giving outcome to some phenomena of emulation.

3. Anorexia Nervosa: Clinical and Ethical Aspects

When confronted with anorexia nervosa, the physician can be torn between his professional conscience that is based on the duty to protect life and the law that demands absolute respect of the patient's autonomy. In fact, anorexia nervosa is a typical example of where there exists a refusal of treatments clearly asserted by the patient. The conflict in this case takes place between two principles of the Anglo-Saxon bioethics: the principle of benevolence and the principle of autonomy. The theory of the respect of autonomy stresses the liberty of the individual and imposes on physician the moral duty to respect the patient's self-determination. In this way, a patient with such capacity has the right to refuse any—even life-saving—treatment. In the approach of benevolence, a physician may act to maximize benefits and goods, even if this might demand acting without the patient's consent.

The use of treatment without consent and the management of treatment refusal are particularly contentious in anorexia nervosa. For example, the force-feeding is in the anorexic patient's best interest because it will keep the patient alive and may help to restore her to a sufficient state of health to engage in other therapies (psychological therapies) necessary to combat anorexia nervosa (Hebert, Weingarten, 2006). So, in the face of treatment refusal, should a compulsory treatment be justified if the treatment is in the patient's best interest?

According to some authors (Tan et al., 2006), there are two arguments against compulsory treatment. One argument is that it is harder, if not impossible, to engage patients in psychological therapies if their treatment is compulsory. The second argument is that re-feeding unwilling patients may lead to short-term weight gain but is ineffective in the long run. But even if the efficacy of compulsory treatment is demonstrated, there remains the ethical issue as to whether or in what circumstances it is justifiable to impose compulsory treatment for a patient with anorexia nervosa.

However, the point at issue is another. Do we consider the anorexic patient competent? Is the anorexic patient's consent valid? The issue of competence is an important and crucial factor in determining when it is generally justified to enforce a treatment on a patient. A person may be able to make a competent decision at one time but not at another, or may at the same time be able to make a decision but not another one. What does "competence" mean?

According to Grisso and Appelbaum (1995), we can speak about competence through the notion of "appreciation." Appreciation means that the patient not only understands the relevant facts but also appreciates that those facts apply to him/her. These authors provide three criteria in judging if patient's appreciation capacity lacks: 1. the patient's belief must be irrational, unrealistic or a considerable distortion of reality; 2 the belief must be the consequence of impaired cognition or affect; 3. the belief must be relevant to the treatment decision.

Buchanan and Brock (1986) think that a competent decision-maker also requires—in addition to the abilities to understand, communicate, reason and deliberate—a set of values or a conception of the good that is at least minimally consistent, stable and affirmed as his/her own. They introduce two important concepts additional to the legal analyses of competence: values and stability of views. This approach derives from the interest in the role of values in rationality (Charland, 2001) and in the "internal rationality." Internal rationality is achieved when a putative decision coheres with an individual's aims and values, it is justified in the light of these values and the proposed justification is deemed appropriate by the third party responsible for assessing competence.

Tan et al. (2006) evidence the difference between so called "factual belief" and "salient belief." Factual beliefs are those beliefs about objective (medical) facts, i.e., the effects on health of severe weight loss. Salient beliefs are beliefs about whether the facts apply to oneself and are the same as Grisso and Appelbaum's concept of appreciation.

Determining whether a patient with anorexia nervosa has capacity, however, is not simple. The problem is assessing if the refusal of treatment formulated by her comes from a decision made in the full understanding and acceptance of the consequences, or if it's the "voice" of disease that is speaking through her (Tan 2003). If the competency includes the following elements—*1.* the subject understands the information; *2.* he/she retains the fact given to him/her; *3.* he/she applies them to his/her decision; *4.* she communicates her choice to the physician— we can conclude that an anorexic patient is perfectly competent. In fact, she is in a position to receive, understand, integrate the information and to give her decision.

But, with regard to clinical studies of anorexia nervosa, cognitive psychology has specially focused on the information process leading to eating disordered behavior and has shown that this process appears dysfunctional at all levels: perception of the input of information, interpretation, decision-making process and output. For example, the interpretation of information is also distorted: "You look good, today" is typically interpreted as "You have put on weight" (Giordano, 2003b). The use of information about food is also dysfunctional. Although people with eating disorders are typically very well informed about food, they seem unable to apply this information. Their capacity to make medical decisions may be affected by fears of obesity or denial of the consequences of actions.

In fact, the study of Tan et al. (2006) demonstrates that competence to refuse treatment may be compromised in people with anorexia nervosa for two reasons: difficulties with thought processing and changes in values. In fact, there are difficulties with concentration, muddled thinking, ambiguity of belief and external influences. Anorexia nervosa can affect thinking in ways that have impact on decision-making about treatment and on competence; i.e., the anorexic patient believes that severe weight loss is dangerous but does not believe that such danger applies to herself. These convictions bring her, depending on the stage of the disease, to deny the possibility of death or to accept it or even desire it. In fact, she may correctly believe that people at her weight are at high risk of serious harm (factual belief) and accept, at least at times, that she may be at risk, but have difficulty in taking such risk seriously when thinking about the need for treatment.

These ambiguities with salient belief are rooted in the experience of anorexia nervosa, which appears to normalize the experience and perception of extreme weight loss and its accompanying decision-making, despite understanding and believing them. And so when making their decision, they could be found incompetent using the usual legal criteria. They are not able to weigh up the key facts in coming decision.

Is the criteria of values sufficient for evaluating competency? The respect for individual autònomy and the freedom to pursue one's life according to one's own values without interference from others are important aspects. But, is it the same when the patient suffers from a mental disorder? Are these values pathological? Does the concept of pathological values, linked to mental disorder, enable such values to be distinguished from the unreasonable, unusual or bizarre values that people are fully entitled to hold, and often do hold, in the course of everyday life?

The physician can wonder whether such a turnaround in the patient's scale of values is not purely and simple distorted by the disease. In other words: are the pathological values "caused by mental disorder?" If a value or a value system can be determined to arise from a mental disorder, then it should be "pathological" and, if this value is determinative of particular decisions, then such decisions are not competent. And if such decisions would lead to significant risk of harm, then it is legitimate to override them in the interests of the patient. There would be even stronger reasons for considering that the values are "pathological" if there were evidence that the person did not hold these values before suffering from the anorexia nervosa; or if the strength with which these values are held fluctuates with fluctuation in the severity of the anorexia nervosa.

According to Tan et al. (2006), from a theoretical point of view, it is insufficient to base incompetence solely on the fact that a value that plays a key role in the decision is caused by, or part of, a mental disorder. Some of the reasons why a patient with anorexia nervosa refuses treatment are not attributable to pathological values. So, even if her decision to refuse treatment can appear unreasonable, the anorexic remains "competent" for a very long time to receive information concerning her state of health and to make up her own mind about what to do next. She may be unable to manage with food; however, she may still be able to decide that she is no longer willing to live under conditions such as these. She may, therefore, be incompetent at the level of diet management but competent at the level of medical decisions. At this level, in fact, she may possess all necessary information about herself and the quality of her life and may use it to take a choice. It may be on the grounds of her considerations about herself and the quality of her life that she may refuse therapy. But should her refusal of treatment be respected?

According to Draper (2000), the refusal of force-feeding under some circumstances should be respected because in these cases—even if the anorexic patient will die because of lack of nutrition—it is not a request for euthanasia. The cause of this affirmation is the paradoxical distinction between passive euthanasia and refusal of treatment (Giordano, 2003b), but the refusal of re-feeding closely resembles passive euthanasia: the doctor is requested to withhold a procedure with the consequence that the patient will die. Moreover, the condition and the death of anorexic patient are avoidable, and physical complications are reversible. We can avoid that she dies simple by feeding her. In this case, does the principle of autonomy preserve intact all its strength? The principle of autonomy stresses that when a competent patient refuses therapy, physicians are ethically and legally bound to accept this refusal. But the fact that the death for anorexia is unavoidable and the physical problems reversible, means that, even if the anorexic patient is making a competent decision, it may not be sufficient to bind physicians to respect refusal of life-saving therapy.

In conclusion, even if there are good reasons why the legal approach to competence focuses on intellectual abilities and eschews a consideration of patient's values (Vialettes et al., 2006), we cannot neglect the effects of a mental disease and the situation characterized by absolute denial of the illness and the refusal to recognize the least seriousness or an eventual risk associated with her condition.

The defence of the physical life is, indeed, priority to the respect of the autonomy, because it is the base of the exercise of autonomy itself. For this reason, it is unacceptable for both the patient bringing damage to her own life and the physician failing in his/her duty to protect the life and the health of an individual who relies upon his/her care, accepting in a passive way, her destructive will. It is, then, necessary to integrate the principle of respect of the autonomy with the duty of responsibility both of the patient and the physician towards the objective good of life. Accordingly, in the face of life-saving treatment refusal, the physician has the duty to seek to obtain the patient's consent but, if he/she doesn't succeed in getting it, he/she has to feel him/herself within the moral obligation to give the patient all the necessary treatments. This is, unfortunately, possible just in the presence of a state of necessity—e.g., the patient has lost consciousness—or in a state of incapacity due to a pre-existing mental disease or to a psychic infirmity caused by the extended fast. However, it is not correct to limit oneself to intervene only under conditions of urgency or state of extreme clinical gravity. It is necessary, instead, that all efforts are made to establish with the anorexic patient a therapeutic relationship with the purpose of helping her to objectively consider her condition and to manage in responsible way her own health, not only in terms of diet and physical exercise (Giordano, 2003c), but also in terms of internal serenity and joy of living.

References

Atkins, L. It's better to be thin and dead than fat and living. *The Guardian*, 2002, July 23. Retrieved 10 March, 2009, from http://www.guardian.co.uk.

Brusset, B. L'Assiette et le miroir. *L'anorexie mentale de L'enfant et de l'adolescent*. Touluse: Privat; 1977.

Buchanan, A.; Brock, DW. *Deciding for others*. Milbank Q., 1986 64 (Suppl. 2), 17-94.

Butler, J. *Gender Trouble: Feminism and the Subversion of Identity*. New York: Routledge, 1990.

Charland, LCE. Mental competence and value: The problem of normativity in the assessment of decision-making capacity. *Psychiatry, Psychology and Law*, 2001 8 (2), 135-145.

Coveney, J. Food, morals and meaning. London: Routledge; 2006

Draper, H. Anorexia nervosa and respecting a refusal of life-prolonging therapy: a limited justification. *Bioethics*, 2000 14, 120.133.

Garner, DM. Pathogenesis of anorexia nervosa. *Lancet*, 1993 341 (8861), 1631-1635.

Giordano, S. Persecutors or Victims? The Moral Logic at the Heart of Eating Disorders. *Health Care Analysis*, 2003a 11 (3): 219-228.

Giordano, S. Anorexia nervosa and refusal of naso-gastric treatment: a response to Haether Draper. *Bioethics*, 2003b 13 (3), 261-278.

Giordano, S. Risk and supervised exercise: the example of anorexia to illustrate a new ethical issue in the traditional debates of medical ethics. *J Med Ethics*, 2003c 31, 15-20.

Gorwood, P; Bouvard, M; Mouren-Siméoni, MC; Kipman, A; Adès, J. Genetics and anorexia nervosa: a review of candidate genes. *Psychiatr Genet.*, 1998 8 (1), 1-12.

Grisso, T; Appelbaum, PS. Comparison of standards for assessing patients' capacities to make treatment decisions. *Am J Psychiatry*, 1995 152 (7), 1033-1037.

Hebert, PC; Weingarten, MA. The ethics of forced feeding in anorexia nervosa. *CMAJ*, 1991 144 (2), 141-144.

Lawrie, Z; Sullivan, EA; Davies, PSW; Hill, RJ. Media influence on the body image of children and adolescents. *Eating disorders*, 2006 14 (5), 355-364.

Lester, RJ. The (dis)embodied self in anorexia nervosa. *Soc Sci Med.*, 1997 44 (4), 479-489.

Pinhas, L; Toner, B; Ali, A; Garfinkel, P; Stuckless, N. The effects of the ideal of female beauty on mood and body satisfaction. *International Journal of Eating Disorders*, 1999 25: 223-226.

Rome, E; Ammerman, S; Rosen, D; Keller, R; Lock, J; Mammal, K; O'Toole, J; Rees, J; Sanders, M; Schneider, M; Sigel, E; Silber, T. Children and Adolescents With Eating Disorders: the State of the Art. *Pediatrics*, 2003 111 (1), e98-e108.

Sgreccia, E. *Manuale di bioetica. I. Aspetti Fondamenti ed etica biomedica*. Milano: Vita e Pensiero; 2007.

Sigel, ED., Eating disorders. In: Hay WW, Hayward AR, Levin MJ, Sondheimer JM (Eds). *Current Diagnosis & Treatment: Pediatrics*, USA: McGraw-Hill Professional; 2002; 162-171

Spettigue, W; Henderson, KA. Eating Disorders and the Role of the Media. *Can Child Adolesc Psychiatr Rev.*, 2004 13 (1), 16–19.

Støving, RK; Hangaard, J; Hagen, C. Update on endocrine disturbances in anorexia nervosa. *J Pediatr Endocrinol Metab.*, 2001 14 (5), 459-480.

Tan, JOA; Hope, T; Stewart, A.; Fitzpatrick R. Competence to make treatment decisions in anorexia nervosa: thinking processes and values. *Plilos Psychiatr Psychol,* 2006 13 (4), 265-282.

Tan, J. The anorexia talking?. *Lancet,* 2003 362, 1246 (letter).

Vialettes, B; Samuelian-Massat, C; Valéro, R; Béliard, S. The refusal of treatment in anorexia nervosa, an ethical conflict with three characters: "the girl, the family and the medical profession." *Diabetes Metab.,* 2006 32, 306-311.

In: Anorexia Nervosa: A Multi-Disciplinary Approach ISBN: 978-1-60876-200-2
Editors: A. Mancini, S. Daini, L. Caruana, pp. 173-186

Chapter 11

SOMATIC SEMANTICS: ANOREXIA AND THE NATURE OF MEANING

Louis Caruana
Department of Philosophy, Heythrop College University of London, UK.

ABSTRACT

This paper explores some ways that perceptual-cognitive accounts of anorexia can benefit from philosophy. The first section focuses on the three dimensions of anorexia most open to a contribution from philosophy: the dimensions of language, perception and cognition. In the second section, I offer a brief overview of what philosophy has to say regarding these dimensions, especially as they relate to two crucial issues: introspection and meaning. I draw from current philosophy of language, especially from the arguments against using internal perception as a model for the way we express our own bodily states. I draw also from current philosophy of interpretation, especially from debates concerning the criteria for handling dialogical misunderstanding. I use these insights to expose some dangers in assuming and working with oversimplified accounts of introspection and meaning. I then suggest refined and updated accounts and examine their applicability and usefulness in the diagnosis and treatment of anorexia.

1. INTRODUCTION

For the diagnosis and treatment of a disease or disorder, the patient's own beliefs about his or her situation are important. This is especially true for anorexia nervosa. Self-induced weight loss, extreme fear of becoming fat, and an insistent pursuit of thinness occur together with a denial of feelings of hunger and a distortion of the patient's own view of her body.[1] In

[1] In this paper, I will be referring to the anorexicanorexic anorexic person as female, but what will be discussed is equally applicable to males. There is an incidence of around 10% males affected, and it appears that this percentage is increasing.

all this, language and interpretation play a central role. Historical records show that even the earliest descriptions of this disorder refer to its elusive and multidimensional nature. In descriptions of medieval fasting saints, the symptoms were recorded as acknowledged signs of sainthood. The cultural and religious context of those times supported this view. In more recent descriptions, from the eighteenth century onwards, the physical aspects of the diagnosis become progressively more and more dislodged from the patient's cultural context. The basic assumption in such relatively recent developments was that medical science needs to disregard the useless cultural coverings so as to arrive at the deeper objective reality of the disorder. This assumption, however, underestimates the essential role in this disorder of language, society and culture. It is wrong to think that the real nature of anorexia lies in biology. Its essential roots lie in society and culture, as well. Keep the same biological characteristics, change the cultural context, and you may end up with a different disorder. Some current studies, in fact, have no problem with claiming that the medieval fasting saints were simply not suffering from the same disorder that anorexics suffer from today. Joan Jacobs Brumberg, for instance, insists that the medieval kind of anorexia, *anorexia mirabilis*, is not the same as *anorexia nervosa*. She gives a warning: "to insist that medieval holy women had anorexia nervosa is, ultimately, a reductionist argument because it converts a complex human behavior into a simple biomedical mechanism. (It certainly does not respect important differences in the route to anorexia.) To conflate the two is to ignore the cultural context and the distinction between sainthood and patienthood" (Brumberg 2000, p. 46). Without getting entangled within the question of which roots are more important, the biological or the cultural, we can at least secure the point that the cultural context for this particular disorder makes a big difference. Anorexia is not all biological. We are dealing with a multidimensional disorder involving biological, psychological, linguistic and cultural issues. The disorder seems to arise because of some particular interaction among these various factors.

Philosophy deals with many topics. Prominent among these are two questions: the question of meaning and the question of interpretation. The diagnosis and treatment of anorexia nervosa is crucially dependent on the meaning of what is said by the patient. It is dependent also on interpretation: the interpretation made by the anorexic about herself and the interpretation that others make of her condition. Because of this, philosophical insights that come from the area of semantic theory can be very helpful. This is especially true for the approach to anorexia that highlights perception, cognition and interpretation. The basic question that will be guiding this inquiry, therefore, can be expressed as follows: how can those who adopt perceptual-cognitive accounts of anorexia benefit from philosophy? In the first section, I will try to determine some major philosophically significant areas in the existing diagnosis and therapy of anorexia. The following section will contain a philosophical evaluation of these areas, an evaluation with the aim of detecting and eventually reducing possible conceptual confusion. In the final section, then, I will address directly the question of what semantic theory can offer in this area, and will conclude with some proposals for further research.

2. PHILOSOPHICAL ISSUES IN ANOREXIA

Many researchers have been aware of the fact that anorexia shows a dependence on semantic, linguistic and cultural factors more than the average dependence one expects for other disorders. One simply cannot avoid studying anorexia via different models of explanation. Following the Brumberg's historical study, let me briefly recall the three major theoretical models employed here: the biological, the psychological and the cultural models. The fact that no one of these models is expected to yield anything better than a partial account shows how complex this disorder is. We are not dealing with easily identifiable causal links. Even cases showing the same symptoms have, in all probability, different causal histories. Anorexia is a clear reminder that some disorders aren't just a physical malfunction. One very often needs to take into consideration a complex interaction of physical state and social perception.

The first model for anorexia is the biomedical model, which involves the empirically accessible data. This model depends on the classic methodological principles analyzed and discussed in philosophy of science. Evidence is collected, some variables are recognized as mutually independent, and then correlations are determined among them. The disorder is then assumed to be totally or very adequately described by these correlations. On this assumption, treatment is devised in terms of the causal chains described in the model. For anorexia, this model is useful but limited. Among other things, it cannot distinguish—or hasn't yet been able to distinguish—between which comes first: hormonal imbalance or starvation. It hasn't any convincing account of why young women are the primary patients. Moreover, this model is blind to the obvious social characteristics of anorexics: they are not found everywhere. They are found among the middle and upper social classes in developed countries in the West and Japan.

The psychological model tries to bring in more than just body-chemistry. It is best seen as a family of related models rather than one monolithic account. These related models derive from psychoanalysis, family systems-theory and social psychology. In the first two, anorexia is seen as a pathological response to the developmental crisis of adolescence. As such, these two approaches focus exclusively on the individual patient. They do not directly consider the effect of the surroundings on the anorexic. So these approaches suffer from incompleteness for the same reasons mentioned above regarding the biomedical model. Models inspired by social psychology are better equipped to include the broader context of this disorder. Since they take perceptual and cognitive disturbances as the main cause of anorexia, they seem robust enough to handle the social and cultural dimension. They do this on the condition that perception and cognition are not considered apart from the community of communicators to which the anorexic belongs. More on this later.

The third model is the cultural model. In this view, anorexia is caused by the powerful cultural obligation insisting that slimness sets the standard for female beauty. This model departs considerably from the biomedical approach. Jennifer Church, for instance, argues that anorexia is not only culture-dependent but also, in some real sense, socially constructed. This doesn't mean, she adds, that the regularities involved in anorexia are not worth studying (Church 2004). It means that they are socially constructed regularities that are more important than clinical studies. This approach is promising because it deals directly with the complex, cultural background of the anorexic. Nevertheless, it still suffers from incompleteness.

Brumberg recalls that, from all the women exposed to the same cultural pressure regarding the importance of being slim, only a few develop the symptoms. Why do cultural imperatives have different effects on similarly situated individuals? There is something going on, therefore, other than direct social or cultural causation.[2]

So what can be learned from this brief sketch of the models used so far? We can retain at least one thing: the physical aspect of the disturbance experienced by the anorexic cannot be detached from the reality of language. Social, cultural and family pressures arise from the way the anorexic, as a person, is perceived by society. This perception cannot be detached from the language in which it is expressed. Moreover, even the anorexic's self-interpretation has a linguistic dimension to it. I will proceed, therefore, by focusing on language and its relation to perception and cognition.

Language

What do anorexics say? Although historical accounts of severe non-eating go all the way back to the Middle Ages, they are unfortunately superficial. They are records of how people saw the anorexic, not how the anorexic saw herself. They do not supply the anorexics' own words. Only in recent times, as medical science gained more respect, were physical diagnosis and somatic treatment recorded together with what the anorexic said about herself. This new kind of evidence tended to make the diagnosis somewhat easy. Because of the anorexic's own evaluation of her condition, biomedical reasons were undermined. What the anorexic said indicated very often that there was no real disorder at all. If you don't eat, you starve. That is clear. So attention was drawn elsewhere. People started seeking the reasons behind the anorexic's unwillingness to eat. Brumberg records some examples from the late 1800s. One anorexic was reported to have refused food "on account of her mother talking to her about being so fat." Another refused food because of a "fear of being seen as a bit heavy." And another stopped eating when she "got the idea that she was too fat after seeing her friends forcing themselves to lose weight" (Brumberg 2000, p. 165). Are these reasons to be taken at face value? In other words, should those engaged in diagnosis and treatment assume that what anorexics say is always true? This point, of course, is not valid only for cases from the distant past. Brumberg, writing in 2000, reported that, among women aged eighteen to thirty-five, 75% regarded themselves as fat even though only 25% were overweight (Brumberg 2000, p. 204). What does this show? Is this a distortion in the perception of oneself or a distortion in the meaning of the word "fat"?

We have, here, an indication of the possibility of semantic distortion or alteration. I want to highlight this point because, in my view, it is the crucial area where philosophy can make a contribution to research on anorexia. The semantic or interpretative alteration I'm referring to is not a shift, on the part of the anorexic, from rational thought to irrational non-sense. It is rather a shift from acceptable rationality to another kind of rationality. There is evidence, at least in some cases, that the anorexic is engaged in reaping some benefits from her condition. She is engaged in non-eating not aimlessly but with a purpose. For instance, according to

[2] For more on cultural and historical accounts of anorexia as a disorder primarily of westernized societies, see: Bemporad (1997) and Bordo (1985-6). Self-destruction, in general, is a very complex affair. It involves social, cultural, psychiatric, psychological, and clinical dimensions. Even for self-destructive tendencies in general, no one dimension should be studied without reference to the others. See Walters (1999).

Brumberg, a typical anorexic of today's culture would often say: "I don't like it when other girls are skinny" (Brumberg 2000, p. 256). The implication here is that the anorexic is coveting the title of "skinny." Such anorexics, therefore, consider themselves engaged in a competition involving the body. They use their bodies to show their success, their endurance, their self-control, their will-power. Their identities are at stake. They are always on the look out to see what is happening not only to their own bodies but also to the bodies of others. Like school children, they want to know what grades they are getting and what grades their companions are getting so as to know where they stand with respect to others. Their aim is to shine, and their means is anorexia.[3]

I take this point about the utility of anorexia to the anorexic as showing that the semantic distortion evident in the anorexic's way of expressing herself should not be seen as an abandonment of logical reasoning. Other interpretations are at work. Any account of anorexia should not underestimate the importance of this point. I move on now to the second and third dimensions, which I will consider together.

Perception and Cognition

A lot of work has already been done in the area of the perceptual-cognitive model of anorexia. Paul Garfinkel and David Garner offer a useful overview of this work in their book *Anorexia Nervosa: a multidimensional perspective*.[4] They adopt a tripartite perceptual-cognitive model, according to which anorexics suffer from the following disturbances in perception and cognition: an inability to perceive the problems with one's own body (body image disturbances); an inability to accurately identify internal sensations such as hunger, or affective states (interoceptive disturbances); and an overwhelming sense of personal ineffectiveness.[5] My contention here is that each of these parts of the model is immersed within important philosophical issues that need to be clarified before further headway can be made in empirical research. Let's consider each part in turn.

Body-image disturbances are often clinically manifested as lack of concern about, or persistent defense of, an emaciated shape. This is not just inability to assess one's own size or weight accurately. It involves, as well, a disturbed attitude towards one's own body in general. A possible theoretical explanation has been proposed for this. The anorexic is trying to avoid biological maturity; this happens in the case of vulnerable adolescents when they cannot face the demands and trouble of adulthood. One can readily notice how, in this view, the question about body-image is being linked to the patient's overall life story. The assumption is, therefore, that the anorexic's relation to her shape cannot be assessed without some idea of her relation to her life story, and this, in turn, cannot be assessed properly without some idea of her relation to her situation in society. The expressed beliefs of the anorexic, distorted as they may be, have a meaning in relation to her other beliefs, those that remain unexpressed, beliefs like those concerning adulthood and social responsibility. This is

[3] For more similar case-studies see Bruch (1978). The anorexicanorexic anorexic may, of course, start with the idea of anorexia as useful and then discover that she had made a mistake; see Hondros & Caroline (2004).

[4] Garfinkel & Garner (1982). See especially chapter 6, entitled *Perceptual and Cognitive Disturbances*.

[5] Garfinkel and Garner are following Hilde Bruch's distinctions, which she had developed in Bruch (1961) and Bruch (1962).

where philosophy comes in. Philosophical analysis of how meaning is related to networks of beliefs rather than to just one isolated belief is crucial.

The second part of the perceptual-cognitive model involves distortions in internal perceptions. For anorexia, the crucial point is hunger-awareness. According to Garfinkel and Garner, hunger-awareness is a matter of perception and cognition. It is something established in early childhood. In normal circumstances, it is established when the mother's reaction to the young child's lack of food corresponds well to the child's actual experience. Perceptual-cognitive confusion arises when, during the crucial learning stage, there is a difference between child and mother. It arises when the time when the child is experiencing food deprivation doesn't correspond to the time when the mother *thinks* the child is experiencing food deprivation. If what the mother thinks the child is experiencing is different from what the child is actually experiencing, then the child doesn't learn well. Those who adopt the perceptual-cognitive model consider this mechanism the main origin of anorexia. But is this kind of reasoning plausible? Embedded within this model, there is a hidden philosophical assumption; and because it is philosophical, it needs to be evaluated through philosophical analysis. The assumption is that internal perceptions function exactly like external perceptions: just as I see the physical objects in front of me, and thereby gain knowledge of them, so also I can see the objects within me, such as my body, and thereby gain knowledge of them. The child is seeing her own body-image from inside, the mother from outside. But there is difficulty here. This assumption is essentially splitting the single individual anorexic into two parts, the internal observer and the internal observed. Is the individual one, or two? Further philosophical analysis is needed to see whether there is here a potential source of confusion.

The third part of this model involves conceptual disturbances. Anorexics have persistent distorted attitudes not only with regard to their body shape, but also with regard to more general attitudes that "seem to affect almost every area of their lives" (Garfinkel & Garner 1982, p. 155). Research has highlighted some of the types of conceptual error involved here. These types include (a) selective abstraction (e.g., "I am special if I am thin"); (b) magnification (e.g., "Gaining five pounds would push me over the brink"); (c) all-or-nothing reasoning (e.g., "If I gain one pound, I'll go on and gain a hundred pounds"); (d) superstitious thinking (e.g., "If I eat a sweet, it will be converted instantly into stomach fat").[6] Anorexics slide into such distorted views of their lives because they assume that weight, shape or thinness can serve as the sole or the predominant basis for inferring self-worth. Moreover, they assume that complete self-control is necessary, and that "absolute certainty" is needed in making decisions. This is where the model leaves us. The philosophical issue underlying this aspect should by now be clear. It is the same issue as the one mentioned with respect to the body-image disturbance. Do the words being used by anorexics mean the same as the same words used by non-pathological people? Researchers would profit from a clearer idea of what constitutes the meaning of assertions and of thinking patterns. What lies in the background is the philosophical question of holism of meaning.

So let me gather the insights gained in these last paragraphs. My first idea was to seek those aspects of the diagnosis and treatment of anorexia that are most open to a possible contribution from philosophy. So I concentrated on language, perception and cognition. Reflecting on language, I concluded that the crucial question of meaning is unavoidable.

[6] Examples are taken from Garfinkel & Garner (1982), p. 157.

Considering then the perceptual-cognitive model of anorexia, I argued that each part of this model is also intimately related to, and even perhaps dependent upon, philosophical issues such as the debate on the multiple-self view of the person, and the debate on holism of meaning. These are the areas, hence, that need further elaboration.

3. A Philosophical Evaluation of Two Crucial Points

We start with the multiple-self view of the person, in its relation to introspection. About 400 years ago, René Descartes launched a new way of doing philosophy that is still with us today. It underlies, in some form or other, much empirical research in current psychology and neuroscience. His views on knowledge and introspection influenced John Locke and gave rise to the idea that introspection should be understood on the model of perception. Just as we perceive things outside of us, like mountains and trees, so also, when we turn our attention inwards, we perceive things inside us, like bodily states, emotions and even thoughts. For Descartes, the self, or the "I," is entirely distinct from the body. So the perception model of introspection is very suitable. We should recall that this is a particular view of the self, one view among possible others. The self eventually came to be seen as an observer who appreciates life as things come in, and eventually move out, of its perceptual field. Life is like a theater with the self watching everything, including all internal states, without itself being watched. There is an inner world and an outer world. I share the outer world with others. They can see what I see. With regard to the inner world, however, I am in a privileged position. Others may get hints of what's going on in my inner world. But there is no comparison between what they can deduce and what I can know about my inner world.[7] Their knowledge of my inner world is fallible. Mine is infallible.

Although this Cartesian view is still assumed to be true by many empirical researchers, many philosophers have identified serious flaws in it. It is founded on an analogy between two human abilities. On the one hand, we have the ability to speak about what we see and about what we hear. We do this because we perceive or observe what is around us. We describe. On the other hand, we have the ability to speak about what we feel, what we think and what we intend. The analogy prompts us to say that the second ability functions like the first. It prompts us to say that the second ability involves description as well. So we say that, in introspection, we perceive inner things. The similarity between these two abilities, however, is too poor to make the analogy useful. One ability involves senses; the other doesn't. We have no internal senses that correspond to our external senses. If we had, the analogy would have functioned well. But since we haven't an inner-eye or an inner-ear, we are not entitled to stretch the analogy too much. We cannot depend on the analogy to claim that introspection is a form of perception. It is much better to abandon the analogy and

[7] Descartes developed his views mainly in Descartes (1641, 1996). For recent work on this issue, see Clarke (2003) and Cassam (1994). *Proprioception* does not mean the same as introspection. Proprioception is the specific faculty whereby a person comes to know whether his or her body, or a part of it, is moving as desired, and where the various parts of the body are located with respect to each other. In more technical terms, it refers to the function of senses within the body that "measure physical properties, such as muscle length, tendon tension, joint angle or deep pressure. Signals from this sensory orchestra are sent by afferent nerves through the spinal cord to the somatosensory, motor and parietal cortices of the brain, where they continuously feed and update dynamic sensory-motor maps of the body." See Smetacek & Mechsner (2004).

consider introspection as a form of reflection on oneself, whereby we pay special attention to our own emotions, attitudes and moods.[8]

This was the first point of special philosophical significance for anorexia. The second deals with holism of meaning. This expression refers to the idea that what a linguistic expression means depends on its relation to many other expressions within the same language. In its extreme form, it takes an expression's meaning to be dependent on *all* other expressions within that language. In recent philosophical work, this idea was systematically studied and usefully applied by Donald Davidson, especially when he discussed interpretation.[9] According to him, the best way to account for what happens when a person *A* is trying to understand another person, *B*, is to think of *A* producing a methodologically correct interpretation of *B*'s utterances. Such an interpretation can only be holistic. In other words, with reference to *B*'s utterances, person *A* can test whole theories only, not singular ideas. Any singular idea is linked to many others. They float or sink together. Even within an individual person, say person *A* taken singly, there cannot be a particular belief on its own. We are entitled to say that an individual has a particular belief only if we attribute to that individual many related beliefs. Davidson writes: "it is necessary that there be endless interlocking beliefs. The system of such beliefs identifies a thought by locating it in a logical and epistemic space."[10] Once we see the plausibility of this account, it is tempting to claim that the meaning of a given sentence is determined by the inferential relations it has with other sentences. For instance, the meaning of "Socrates is mortal" is determined by the meaning of "All men are mortal" and of "Socrates is a man." But this cannot be true. To conceive of inferential relations at all, we need first to have meanings. So meaning cannot be determined by inferential relations. We need to look for something else, something that constitutes the interdependence of expressions. This something else is the set of non-semantic properties of these expressions. In other words, what constitutes the interdependence of expressions is ultimately a set of interlocking non-semantic properties associated with those expressions. For Davidson, these properties refer to what speakers do in practice. Speakers show in their behavior what expressions they are holding to be true. They behave meaningfully. So holism of meaning reflects the complexity of human behavior patterns.

Enough has been said at this point about the two common assumptions related to anorexia, one related to introspection and the other to meaning. Having clarified these concepts to some extent, we can now examine the implication of these refinements to the debate on anorexia.

4. New Directions

With regard to the refined version of introspection, we start by focusing our attention on the perceptual-cognitive model. My source was the work of Garfinkel and Garner, but even they express some concern about the completeness of the approach of their own source; Hilde Bruch: "while the empirical research on body image, interoception, and conceptual deviations

[8] For further clarification, see Bennett & Hacker (2003), especially pp. 90-92.

[9] See especially his two ground-breaking papers *Truth and meaning* and *Radical Interpretation,* both reprinted in: Davidson (1984).

[10] Donald Davidson, *Thought and Talk,* in Davidson (1984), p. 157. For an up-to-date overview of meaning holism, see Pagin (2006), pp. 213-233.

will be reviewed, we believe that a clear understanding of the development of these disturbances is not possible at present" (Garfinkel & Garner 1982, p. 124). What I argued with regard to introspection could be a good basis on which to build a more complete approach. In the following few paragraphs, I would like to present some possible new directions for a better understanding of the disturbances under investigation by the perceptual-cognitive model.

First of all, consider the proposal of the childhood origin of anorexia. This proposal depends on the interaction between mother and child. How does a mother correctly determine what her child is experiencing? The mother-child interaction, in this case, can be understood as a special case of rule-following. The mother may be taken to accept simple, generalized norms of the kind: "When I see such-and-such behavior, I proceed in such-and-such a way." In general, with regard to new rules, teacher-learner interaction depends a lot on behavioral manifestations, including linguistic expression. But the manifestations are never enough, strictly speaking, to determine which rule is indicated in that specific case. For the case discussed here, the manifestations on the part of the child are never enough to completely determine which of the mother's various generalized norms concerning her child is correct. Even though most cases of learning a new rule are successful, there is always some room for error. Anorexia may indeed be due to such an error. A slight error in childhood could then grow into a distortion during teenage life. If this analysis is correct, there is a way to prevent this possible imbalance. The longer the mother-child interaction, the less the chance of giving rise to dissonance between mother and child. A child that does not interact often with its mother (as happens when the mother has a job somewhere, leaves her child with various child minders, etc.) has a higher chance of lacking the normal understanding of her own bodily states via confirmation with its mother.

The second observation concerns the very idea of distorted, internal perceptions. When discussing body-image, I mentioned that the perceptual-cognitive model could be harboring a hidden assumption involving inner-senses and inner-observation. Let us consider again the distance arising in early childhood between the mother's realization of the child's hunger and the child's own awareness of her hunger. On this view, the child is assumed to have privileged access to the internal state of her body. This idea, implied at various points by Garfinkel and Garner, is a potential source of confusion. Strictly speaking, the idea of internal perception functions properly only if we adopt the theater-account of the mind. It functions properly when we assume that, just as I see the physical objects in front of me, so also I can see the objects within me, namely the workings of my body from the inside. But, as explained above, when I say, "I am in pain," I am not reporting a perception, as if I had a look inside myself and then discovered a state I refer to by the word "pain." When I say, "I am in pain," it's a polite or refined way of groaning, crying out, or wincing (Bennett & Hacker 2003, p. 93). The utterances of anorexics about themselves function like the expression "I am in pain." So, if this reasoning is correct, the anorexic should not be taken to be reporting an inner perception. When she says, "I'm not hungry," she is making the linguistic-behavioral equivalent of pushing the plate away, as little children do. Notice how Garfinkel and Garner describe this point: "Accurately recognizing hunger, satiety, and other bodily sensations or feeling states is thought to be acquired by learning and, according to this viewpoint [i.e., Bruch's], people who develop anorexia nervosa have never learned the connection between basic drives and appropriate biological or environmental stimulus situations, which lead to drive reduction." I would say that the overall point here is correct and certainly very useful for research. There is, however, the danger of dissociating the person from the person's state, as if what the young child needs to learn is to recognize correctly which bodily state goes with what descriptive term (terms like "hungry," "full," "thin," "fat"). I recommend, on the contrary, that what the child needs to learn is how to express herself in words and to do that correctly. This new account is meant to reduce the artificial conceptual gap between the anorexic and her body.

Moving on now from the introspection, let us consider how the diagnosis and treatment of anorexia may benefit from a refined theory of meaning. Anorexics express many beliefs, mainly about themselves; these beliefs often leave their caretakers, nurses and doctors baffled. Given the point highlighted by Davidson concerning meaning holism, such expressed beliefs should be seen as only the tip of the iceberg. The anorexic expresses a given particular belief only insofar as she has accepted many other beliefs that are in relation to that one expressed belief. Moreover, what determines how these many beliefs are related to one another, in other words what determines how they form a consistent whole, is the way that the anorexic is situated within her world—within her world of objects, persons, relations and culture in general. The entire iceberg, one might say, is the entire worldview adopted by the patient, a view molded into a specific shape as a result of social, psychological and religious pressures. Within that world, she holds some propositions as true and others as false. There is some evidence that anorexics are sometimes aware of the fact that they live in their own special world, a world that is different from the normal one. The once-anorexic Catherine Garrett writes from personal experience: "Eating problems are not about vanity, but a way of coping with trauma [including, in her case, unresolved grief]. To resolve the eating disorder, we must find other, less damaging ways of dealing with past hurts. 'Knowing' about the causes of anorexia is not enough; it can merely confirm an anorexic 'identity.' Anorexia is a negative, protective ritual; its resolution requires different, positive rituals of engagement with the world" (Garrett 1998, p. 85).

To what extent is the anorexic's world accessible to others? One way to describe the body-image disturbance is to say that the anorexic cannot, or will not, accept what others are saying about her. The anorexic has some personal semantic space of her own, a corner to which she can retreat.[11] As was said above, the meaning of words is determined primarily by the common practice of language-users. So if we assume that the anorexic has established a personal semantic space, we can describe what's happening by saying that some of her crucial words constituting the body-image, such as "thin" and "fat," became detached from the linguistic practice they normally belong to. The anorexic reassigns the meaning of these words. She remains semantically attached to the community for most areas, but not for all. And because of holism of meaning, such compartmentalization of linguistic meaning is bound to create tensions arising from internal inconsistency. This point has been recognized to some extent by ex-anorexics like Garrett. She insists that the fact that anorexics see themselves in the mirror as fatter than they are should not be taken to be a problem with perception. She

[11] Karl Jaspers (1963, pp. 356-7) defends the view that a person can never be fully and finally understood. This is entirely in line with what I'm calling a personal semantic-space. One of Jaspers's proposed laws of psychological understanding is that understanding occurs in a hermeneutic circle. To understand a given singular experience, described by the individual patient, the therapist needs to move to the whole personality. It is only in the context of the whole that the meaning of the individual experience can be appreciated. The whole, however, is also inaccessible. The therapist thus needs to repeatedly go through the circle of understanding the whole in terms of the parts and the parts in terms of the whole.

recalls: "when I was anorexic, I knew very well that I was thin; this did not stop me from *feeling* fat—in relation to my ideal, not to objective visual reality" (Garrett 1998, p. 50). She is referring to an *internal* criterion of meaning. Although the normal criterion of meaning is external, in the sense that meaning is determined by the practice of a community, here we have a criterion of meaning that is internal. The anorexic has a means of determining correct and incorrect feelings with respect to a standard, an ideal, that is accessible only to herself—or so it seems. The establishing and consolidation of the anorexic's personal space may be described in existentialist terms as a form of self-realization: the anorexic wants to realize herself; she wants to create her own self independently of the linguistic community in which she was brought up.

Philosophers will be quick here to recognize that special care is needed when one starts talking of an internal criterion of meaning. It would be a mistake to say that the anorexic has a private-language, accessible only to herself. The idea of a private-language, strictly speaking, is inconsistent. A private ostensive definition cannot determine a rule for the use of a word and, thus, a norm for its correct application.[12] Garrett is suggesting that a bodily-state (e.g., being extremely thin) was an ideal for her, known only to herself. This cannot be taken to mean that the way she would talk about that ideal, if she wanted to, would be inaccessible to others. Access to the personal semantic space is indeed possible, but often difficult.

Let us move on now to the therapist. The therapist is in the business of interpreting the anorexic's expressions, and of acting on the basis of the knowledge he or she discovers. In line with the refined account of meaning adopted here, the therapist is obliged to attend not only to the patient's utterances but also to the hidden background to these utterances, the far-reaching background made up of the network of the anorexic's interrelated beliefs. This is a challenge; and it is compounded by the fact that the anorexic has established some personal semantic spaces that are accessible to outsiders only with great difficulty. In a sense, the therapist, in such a situation, is somewhat similar to an anthropologist who is trying to understand the linguistic behavior of a tribe that he had never met before. In this imaginary scenario, the anthropologist seeks some correlation between the sounds made by the natives and elements of their behavior that he can recognize. Once some correlation is available, the anthropologist will start building a simple vocabulary, establishing one meaning after another, each new meaning depending on his previously established meanings. In the 1960s, this procedure underwent considerable analysis by many philosophers. Some drew the conclusion that such radical interpretation is always doomed to failure, because there is never enough data available to determine one correct initial vocabulary list.[13] If this is true, a therapist dealing with an anorexic would be, in principle, incapable of ever understanding what the patient really means by her utterances.

The problem here can be resolved to some extent by referring back to Davidson's insights on meaning holism. The process of interpretation does not involve just two expressions, the one expressed by the anorexic and the one proposed by the therapist as a possible candidate for the anorexic's meaning. It involves also the background beliefs on both sides: the background beliefs of the anorexic and the background beliefs of the therapist. To deal with this situation, Davidson insists that, in the process of interpreting others, most of the beliefs of

---

[12] The original arguments on private language are in Wittgenstein (1953, 1967), §§ 243-315. For a good collection of papers showing the many possible interpretations of these arguments, see Canfield (1986).

[13] See Quine (1960), chapter 2; and his more recent paper Quine (1987). For an important philosophical development of this, see D. Davidson, *Radical interpretation*, in Davidson (1984), pp. 125–139.

the people whose language is being translated should be taken to be true, or, at least, intelligible. We cannot attribute massive irrationality to the one we are trying to interpret. If we do that, we are essentially already assuming that the enterprise is impossible.[14] Anorexia involves patient-therapist communication that is particularly sensitive to the fragility of interpretation. These points are, therefore, very relevant, but the philosophical literature on interpretation is vast. The least that can be said here is that, although the therapist knows that what the anorexic says is false if taken literally, he or she should be encouraged to use it to reach down into the anorexic's personal semantic space so as to see how that false expression is justified, is indeed true, within the reasoning of the anorexic. A clear example of such reaching down occurs when the therapist tries to appreciate the possible utility of the disorder from the anorexic's point of view, as mentioned above.[15]

CONCLUSION

At the beginning of this paper, the original question was: how can those who adopt perceptual-cognitive accounts of anorexia benefit from philosophy? The first section focused on language, perception and cognition; these three dimensions of anorexia were deemed most open to a contribution from philosophy. In the second section, I offered a brief overview of the philosophical background for two crucial issues: introspection and meaning. I concluded that accounts of anorexia would suffer if they did not adopt refined versions of introspection and of meaning. The first recommendation was to work within the parameters of a refined account of language-acquisition rather than an oversimplified one. When dealing with expressions involving bodily states, one should not adopt an internal-perception model. The second recommendation dealt with the subtle features of interpretation. These were shown to be indispensable. The anorexic is neither fully rational nor fully irrational. The best procedure seems to be to maximize not the truth but the intelligibility of the anorexic's expressions. Having drawn these modest conclusions, I am not suggesting that anorexia can be understood and resolved exclusively as a philosophical problem of meaning. We should not underestimate the deterministic nature of the mechanism involved (Lucas 2008, p. 133). Once the biological mechanism has triggered off, the anorexic will have less mental control over her condition. Therapists can help patients come to grips with their emotional conflicts. Talking about these conflicts is often therapeutic in itself, because it helps the patient understand herself, her motivations and her reasons. But once the physical changes associated with anorexia have set in, they take on a life of their own.[16]

[14] For Davidson's views on the principles involved in interpretation, see especially his two papers *Radical interpretation* and *Thought and talk*, both included in Davidson 1984.

[15] The "benefits" of anorexia have indeed started to receive some attention from researchers recently. In one such study, the following positive functions associated with anorexia have been determined: it makes anorexicanorexics happy; it helps them feel safe and in control; it helps them be more popular, different from the rest, or noticed; it helps them avoid growing up. See Tan et al. (2006) and Rosenberg (1965).

[16] I owe a special thanks to Peter Hacker, Roger Dawson, both of Oxford University, and to Alison Mantell of The Hampshire Clinic, UK, for useful comments on previous drafts of this paper.

REFERENCES

Bemporad, Jules R. (1997), "Cultural and Historical Aspects of Eating Disorders," *Theoretical Medicine* 18(4): 401-420.

Bennett, M.R. & Hacker, P.M.S. (2003), *Philosophical Foundations of Neuroscience*, (Oxford: Blackwell)

Bordo, Susan (1985-86), "Anorexia Nervosa: Psychopathology as the Crystallization of Culture," *Philosophical Forum* (Boston) 17: 73-104.

Bruch, Hilde (1961), "Conceptual confusion in eating disorders," *Journal of Nervous and Mental Disease* 133: 46-54.

Bruch, Hilde (1962), "Perceptual and conceptual disturbances in anorexia nervosa," *Psychological Medicine* 24: 187-194.

Bruch, Hilde (1978), *The Golden Cage: the enigma of anorexia nervosa* (Cambridge Mass., Harvard University Press).

Brumberg, Joan Jacobs (2000), *Fasting Girls: The History of Anorexia Nervosa* (New York: Vintage).

Canfield, J.V. (ed.) (1986), *The Philosophy of Wittgenstein, vol. 9, The Private Language Argument* (New York: Garland,).

Cassam, Q. (ed.) (1994), *Self-Knowledge* (New York: Oxford University Press).

Church, Jennifer (2004), "Social Constructionist Models: Making Order out of Disorder – On the Social Construction of Madness", in: *The Philosophy of Psychiatry: A Companion*, Jennifer Radden (ed.) (Oxford: Oxford University Press), pp. 393-406.

Clarke, Desmond (2003), *Descartes's Theory of Mind* (Oxford: Oxford University Press).

Davidson, Donald (1984), *Inquiries into truth and interpretation* (Oxford: Clarendon Press).

Descartes, René (1641, 1996), *Meditations on first philosophy: with selections from the Objections and replies*, trans. and ed. by J. Cottingham (Cambridge: Cambridge University Press, 1996).

Garfinkel, Paul E. & Garner, David M. (1982), *Anorexia Nervosa: a multidimensional perspective* (New York: Brunner/Mazel, Inc.).

Garrett, Catherine (1998) *Beyond Anorexia: Narrative, Spirituality and Recovery* (Cambridge University Press).

Hondros, M. and Caroline, E. (2004), "Anorexia Nervosa: The Illusion of Power, Perfection, and Purity," *Philosophy in the Contemporary World* 11(1): 19-26.

Jaspers. Karl (1963), *General psychopathology*, trans. J. Hoenig and M.W. Hamilton (Manchester: Manchester University Press).

Lucas, Alexander R. (2008), *Demystifying Anorexia Nervosa: an optimistic guide to understanding and healing* (Oxford: Oxford University Press).

Pagin, Peter (2006), "Meaning Holism," in: E. Lepore & B. Smith (eds.), *The Oxford Handbook of Philosophy of Language* (Oxford: Clarendon Press), pp. 213-233.

Quine, Willard van Orman (1960), *Word and Object* (Cambridge, MA: MIT Press).

Quine, Willard van Orman (1987), "Indeterminacy of translation again," *The Journal of Philosophy* 84(1): 5–10.

Rosenberg, M. (1965), *Society and the adolescent self-image* (Princeton, NJ: Princeton University Press).

Smetacek, Victor and Mechsner, Franz (4 November, 2004) "Making sense," *Nature*, vol. 432: 21.

Tan, Jacinta O.A., Stewart, Anne, Fitzpatrick, Ray, & Hope, Tony (2006), "Competence to make treatment decisions in Anorexia Nervosa: Thinking processes and values," *Philosophy, psychiatry and psychology* 13/4: 267-282.

Walters, Glenn D. (1999), "Human Survival and the Self-Destruction Paradox: An Integrated Theoretical Model," *Journal of Mind and Behavior* 20(1): 57-78.

Wittgenstein, Ludwig (1953, 1967), *Philosophical Investigations* (Oxford: Blackwell, 3rd edition).

In: Anorexia Nervosa: A Multi-Disciplinary Approach ISBN: 978-1-60876-200-2
Editors: A. Mancini, S. Daini, L. Caruana, pp. 187-201

Chapter 12

ANOREXIA NERVOSA: A CASE OF SELF-DECEPTION?

Mark Sultana

Department of Fundamental and Dogmatic Theology, University of Malta, Republic of Malta

ABSTRACT

Anorexia nervosa readily reminds one of the phenomenon of self-deception. After all, it is characterized by body image distortion and denial of illness. In this paper, after a very brief presentation of the philosophical paradoxes that appear to afflict our accounts of self-deception, a conceptual analysis of "self-deception" is carried out with the purpose of clarifying our use of the term. The result is the emergence of four criteria delineating the meaning of self-deception together with an examination of their applicability to *anorexia nervosa*. Finally, the question whether *anorexia nervosa* is really a case of self-deception or delusion is investigated, with specific reference to the relation between the anorexic's self-image and the self-deceptive beliefs that may be pervasively present in a society.

INTRODUCTION

Anorexia nervosa is a curious condition that has challenged clinicians for over two centuries. Indeed, it is characterized by an extremely odd cluster of symptoms. Despite having lost at least 15% of their body weight, people with *anorexia nervosa* minimize and forestall eating. They often feel boundless energy and exercise vigorously (Garfinkel and Garner 1982; Beumont et al. 1994). But perhaps the strangest and most striking symptom is that they see themselves as in good health—and even as overweight—when they are dangerously thin.[1]

Before this peculiar cluster of symptoms, both the clinician and the person with *anorexia* want to ask questions like: why do they think they are fat when everyone else, including their

[1] *DSM-IV-TR* reports a disturbance in the way in which one's body weight or shape is experienced (see *DSM-IV-TR*, 307.1), whereas *ICD-10* reports a body-image distortion (see *ICD-10*, F-50).

loved ones, are frightened by their weight loss? Why do they exercise so strenuously? And why does abstaining from food appear so easy and even virtuous (Chisholm 2002)?

In the literature, it is emphasized that *anorexia nervosa* manifests itself in the context of a complex interplay among environmental, genetic and other factors. The condition has been described as a biological, social, psychological, philosophical and even moral phenomenon.[2] However, even if the literature is very extensive and complex, one can detect a clear conceptual divide in the focus of different clinicians. Indeed, some would emphasize that *anorexia nervosa* is an addiction in the hard or strong sense, meaning that such persons cannot control their behavior. Such clinicians would maintain that neuro-endocrinal factors are *causing* the person's behavior in such a way that the eating-disorder behavior is out of the person's control (Halmi 1992, p. 83; Guisinger 2003). And to be sure, anorexic persons do "report enormous difficulty eating and refraining from exercise, as though something other than their conscious will were in charge of their behavior, sensations and cognitions" (Guisinger 2003, p. 747). Conversely, other clinicians would emphasize that, in an important sense, *anorexia* is a self-imposed condition. They would point out that people with eating disorders do not complain about their eating habits but either hide them or defend them or both, even in the face of advanced emaciation. And indeed, the *DSM-IV-TR* assumes that the anorexic person eats little and exercises much because of her "refusal to maintain [normal] body weight" (DSM-IV-TR 2000, p. 583). The *International Classification of Diseases* concurs in describing the central feature of the condition as being "deliberate weight loss, induced and sustained by the patient" (ICD-10 1992, F10-19). This would mean that *anorexia nervosa* is a progressive pursuit of bodily lightness though different methods such as control of food intake and exercise (Giordano 2005, p. 94). This would, in turn, mean that, although *anorexia* is a complex or multifactorial condition, with genetic, environmental and social influences being involved, of vital importance is the fact that the anorexic person is *active*: in some way, and to some extent, she wants and accepts her condition.

In this latter regard, it has been noted that the anorexic person does not appear to have an identity apart from not-eating (Evans 2001, p. 3). She is typically a socially compliant, perfectionist, high achiever and would not recognize the condition as some entity distinct from herself (Garfinkel and Garner 1982). A recent study published the replies of eating disorder patients to the question: "Do you think you would make [*anorexia nervosa*] magically disappear if you could?"

> If I knew I would be happy—but it would be a completely different me, it would be a completely different way of thinking, because I don't think I could be the person I want to be, at the moment, without anorexia, because it's a part of me; so if I could change the kind of person I wanted to be, then yes, I would take that pill, but until then I probably wouldn't … I wouldn't know who I was. And I would be completely and utterly lost in what I was doing.[3]

Such statements, together with the sincere conviction of anorexic persons that they are well, even overweight, when they are dangerously thin, remind one of the phenomenon of self-deception. After all, *anorexia nervosa* is characterized by body image distortion and denial of illness and, already in 1873, Laségue wrote of the "inexhaustible optimism against

[2] See Kaplan and Garfinkel (1993) and Strober (1991). The moral side of *anorexia nervosa* has been well brought out by Duker and Slade (2003) and Giordano (2005).

[3] Tan et al., (2003), pp. 533-548, as quoted in Giordano (2005), p. 231.

which supplications and menaces are alike of no avail" expressed by anorexic patients (Lasègue 1873, p. 266). In line with this view, it is cognitive behavior therapy that is generally considered to be the first-line treatment of choice for *bulimia nervosa* (Thompson-Brenner et al. 2003), and which has also been applied to *anorexia nervosa* (***Vitousek 2005).***

Now, the accusation that the anorexic person might be deceiving herself is scarcely a novel one. However, there are two points that require closer examination here. First, self-deception tends to present a rather tricky, and paradoxical, air: it would seem impossible that the self could be, at a time, both deceiver and the deceived, since it would either have too little knowledge to play the former role, or too much to yield to the latter. Secondly, what is involved in *anorexia nervosa* often is an extreme departure from reality; so extreme, indeed, that one has to examine whether it is truly a case of self-deception.

With respect to the first query, a number of accounts proposed in recent years have focused on offering an explanation that abandons some feature of the analysis of self-deception along the lines of lying. In particular, it is often suggested that one should abandon the idea that self-deception has an intentional component and see the beliefs involved in the self-deceived state as motivated, *not intended*.[4] However, such accounts seem to trivialize somewhat the concept, doing less than justice to the accusation of intellectual deceit than is implicit in the charge of self-deception. They do not appear to cover the strong sense of the term which, one feels, is an accurate, and yet apparently self-contradictory, description of certain human situations.

Other accounts have attempted to circumvent the apparent contradiction by supposing that, indeed, there are different cognitive systems at work in the mind of the self-deceiver, where one system is able to conceal or misinterpret reality purposely in order to trick the other system into holding the mistaken, but preferred, belief.[5] The problem here is that what one seeks to know is, precisely, how such a phenomenon could occur in a single person, not how the single person could be carved up on the model of two or more people.

One, therefore, needs a new, more fruitful line in enquiry. In this paper, I would like to examine the first query noted above by *looking* at the use of the concept "self-deception" and *seeing* when one would say "I deceived myself" or "He is deceiving himself." The outcome of the surview of the grammar of the concept "self-deception" will be the elucidation of four criteria that will enable one to understand the concept more clearly.

Now, when one looks and sees what happens when an agent speaks out, one notes different kinds of situations: for instance, one could take the case of someone confessing to being quite tired, whereas her companion, who knows her extremely well, can clearly see that she is petrified of something. Here, the person is surprisingly wrong in what she says but what she says and does is not that obscure. Now, it would often be the case that she might immediately agree with her friend's interpretation of her state of mind as soon as this is proffered, recognizing her past account as "mistaken." Nevertheless, it could also be the case that she does her best to explain away, often in a rather "irrational" and strong manner, what her friend might point out.

Another kind of situation could be that where one describes his wife as extremely faithful, when it is perfectly clear to his interlocutor that she is developing an increasingly

---

[4] See: Mounce (1971); Bach (1981). Alfred Mele has notably presented this model in a number of places, for instance, in Mele (1983); (1987a); (1987b); (1997); (2001). See also: Johnston (1995); Nelkin (2002).

[5] Such accounts include those of Demos (1960); King-Farlow (1963); Rorty (1972); Audi (1982); Pears (1984); Davidson (1985); Talbott (1995).

warm relationship with another man, and moreover, that this should be evident to the husband. Now, such a circumstance, where the person is seemingly blind to the obvious, appears to be surprisingly irrational, but is not unintelligible at all. Once again, the cuckold might listen to his friend on being told the latter's diverse interpretation of the situation. Nevertheless, it could turn out that he angrily dismisses any insinuations contrary to his description of the relationship.

In the case of the person who does not appear to notice her own fear, she is expressing or reporting her self-consciousness in what she does say. Of course, she might be pretending. More interestingly, if she were to report sincerely "I believe I am not tense, but my belief could be wrong," one feels that there is a contradiction of sorts. One would feel that, if the avower were right about not being afraid, the first phrase would be verified and the second falsified, and if she were wrong, the opposite would be the case. However, one would also say that such a situation would not constitute the type of contradiction decried by Aristotle in the latter chapters of *Book Γ* of his *Metaphysics*. For, if one were to say "'I believe I am not tense," *someone else* might contemporaneously know that such is not the case. Moreover, one knows that one might be conceivably wrong in one's beliefs, even when one is confident in one's beliefs and even though one is mostly right. However, such a general acknowledgement does *not* mean, of course, that one is wrong in any particular case. It would be absurd to put "unless I am wrong" after every statement of belief, for *there is no way of distinguishing the right from the wrong cases* here. One could only distinguish when, for some particular reason (such as, when someone else says so), there is some room for doubt about one's expression or report. In a similar fashion, the form of words *reporting* "I am currently self-deceived" is excluded from our language. Their sense is senseless. It is only when grounds for doubt are available that one could speak of knowledge, self-knowledge and self-deception.

Accordingly, it is instructive that, while the fearful person is not offered another interpretation of her reactions by her friend, one would hesitate to call her "self-deceived." One could consider describing her as self-deceived if one held that she has access to another account of herself or of events affecting her but sees that she brushes it away, without allowing for it.

In this light, the first criterion (C1) characterizing the concept of "self-deception" is that it is used when one is deemed to have access to the true belief such that one is considered to be able to *know* the true belief. There can be no self-deception where there can be no distinction between "One knows ..." and "One thinks one knows ...."

Now, of course, the case of the poor cuckold is a classic case of self-deception. The poor man has all the evidence he might need in order to realize that his wife is betraying him. Naturally, he might be living extremely unreflectively, so that he does not *know* his convictions and, therefore, error would not be intelligible. However, such a scenario appears extremely unlikely. For, the doubt about his wife's fidelity is not a piece of empty nonsense but has real, live content. One would ask oneself how it could be possible that he does not see what is staring him in the face. It is likely that it is such stupefaction before the irrational occurrence of self-deception that fuels explanations modeled on inter-personal lying and postulating splits within the self. In the case of the anorexic person, one would ask how it could be possible that she looks in the mirror and sees "fat" when it is obvious that she is dangerously thin and that, moreover, her family and loved ones are frightened by her weight loss (Roukema 2003, p. 147).

At this stage, I want to examine a second criterion (C2), by refining, further, the first criterion. I want to say that the concept "self-deception" is only attributed where the circumstances are such that the subject is expected to speak or act in knowledge, that is, when he is expected to be able to give reasons for his beliefs, judgments, intentions, thoughts, desires, actions and so forth but is seen to be wrong in such a manner that, at the time, he proves resistant to correction. Such a person treats a belief, that is recognized as mistaken by those around him or, possibly, by himself afterwards, as a certainty without being able to consider, at the time the description of self-deception is attributed to him, that such belief is mistaken.

The unrepentant cuckold is, in effect, acting out his conviction that he cannot be wrong. Sadly, however, he is wrong and this is concerning something he has the capacity and possibility to be right about. For the grounds for the right interpretation of his situation are available to him and, normally, are within his grasp. That is, his is not one of the cases where one could not understand his situation or his reasoning, or where the hypothesis he believes cannot be logically sustained in that one would not be able to understand what sustaining such a hypothesis would be, or where the mere occurrence of accepting his conviction destroys the entire practice of judging anything. His is a case, however, where any evidence he might see—any grounds, reasons or arguments one could offer—pass him by; they do not convince him. Indeed, one feels that one cannot refute such a man.

The fact is that the self-deceived person is convinced that, in his case, he cannot be making a mistake. Indeed, *he is not making a mistake*; he is insisting: "I know that my wife is faithful" where "I know ..." is logically equivalent to "I swear ..." He lives with a kind of certainty that is rooted very profoundly in his life and lies beyond being justified or unjustified. His logical situation can be expressed in the words: "I cannot be making a mistake, but I may sometime come to believe, rightly or wrongly, that I was not competent to judge" (Wittgenstein 1977, §645), where this not a contradiction since there is a distinction between the certainty that cannot be called a "mistake" and the ever-present abstract possibility that one may be mistaken. In self-deception, certainty is defended in the face of very legitimate doubt.

Here, one must point out that the majority of authors writing on self-deception tend to characterize the phenomenon in terms of *isolated beliefs*. Thus, they would try to explain how the true and the false belief could live together within the same agent, or how the true belief is put aside and ignored in favor of the false belief. It is important to note that one must, rather, talk more of a nest of beliefs with partly fluid and partly stable characteristics. Thus, for instance, the cuckold's confidence in his wife's fidelity is not an isolated certainty but is firmly embedded in his way of acting. His very way of conducting his life shows that the sure judgment that is not called into question is an intrinsic part of the nest of convictions that shape his life. This also clearly appears to be the case in anorexic patients: "[p]eople with eating disorders appear to attach the value of absolute and unquestionable truth to their beliefs" (Giordano 2005, p. 223), sometimes evidently false beliefs like superstitious thinking of the sort that "if I eat this, it will be turned into fat on my buttocks immediately" or dichotomous reasoning like "gaining 500 grams has made me unattractive." Indeed,

> the fact that the person gives that interpretation means that the person is active in this process. The fact that the eating-disordered person believes that if she goes to the restaurant one day she will get fatter is not something that "just happens to her" because she has some mistaken

> information, but is part of … her system of thought, her fears, her emotional life, her feelings, and her objectives. [Such beliefs] are "a part" of that person, part of what being that particular person means to the person herself (Giordano 2005, p. 230).

At this point, it would be extremely helpful to clarify the concept of self-knowledge, since it is logically intertwined rather intimately with self-deception.

Self-knowledge is *not* knowledge of a self, but it is knowledge that one holds of oneself. Indeed, a moment's thought will show that to turn one's attention upon one's own consciousness is vastly different from one's being conscious of something like the chiming of bells. For self-consciousness is a disposition or capacity to have "I" thoughts of this object here about which I can *find out* (if I do not already *know* it), *not that it is "me,"* but that it is Mark Sultana and about which I *learned* that it is a human being (Anscombe 1981, 34). Now, one can, of course, attend to many things about oneself, ranging from what one is imagining, to states of consciousness like one's sensations, to the specialized use of descriptions of one's hopes. None of this attendance, however, is perceptual. Self-consciousness, seen as consciousness of, or about, a self, is an illusion stemming from a superficial (mis-)use of words.

Now, knowledge can be had where doubt makes sense and error is conceivable. That is, one can claim "I know …" where one can give grounds or demonstrate the truth or falsity of the assertion (Wittgenstein 1977, §11). This is no exception for self-knowledge.

Hence, self-knowledge is constituted by the "I" thoughts for which one can give justification, reasons or grounds for one's claims about oneself. That is, spontaneous cries of pain are not part of one's self-knowledge (and neither could one be deceiving oneself). Conversely, descriptions of oneself such as about one's body shape or weight, which may involve surmising, doubt, interpretation, a striving for accuracy, the ability to correct oneself, and so forth, constitute part of one's self-knowledge.

Such descriptions of oneself are constituted by what one claims for oneself. What is interesting about such utterances is that they constitute matters that are necessarily ones in which observation is crucially significant. That is, "I am seated" or "I was extremely angry today" or "I am too fat" are all true if and only if the corresponding second- or third-person assertion is true. It is interesting to note here that the ICD-10 reports that people with eating disorders experience a body-image distortion (*ICD-10*, F-50), whereas the DSM-IV-TR states that the person with *anorexia nervosa* suffers from a "disturbance in the way in which one's body weight or shape is experienced" (*DSM-IV-TR*, 307.1). *The National Association of Anorexia Nervosa* provides a more graphic description of the situation:

> When a person with anorexia looks into a mirror he/she does not often see an accurate reflection. A person with anorexia sees him/herself as fat, even if he/she is dangerously thin. This is a very frightening experience and feels very real—driving the person to diet. Sometimes, a person with anorexia can accept that he/she is very thin but cannot accept how dangerous the situation really is. It is difficult for him/her to understand that a very low weight and dangerous dieting habits can actually be fatal.[6]

---

[6] *The National Association of Anorexia Nervosa*, http://www.anad.org/22385/22427.html (accessed 26th January 2009).

Now, one only attributes the concept "self-deceived" to someone who, one knows, has all the evidence "before him" but who, to an outside observer, is clearly mistaken. The concept is used when an utterance or an action of the self-deceiver's is incorrect and can be seen and shown to be so—as is clearly the case with the anorexic person.

Throughout the discussion, one could see that self-knowledge and self-deception cannot be described as logically independent of agency; one cannot describe someone as being self-deceived, without also describing him or her as doing (or saying) things in accordance with her self-deception. Naturally, one is, here, saying that self-deception, self-knowledge, and one's knowledge are *logically* related to one's practices; one is *not* claiming that every belief one may have must be accompanied by some action. Indeed, it is logically quite possible for one to know one's beliefs and practices, as it were, from a third-person point of view, and see oneself "in a different light."

Such a third-party point of view may be seen in one's reflective utterance averring: "I know that it is true, but I can't believe it." Here, one is describing the degree of one's commitment to, or competence in, a particular way of acting. One may, for instance, confess that one cannot take to heart and act on what one knows to be the case in one's more reflective moments. Or, one might note that even such reflective utterances might be inaccurate, exaggerated, or understated; one might scrutinize them oneself and notice errors or biases. Hence, it is always possible for the cuckold to reflect upon his life and *see* that he is being gullible. Such a realization, however, is dependent on his being able to step outside and modify his nest of convictions, and this is normally only possible if he allows himself to be rather badly shaken by certain bits that do not fit and that he perennially had tried to explain away. More usually, this is possible if he listens to someone whom he trusts, who gives him a third-person description that, at first, might seem completely alien but that he strives to take on board, on a first-person level, until his own way of acting is changed sufficiently in that his beliefs and his life become different. What happens in cases like the latter is that someone seeks to cure or convince the self-deceiver initially by offering reasons, but where at the end of reasons comes persuasion; at the end of argumentation comes trust.

In defending an account of self-deception that is intentional, perhaps one of the main obstacles is the presupposition that intentional self-deception requires an intention to deceive oneself, where this is seen as incoherent for two main reasons: first, that one cannot intend to bring it about that one simultaneously entertains contradictory beliefs, and, secondly, that any intention to deceive oneself necessarily falls prey to the paradox questioning the possibility of one's getting oneself to believe a belief one knows to be false.

The account advanced in this paper, however, does not fall prey to such strong objections, for it elucidates self-deception not as being a question of wanting to deceive oneself or a question of intentionally getting oneself to believe what one knows to be false but, rather, as a question of *accepting* certain judgments as beyond doubt. Indeed, the ways in which we use the terms related to the concept clearly manifest that our verdict on the self-deceiver is that he *does not want to doubt* such-and-such despite grounds for doubt that are available and that should be clear to him. We see that the self-deceiver has a stake in this, and it also appears clear to him when he recognizes himself as having been self-deceived: he might feel that he was not strong-willed enough to face reality but, perhaps paradoxically, what may have rather happened was that he was *too strong-willed* to admit reality. This appears to be the case with anorexic patients who "are often hungry, even frantically obsessed about food, but consider self-denial and discipline the highest virtue and condemn satisfying their needs and desires as shameful self-indulgence" (Bruch 1978, x). Indeed, the third criterion (C3), for the use of the term self-deception is that the concept is used when one sees that the agent *does not want to doubt* such-and-such despite the fact that it should be clear to him or her that there exist grounds or reasons for doubt.

To be sure, if the agent decides that such a judgment be removed from the games of doubt and query and shunted onto, as it were, a siding, the judgment in question would *indeed* have a peculiar logical role: it would constitute, for the agent, an issue that does not arise. Such a decision is not normally taken in some kind of quintessential moment of decision in which the agent hesitates before the options, thinks, then chooses what to believe. On the contrary, it is more a matter of its being acted out and manifested in the agent's intentional words and deeds in such a manner that it becomes obvious to him or her to judge in *this* way so that, normally, he never hesitates as to whether or not his wife is still faithful to him. Of course, even in such a situation, the agent still has a choice; only, it becomes very difficult to come to see things otherwise. As it were, certain "comfortable certainties" come to constitute matters that form part of the context, to the way the agent speaks, thinks and gives as "good reasons," and within which doubting and enquiry can take place. The ways of speaking, arguing and acting of the agent show the stable axes around which the—logical—possibility of their occurrence revolves, where the foundation-walls that these axes constitute are carried by the whole house (Wittgenstein 1977, §248). This inversion of architectural foundationalism is shown clearly in that the self-deceiver protects his or her "comfortable certainties" through ways of arguing and acting that ensure that such certainties are not touched in the least. The self-deceiving cuckold would never want to hire a private detective; he simply does not want to act in such a way that could introduce serious doubt into his life about the matter. Conversely, the agent's world-picture[7] is manifested in what he takes as an explanation. If he accepts, as reasons for his wife's fidelity, occurrences and factors that are real but that others would not think are of major importance while refusing to consider or even to check factors that would normally be crucial in enabling his seeing that his wife is no longer faithful to him, this shows that his belief in his wife's fidelity has taken on the peculiar logical role mentioned above. In the case of *anorexia nervosa*, a sense of virtue in ignoring hunger pangs is often present. Anorexic saints believed that their ability to fast, even when hungry, was a sign of their piety (Bell 1985) and, even in the case of clinical anorexia, there is often a quasi-religious thrill experienced in abstaining from food and pushing oneself to exercise harder and harder (Hornbacher 1998). Clinicians have described the pursuit and adoration of thinness as a desperately held and absolute imperative, even if with potentially fatal consequences (Bloom et al. 1994).

Here, it is not a question of the self-deceiver picking and choosing what to believe. It is, rather, that the logical order of one's beliefs manifests what one's purposes, interests and wants are; there are important connections between the ultimate "beliefs for the sake of which" that grant intelligible order to the agent's life and the "hinge those for the sake of which" that are the agent's ultimate wants. For one's ways of acting and judging, within which reasons are given for and against courses of action, constitute a kind of second-order

[7] What Wittgenstein called one's "world-picture" can be "described" as the inherited background where there is no such thing as doubt and against which one distinguishes between true and false (see Wittgenstein 1977, §94). The "world-picture" is what normally goes unmentioned in one's life and yet is part of what gives one's way of looking at, and going about, things its form (*Ibid.*, §211), so that one would not know and believe what one does, and act as one does, and be in doubt about *that*.

ranking of one's beliefs and judgments, where such an ordering is an active, intentional practice and where one does not have any reason for *accepting* such-and-such as reasons or grounds for the said ranking. Indeed, this ordering is a function of the interests and purposes of the society and the individual. What one does have is one's—deep—decisions to approach reality the way one actually does, where the ultimate practical "those for the sake of which" are present in and *inform* the whole order of beliefs and conceptually connected actions. In *anorexia nervosa*, "the disorder is seductive. Some patients relapse ... for the high. When an anorexic model sometimes feels like superwoman and looks like a supermodel, a more cogent question may be how any are able to give up the disorder. It is also narcissistically appealing to see oneself as uniquely able to ignore appetite, hunger and pain" (Guisinger 2003, p. 757).

The self-deceiver *is able to say without the need for observation* what the axes, around which his life rotates, are. This does not mean, of course, that, while acting, the agent is conscious of what the beliefs, for the sake of which he or she is acting in such-and-such a manner, are: beliefs and intentions are not states of mind or processes within the mind. Rather, it means that the said agent is able to say what they are on being asked. And one can do so, not by peering deeply beneath one's deeds to see what lies at their bottom but, rather, by seeing, in one's ways of thinking, speaking and acting, where the explanations for their intelligibility stops. Indeed, there is nothing mysterious about the comfortable certainties: they are expressed in the actions and manners of speech of the agent, even if the latter may be reluctant to acknowledge them. Such "comfortable certainties" are present in the agent's beliefs and actions and show forth a way of treating the world that includes recognizing such-and-such as reasons and determining what the relevant facts are in the given situation.

The centrality of the agent's intention in self-deception is also clear in the possible cures the agent may *choose*. What is important, here, is that the choice of the agent means that the comfortable certainty is *abandoned,* not falsified. Only once cured does the agent see it as false. It is not a question of a conceptual shift; *indeed* the poor, self-deceived cuckold uses the same concept of marital fidelity as anybody else in his social milieu and, once he has been rid of self-deception, no change in meaning is involved. Rather, the change is more like an initiation than the correction of a mistake. It is question of a shift in background; it is a change in the way in which the agent lives his life. When asked what would change, if the person had the power to swipe *anorexia nervosa* away with a magic wand, the rather startling reply was "Everything. My personality would be different. It's been, I know it's been such a big part of me, and—I don't think you can ever get rid of it, or the feelings, you always have a bit—in you" (Tan et al. 2003, as quoted in Giordano 2005, p. 231).

In order to facilitate such a shift, the agent can well change the circumstances in which he lives; of course such changes could *happen* to him but this does not exclude the agent's decision concerning new ways of acting. Alternatively, one could intentionally change some ways of thinking and acting that—perhaps indirectly—impinge on the immobility of the comfortable certainty in such a way that one's world-picture is transformed. In the case of *anorexia nervosa*, the self-help advice given includes acknowledging that one may not be the best judge of whether one is eating enough or is at a healthy weight, identifying situations that are likely to trigger thoughts or behavior that may contribute to one's anorexia so that one can develop a plan of action to deal with them, looking for positive role models, and not visiting pro-anorexia websites or calling anorexia one's friend.[8] Then again, one could consult a trusted friend and choose to abide by the latter's judgment. One of the most difficult, yet essential, aspects of treatment, in the case of *anorexia nervosa*, is that clinicians be supportive of the patient's efforts throughout treatment, even if she has been hospitalized against her desires. Indeed, building a trusting and supportive relationship with her is deemed to be one of the most important parts of treatment.[9]

At this stage, I want to examine a fourth criterion (C4), which will prove important to the second query raised at the beginning of this paper: the question whether *anorexia* is really a case of self-deception or delusion. For one would use the concept "self-deception" in the case of one who possesses the same system of knowledge, and who uses concepts in the same manner, as one's community of linguistic practices even if he shows himself to be strangely resistant to some patent truth. This point is important, since what is involved in *anorexia nervosa* often is an extreme departure from reality; so extreme, indeed, that one needs to examine whether it is truly a case of self-deception or delusion.

Thus, one would *not* use the concept "self-deception" of persons who share the same world-picture with others around them, yet possess a system of knowledge—say, concerning human relationships or about food and nutrition—that is much poorer than is the norm in persons around them. One would, rather, say that one is in the presence of a form of ignorance like that of a child. The cure consists in a form of teaching, leading to a change in opinion. This does not appear to be the case in *anorexia nervosa*, where the person is normally very well informed about food and nutrition and where unrealistic perceptions of hunger and satiety cannot be corrected by teaching the person because "[i]t seems that the person at some level 'wants to believe what she believes' in order to support her modality of behavior" (Giordano 2005, p. 260). Nor would the concept "self-deception" be used in situations where the person uses concepts in a very different way than that of his or her linguistic community, perhaps after having grown up in quite exceptional circumstances: one who upheld "free love" would have a radically different concept of "love" from that of, say, a community of linguistic practices where absolute fidelity is upheld. Of course, the classic example of delusion is that of a person who refuses to accept, even after having been present at the funeral, that a loved one has died. Such a person, in delusion, might continue to speak to her husband and explain to a friend that: "I *know* that he is still alive … and even you cannot explain everything."[10]

Here, what is happening is that such a person, in delusion, is seeing an aspect that is simply *not there at all*. She is making a judgment against and within the background of a different world-picture; one that is intellectually and practically so distant from ours that her very concepts of death and of what it means to be present to someone are very different from ours. Clearly, she is seeing something under a description; that is, for her, her husband is still alive, and she is acting accordingly. Evidently, there is an intentional aspect to her thoughts, words, and actions that manifests the *description under which* she is judging and acting. Nevertheless, this intentional aspect is not intelligible at all; the description under which the agent judges and acts is not a description that is conceivable of what is seen *at all*. Perhaps

---

[8] See *Mayo Foundation for Medical Education and Research*, http://www.mayoclinic.com/health/anorexia/DS00606/DSECTION=coping-and-support (accessed 26th January 2009).

[9] See *Psych Central*, http://psychcentral.com/disorders/sx2t.htm (accessed 26th January 2009).

[10] See: Wittgenstein (1977), §108. Béla Szabados uses the same kind of argument in order to elucidate the distinction between self-deception and delusion (Szabados, 1985).

the person in delusion is even totally hallucinating and speaking to someone in a hallucinatory scene; whatever the case, this person in delusion is in a situation wherein one would say that whom she is speaking to is no one.[11]

The case of self-deception is clearly quite diverse. For in self-deception, the feeling of a vast intellectual distance between the observer and the self-deceiver is not present. What is more present is the feeling of frustration at the seeming lack of cognizance on the part of the self-deceiver. For one sees that the self-deceiver is one of us; he or she is using concepts—say of fatness, hunger, and satiety—just as we do. One sees that he or she ought to see what one can see and, indeed, that he or she usually does; and yet, one also sees that the self-deceiver, as it were, refuses to see what is quite visible. Indeed, self-deception is a prime example of the tangled nature of each of the concepts of seeing, judging, thinking and believing; these concepts are not as unitary or simple as they appear to be.

One must, here, investigate whether the case of *anorexia nervosa* is more like the situation of the cuckold or like that of the person who denies that a loved-one has died. Here, perhaps it would be best to give the word to a former anorexic person:

> Contrary to popular belief, I saw myself as thin, although I told people that I was "fat." For me, the word "fat" took on a whole new meaning. I had a different standard for myself and for the outside world. For example, I might see someone on the street corner who weighed much more than I did, but was still thin, and say, "Gee, that person is awfully thin." When I looked at myself in the mirror, I saw the protruding bones and the greyish blue skin. In my mind, I was still "fat" because I was still less than perfect and still unhappy. For me, it became a "numbers game." The only way to "win" was to watch the numbers go down on the scale. I once told my mother that I wouldn't be happy until I reached "zero" (knowing full well that I would be dead long before that point in time). During much of my illness, the misery was such that death often seemed like a more desirable option (that way, the suffering would be over with). Anorexia nervosa is a horrible state of existence. Hopefully you can see by the reasoning provided above that it would be fruitless to try to "talk sense" into someone with anorexia and "convince them that they are really not "'fat'"[12]

Such a statement is confirmed by studies indicating that anorexic patients typically manifest body image distortion and denial of illness in a manner that is startling to most members of their culture. As mentioned above, in 1873, Laségue had already described anorexics' serene obliviousness to their ever-thinner stature (Lasègue 1873, p. 266). In this light, it may be thought evident that such persons are suffering from delusion, not self-deception: their distorted body image often represents such a grave departure from reality that it has often been seen as an indication that such patients are more disturbed than their premorbid history and their competence in other spheres of life may indicate (Guisinger 2003, p. 753). It seems obvious that the anorexic person has a different world-picture and is using concepts in a rather different manner from that of her linguistic community.

However, it must also be said that, while *anorexia nervosa* was first reported by Richard Morton in 1689, and was recognized as a pathological eating disorder in 1873, within the past

---

[11] I am writing in this roundabout fashion because it is clearly false that the person in delusion is speaking to no one, for that would imply that the sentence "She is speaking to someone" is not, in any sense, true.

[12] Judy Sargent, http://www.angelfire.com/ms/anorexianervosa/questions.html (accessed 26th January 2009).

twenty years, incidence has increased so rapidly that it has been termed a social epidemic.[13] In addition, women and girls are far more vulnerable to the syndrome[14] and its highest incidence remains in Western societies (Gordon 2000). Such observations appear to show that there is a marked social dimension to *anorexia nervosa*. In this regard, it is obvious that there is much modern pressure on women to diet (Garner and Garfinkel 1980, pp. 647-656). The fashion and entertainment industries promote a physique that is impossible for most women to attain.[15] Indeed, 78% of U.S. women—or three times what the health charts actually indicate—saw themselves as overweight (Jacoby 1990, as quoted in Evans 2001, p. 1). For many women, chronic dieting, often including excessive exercising, is considered a normal experience (***Polivy*** and ***Herman 1985***). Thus, these social observations do help to explicate *anorexia nervosa*'s etiology even if they do not satisfactorily explain anorexia's distinctive delusional symptoms.

CONCLUSION

In the light of the foregoing arguments, even if one were to maintain that the anorexic person is deluded not self-deceived, the personal level is not the only pertinent plane of possible self-deception. Of course, the anorexic person is deluded in grossly overestimating her body weight and health condition and distorting her body image. However, when such a person is urged to recognize her delusion and acknowledge honestly what she is, it is precisely the rigid image of the ultra-thin physique that she is asked to embrace. Several suggestions have been put forward for the way in which the dealings of our Western culture with the feminine gender could be central in understanding and treating eating disorders. It has been proposed that *anorexia nervosa* might be a means to assert one's intellectual and managerial capacities by achieving a more androgynous look (Gordon 2000, pp. 137-138), or that anorexia is an attempt to demonstrate power over one's own body (MacSween 1995, pp. 247-254), or that it gives the person the feeling that she is gaining power over others (Bruch 1980, pp. 72-90; Orbach 1986), or that it constitutes an avoidance of sexual experience or exploitation (Wooley 1995, pp. 294-298). It has also been noted that food-restriction is an attempt to regress to a pre-pubertal state (Crisp 1980) and that self-starvation becomes a defense against sexuality or as an ascetic repudiation of bodily urges (Casper 1983). While it has been proposed that "three characteristics ... are particularly marked in any sufferer: [t]hese are an intense morality, an extreme sensitivity, particularly to the needs and sufferings of others, and a profound sense of worthlessness," it has been noted that "it is the continuity between the sufferers' moral attitude and that of their social group or culture that again explains why the condition can be lethal" (Duker and Slade 2002, pp. 108-110).

Indeed, it appears that ideas such as the great aesthetic and social desirability of a thin body, the idea of the body—and particularly the female body—as the locus of corruption, the

---

[13] See Gordon (2000). Since 1960, incidence of *anorexia nervosa* appears to have increased in Europe and the United States and lifetime prevalence among women is now 0.5% (Guisinger 2003, p. 745).

[14] It is estimated that 90% of *anorexia nervosa*'s victims are women and girls (see http://emedicine.medscape.com/article/286063-overview [accessed 26th January 2009]).

[15] Until a few months ago, many fashion houses did not hire women as models unless they were thinner than 95% of their age mates. Indeed, female fashion models generally weighed about 85% of ABW (Seid 1994), thus meeting part of the *DSM–IV–TR*'s first criterion for *anorexia nervosa*.

view of women as being especially emotional beings in need of much control and discipline, and the emphasis on narcissism fuelled by the fashion industry are all are very present, though often unacknowledged, in our society. We all habitually refuse to see ourselves except in this manner. Indeed, it appears that when anorexic patients are urged to recognize and acknowledge their condition, it is precisely the image of the "ugly," "shameful," "corrupt," and "overly-emotional" self that they are asked to embrace. They are asked to abandon one false self-image for another. We rightly criticize their delusion, but ask them to abandon it for what can be seen as self-deception pervasively present in a society captivated by a particular way of seeing persons—particularly female persons—and their bodies. Perhaps we should all embark on the journey of acknowledging that anorexic persons unconsciously express a widespread cultural bias. To the extent to which we propagate these myths through our ways of life and popular culture, we are arguably all self-deceived. Such social myths serve to reinforce the role of food-restriction and emaciation in the anorexic's life. It is, indeed, no wonder that anorexics find it especially hard to escape their delusion. If they acknowledge it for what it is, they would be asked to accept an image of themselves and of their lives which is itself self-deceptive and which, moreover, tends to increase the power of *anorexia nervosa* over them. Given our "societal" self-deception, in which each of us plays some part, perhaps anorexic persons are less deluded than we might want to think.

REFERENCES

Anscombe, Elizabeth (1981), "The First Person," in *Collected Philosophical Papers*, III (Oxford: Basil Blackwell).

Audi, Robert (1982), "Self-Deception, Action and Will," *Erkenntnis* 18: 133-158.

Bach, Kent (1981), "An Analysis of Self-Deception," *Philosophy and Phenomenological Research* 41: 351-370.

Bell, Rudolph (1985), *Holy Anorexia*. Chicago: University of Chicago Press.

Beumont, P.J.V., Arthur, J.B., Russell, D. and Touyz, S.W. (1994), *Excessive Physical Activity in Dieting Disordered Patients*, in *International Journal of Eating Disorders* 15: 21-36.

Bloom, Carol, Gitter, A., Gutwill, S., Kogel, L., and Zaphiropoulos, L. (1994), *Eating Problems*. New York: Basic Books.

Bruch, Hilde (1978), *The Golden Cage*. Cambridge Mass.: Harvard University Press.

Casper, R.C. (1983), "On the Emergence of Bulimia Nervosa as a Syndrome: A Historical View," *International Journal of Eating Disorders*, 2: 3–16.

Chisholm, K. (2002), *Hungry Hell: What It's Really like to be Anorexic*. London: Short Books.

Crisp, A.H. (1980), *Anorexia Nervosa — Let Me Be*. London: Academic Press.

Davidson, Donald (1985), "Deception and Division," in *Actions and Events: Perspectives on the Philosophy of Donald Davidson*, edited by Ernest Lepore and Brian McLaughlin. Oxford: Basil Blackwell, pp. 138-148.

Demos, Raphael (1960), "Lying to Oneself," *Journal of Philosophy* 57: 588-594.

DSM-IV-TR (2000), Diagnostic and Statistical Manual of Mental Disorders, 4th Edition Text Revision. Washington DC: American Psychiatric Association.

Duker, M. and Slade, R. (2002), *Anorexia Nervosa and Bulimia.* United Kingdom: Open University Press.

Duker, Marilyn and Slade, Roger (2003), *Anorexia and Bulimia: How to Help.* Buckingham: Open University Press.

Evans, Gloria J. (2001), *The Relationship of Attachment and Shame to Anorexia: A Case Study Comparing Restrictive and Normal Eaters* (unpublished Ph.D. Dissertation, University of North Texas).

Evans, Gloria J. (2001), *The Relationship of Attachment and Shame to Anorexia: A Case Study Comparing Restrictive and Normal Eaters*. University of North Texas: unpublished Ph.D. Dissertation.

Garfinkel, P.E. & Garner, D.M. (1982), *Anorexia Nervosa: A Multidimensional Perspective* New York: Brunner/Mazel.

Garner, D.M. and Garfinkel, P.E. (1980), "Sociocultural Factors in the Development of Anorexia Nervosa," *Psychological Medicine* 10: 647-656.

Giordano, Simona (2005), *Understanding Eating Disorders.* Oxford: Oxford University Press.

Gordon, Richard A. (2000), *Anorexia and Bulimia: Anatomy of a Social Epidemic.* Oxford: Blackwell Publishers.

Guisinger, Shan (2003), "Adapted to Flee Famine: Adding an Evolutionary Perspective to Anorexia Nervosa," *Psychological Review* 110: 745-760.

Guisinger, Shan (2003), *Adapted to Flee Famine: Adding an Evolutionary Perspective to Anorexia Nervosa*, in *Psychological Review* 110: 748-752.

Halmi, K.A. (1992), *The Psychobiology of Eating Behavior*, in K. A. Halmi (ed.), *The Psychobiology and Treatment of Anorexia Nervosa and Bulimia Nervosa.* Washington DC: American Psychiatric Press.

Hornbacher, Marya (1998), *Wasted: A Memoir of Anorexia and Bulimia.* New York: Harper Collins.

ICD-10 (1992), *International Classification of Diseases.* Geneva: World Health Organisation.

Jacoby, S. (1990), "*The Body Image Blues*," in *Family Circle*, pp. 41-47.

Johnston, Mark (1995), "Self-Deception and the Nature of Mind," in *Philosophy of Psychology: Debates on Psychological Explanation*, Cynthia Macdonald (ed.). Cambridge: Blackwell.

Kaplan, Allan and Garfinkel, Paul (1993), *Medical Issues and the Eating Disorders: The Interface*. New York: Brunner/Mazel.

King-Farlow, John (1963), "Self-Deceived and Sartrean Seducers," *Analysis* 23: 131-136.

Lasègue, C. (1873), "On Hysterical Anorexia," in *Medical Times and Gazette* 2: 266.

Macsween, M. (1995), *Anorexic Bodies: A Feminist and Social Perspective.* London: Routledge.

Mele (1987a), *Irrationality: An Essay on Akrasia, Self-Deception and Self-Control.* Oxford: Oxford University Press.

Mele (1987b), "Recent Work in Self-Deception," *American Philosophical Quarterly* 24: 1-17.

Mele (1997), "Real Self-Deception," *Behavioural and Brain Sciences* 20: 91-102.

Mele (2001), *Self-Deception Unmasked.* Princeton: Princeton University Press.

Mele, Alfred (1983), "Self-Deception," *Philosophical Quarterly* 33: 366-377.

Mounce, H.O. (1971), "Self-Deception," *Proceedings of the Aristotelian Society*, 45: 61-72.

Nelkin, Dana (2002), "Self-Deception, Motivation and the Desire to Believe," *Pacific Philosophical Quarterly* 83: 384-406.

Orbach, Susie (1986), *Hunger Strike: The Anorectic's Struggle as a Metaphor for our Age.* New York: Norton.

Pears, David (1984), *Motivated Irrationality.* Oxford: Clarendon Press.

Polivy, J., and ***Herman***, C.P. (***1985***), "Dieting and Binging: a causal analysis," *The American Psychologist* 40: 193-201.

Pugmire, David (1969), "'Strong' Self-Deception," *Inquiry* 12: 339-361.

Rorty, Amélie O. (1972), "Belief and Self-Deception," *Inquiry* 15: 387-410.

Roukema, Richard W. (2003), *What Every Patient, Family, Friend, and Caregiver Needs to Know about Psychiatry.* Arlington VA: American Psychiatric Publications.

Seid, R.P. (1994), "Too 'Close to the Bone': The Historical Context for Women's Obsession with Slenderness," in P. Fallon, M. A. Katzman, and S. C. Wooley [eds.], *Feminist Perspectives on Eating Disorders.* New York: Guilford Press, pp. 3-17.

Strober, Michael (1991), *Disorders of the Self in Anorexia Nervosa: An Organismic Developmental Paradigm*, in Craig L. Johnson (ed.), *Psychodynamic treatment of Anorexia Nervosa and Bulimia.* New York: Guilford, pp. 354-373.

Szabados, Béla (1985), "The Self, its Passions and Self-Deception," in *Self-Deception and Self-Understanding: New Essays in Philosophy and Psychology*, ed. Mike W. Martin. Lawrence/KS: University Press of Kansas, pp. 159-160.

Talbott, W.J. (1995), "Intentional Self-Deception in a Single Coherent Self," *Philosophy and Phenomenological Research* 55: 27-74.

Tan, Jacinta O.A., Hope, Tony, and Stewart, Anne (2003), *Anorexia Nervosa and Personal Identity: The Accounts of Patients and their Parents*, in *International Journal of Law and Psychiatry*, 26: 533-548.

Thompson-Brenner, H., Westen, D. and Glass, S. (2003), "A Multidimensional Meta-Analysis of Psychotherapy for Bulimia Nervosa," *Clinical Psychology: Science and Practice* 10: 269-287.

Vitousek, K. ***(2005)***, "Cognitive–Behavioral therapy for ***Anorexia*** Nervosa," in C. G. Fairburn & K. D. Brownell (eds.), *Eating Disorders and Obesity.* New York: Guilford Publications, pp. ***308-313.***

Wittgenstein, Ludwig (1977), *On Certainty*, edited by G. E. M. Anscombe and G. H. von Wright, translated by Denis Paul and G. E. M. Anscombe. Oxford: Basil Blackwell.

Wooley, S. (1995), "Feminist Influences on the Treatment of Eating Disorders," in K. D. Brownell and C. G. Fairburn (eds.), *Eating Disorders and Obesity.* New York: Guilford Press, pp. 294-298.

In: Anorexia Nervosa: A Multi-Disciplinary Approach ISBN: 978-1-60876-200-2
Editors: A. Mancini, S. Daini, L. Caruana, pp. 203-223

Chapter 13

NIETZSCHE'S ASCETIC IDEAL AND THE ANOREXIC CONDITION

Terrance Walsh
Department of Philosophy, Heythrop College University of London, UK.

ABSTRACT

This paper examines the correspondence between the symptoms and etiology of anorexia nervosa and Nietzsche's theory of the ascetic ideal and his consequent analysis of the will. Nietzsche's theory of the manifold and destructive ways that human beings seek release from the suffering and aimlessness of existence illuminates not only the cultural conditions under which anorexia thrives, but also the paradox of a will that seemingly wills to act against its own well-being. In light of Nietzsche's analysis of the ascetic ideal, anorexics are ascetics without an otherworldly ideal as their goal; it was the ideal that kept the nihilistic tendencies of the ascetic in check, kept him or her willing and striving in pursuit of an end. The anorexic, who lives in a culture where these higher ideals have lost credibility engages in the self-abnegating practices of the ascetic without the corresponding goal of another, truer world beyond the body. What happens when the ascetic does not have a spiritual ideal to sustain her will? Nietzsche, the philosopher, leaves us with a philosophical problem, which, he concluded, could have no philosophical answer, but had to be worked out by the afflicted person "experimentally."

INTRODUCTION

There is only one world, and this is false, cruel, contradictory, seductive, without meaning ... We have need of lies in order to conquer this reality, this "truth," that is, in order to live—that lies are necessary in order to live is itself part of the terrifying and questionable character of existence. The human being must be a liar by nature; he must be above all an artist. And he is one: metaphysics, religion, morality, and science—all of them only products of his will to art, to lie, to flight from "truth."

> Nietzsche, Draft for a preface to the new edition of *The Birth of Tragedy* (1887).

> To tolerate life remains, after all, the first duty of all living beings. Illusion becomes valueless if it makes this harder for us.
> Freud, *Our Attitude toward Death* (1915).

> That a psychologist without equal speaks from my writings is perhaps the first insight reached by a good reader—a reader as I deserve him, who reads me the way good old philologists read their Horace.
> Nietzsche, *Why I Write Such Good Books* (1888).

Silently and invisibly, beneath the symbolic discourses and affirmations of Western culture, we have come to accept that we are bodily beings, purely natural phenomena, for whom words such as "soul" and "spirit" are references to the concrete, material reality of bodily or psychological existence. When we speak about spiritual values of self-fulfillment or well-being, we are, in fact, thinking about bodily satisfactions. Nietzsche was the first to recognize and analyze this watershed in valuation and self-understanding of our culture as the first sign of nihilism—which he thought had not yet reached its final stage in the late 19th century. He thought that European culture, which had been shaped and determined by two supreme teleological forces, Greek rationalism and Christian morality, was still in the grip of a powerful and inescapable self-denial about its nihilistic essence. The persistent refusal to recognize the consequences of our own development as a culture, Nietzsche argued, would inevitably lead to a catastrophic breakdown of the will; in fact, its first manifestations were already at work in science, technology, and politics. There is something fatally destructive about a culture that entertains elaborate claims of self-fulfillment in space and time, but has not faced up to how these claims could possibly be fulfilled by the body alone. Moreover, there is an implicit contradiction in Western culture that only now, after two millennia, is coming to a head: the individual fragile and imperfect body must bear the onus we place upon it of being both the end of existence and the means to that end. There is something incoherent about such an understanding of the self, the world, and the conditions of willing something as both means and end. Nietzsche was the first to bring this conflict to light by means of a new method of critical insight, which, in contrast to academic philosophy, he called "psychology."[1] The Nietzschean-inspired psychological analysis of the will that I propose in this paper reveals a culture that posits as the purpose of its striving a certain state of the body, symbolized by the perfection of the body (its size, shape, and tone), while in fact never clearly articulating exactly how the body could possibly satisfy incorporeal desires for well-being, peace of mind, self-acceptance, and purposefulness—to be realized by the body and for the body.[2] In a passage from his *Notebook* written in 1888, Nietzsche outlines the psychological effects of becoming aware of the futility of pursuing meaning in self-posited ends:

> Nihilism as a psychological state will have to come about firstly when we have sought in everything that happens a "meaning" it doesn't contain, so that in the end the searcher loses

[1] Nietzsche (2002), §23. For a recent interpretation of Nietzsche's "psychology" see Pippin (2009).

[2] Kant defines persons as beings whose value is not simply as a means, but as ends in themselves (Kant 1997, Section II, p.45).

courage. Nihilism is then the becoming conscious of the long squandering of our strength, the torment of the "in vain" —being ashamed towards oneself as if one had deceived oneself for far too long ...What all these kinds of ideas share is that the process aims to achieve something; and now it is realized that becoming aims for nothing, achieves nothing ... Hence disappointment about a supposed purpose of becoming as a cause of nihilism.3

The pathological condition that Nietzsche perceived in the late 19th Century seems full-blown in contemporary young women in the process of starving themselves to death. Below, an excerpt of a support group exchange among three anorexic women displays remarkable similarities to psychological nihilism:

Layla: How would I ever ... can explain it ... To know that my stomach was empty gave me such a good feeling, but now I can see that these are just the surface ...surface decorations of it that I used to be in something ... socially acceptable so that I could live in that misery, and I wouldn't see it as just a way of avoiding thought. It had to be, it had to convey some messages or, how to say, I mean I had to convince myself that it was good. So I think that my mind has worked in that way so that I could be happy in that.

Zoe: I think I would say it's just not worth it ... like I really think it comes from being insecure ... and I think also it's, that also tends to be a way where like: Wow! Everyone expects so much of me. I don't know if I can do all this. At least this one way I can succeed and be successful.

Cathy: Now, I think I have to say that for most people, I think when I say this I do represent most people, is that you feel so alone. I don't think there is any vocabulary to really express just how alone you feel. Um ... nobody in the world understands you. Nobody cares. You feel as if ... um, you're in a bubble and nobody can get in and you can't get out (Malson 1998, p. 2-3).

In his classic treatment of the nihilistic will of the ascetic, who needs to create an other-worldly ideal to strive for even if it entails a weakening or disappearing of the self, Nietzsche writes: "It was precisely here that I saw the great danger to mankind, its sublimest enticement and seduction—but to what? To nothingness? It was precisely here that I saw the beginning of the end, the dead stop, a retrospective weariness, the will turning against life, the tender and sorrowful signs of the ultimate illness."[4] Our final illness is nihilism, and its cultural disguise is the ascetic ideal.

This paper examines what I think is both an interesting and important correspondence between the symptoms and etiology of anorexia nervosa and Nietzsche's theory of the ascetic ideal and his consequent analysis of the will. Although there are important disanalogies between the pathology of the ascetic ideal and anorexia, I will argue that Nietzsche's theory of the manifold and destructive ways that human beings seek release from the suffering and

---

[3] *Notebook* (1887-1888), 11 [99]: nihilism as a "psychological state" (Nietzsche 2003).

[4] Nietzsche 1967, Preface §5. And at the very end of the book Nietzsche concludes: "man would rather will nothingness than not will" (III, 28).

aimlessness of existence illuminates not only the cultural conditions under which anorexia thrives, but also the paradox of a will that seemingly wills to act against its own well-being.[5]

I will argue the following thesis: In light of Nietzsche's analysis of the ascetic ideal, anorexics are ascetics, but without an other-worldly ideal as their goal; it was the ideal that kept the nihilistic tendencies of the ascetic in check, kept him or her willing and striving in pursuit of an end. The anorexic, who lives in a culture where these higher ideals have "devalued themselves," engages in the self-abnegating practices of the ascetic without the corresponding goal of another true or real world beyond the body. What happens when the ascetic does not have the fantasy of a spiritual ideal to sustain her will? Nietzsche expressed this impasse as a tension between two wills in us: a will to knowledge and rational control of the body, and a will to truth—seeing things, especially ourselves, honestly and fearlessly like people who have nothing to lose. The traditional interpretation states that the will to power is the answer to such a problem. This is, unfortunately, not the case. Nietzsche, the philosopher, leaves us with a philosophical problem, which, he concluded, could have no philosophical or a-priori answer, but had to be worked out by the afflicted person "experimentally."

ART, ILLUSION, AND METAPHYSICS: THE PATHOLOGY OF THOUGHT

At the beginning of his first book, *The Birth of Tragedy* (a project Nietzsche criticized, rethought, and revised for the rest of his active life, without ever totally renouncing), Nietzsche recounts the Greek legend of King Midas' search for Silenus, a forest daemon with composite human and goat-like properties and companion to Dionysos:

> When Silenus had finally fallen into his hands, the King asks what is the best and most excellent thing for human beings. Stiff and unmoving, the daemon . . . finally breaks out in shrill laughter and says: "Wretched, ephemeral race, children of chance and tribulation, why do you force me to tell you the very thing which it would be most profitable for you not to hear? The very best thing is utterly beyond your reach not to have been born, not to be, to be nothing. However, the second best thing for you is: to die soon."[6]

Nietzsche means for us to draw three lessons from this stark response: (1) Silenus' is a cold-eyed, not fully human, perspective on the truth of existence, a truth, once stripped of wishful-thinking and fanciful adornment, it would be best for humans not to hear; (2) the best advice that Silenus offers is, of course, impossible to put into practice, not to have been born, to be nothing; (3) yet, the second best advice, to die as soon as possible, is almost universally ignored, repressed, or in Nietzsche's view sublimated by a vision of the beautiful, a desire for appearance for appearance's sake, especially on the part of the Greeks, whom Nietzsche admired above all ancient and modern peoples. In *The Birth of Tragedy,* Nietzsche argues that

---

[5] Joan Jacobs Brumberg's argument that anorexia is not a modern version of anorexia mirabil is widespread among medieval religious women is important historical support for my own thesis (Brumberg 1988, especially pp.43-48).

[6] Nietzsche 1999, §3, pp. 22-23. For the German text, I have used Nietzsche 1972. The most stimulating recent discussion of the text is Porter 2000. Porter argues for a deep consistency between Nietzsche's early essay with his later writings. Although I agree that this is, in fact, the case and needs to be underlined, I think his position on the identity of Nietzsche's early and late views is extreme and not in a position to explain fully Nietzsche's criticism of metaphysics and the ascetic ideal in the 1880s.

the unpleasant truths of existence were neither ignored nor repressed by the Greeks, but embraced in such a way as to become their incentive *for* life: "The Greeks knew and felt the terrors and horrors of existence; in order to live at all they had to place in front of these things the resplendent, dream-born figures of the Olympians . . ."

> How else could that people have borne existence, given their extreme sensitivity, their stormy desires, their unique gift for suffering, if that same existence had not been shown to them in their gods, suffused with a higher glory? The same drive which calls art into being to complete and perfect existence and thus to seduce us into continuing to live, also gave rise to the world of the Olympians in which the Hellenic "will" held up a transfiguring mirror to itself. Thus gods justify the life of men by living it themselves [...] (Nietzsche 1999, §3, pp. 23-24).

There is, without doubt, a brilliance to this interpretation of the meaning of Greek art and religion as idealizations of existence, which, in Nietzsche's eyes, amounted to the "only satisfactory theodicy" (by which he meant that we need gods to justify to ourselves our own existence; in order to see that our lives have value, we have to experience them as spectators).[7] At the same time, however, there is something troubling and problematic about the claim, for how could a culture that knew the "truth" about the pointlessness of existence settle for the appearance of a glorified fiction? They knew the image of reality presented by their "transfiguring mirror" lied, yet they took it for a reason to affirm life—a lie accepted as a reason to live—is this cowardice, a bizarre self-deception, or some new type of wisdom? The inspiration for this dream-like existence is the god, Apollo, the diviner of dreams, out of which developed the Olympian divine order of joy: "It is an illusion of the kind so frequently employed by nature to achieve its aims. The true goal is obscured by a deluding image; we stretch out our hands towards the image, and nature achieves its goal by means of this deception."[8] For a period of time, the Apolline dream-illusion of beauty, truth, and rational order gained the upper hand over the darker vision of chaotic appearance and destruction: "... by employing powerful delusions and intensely pleasurable illusions [Apolline culture] gains victory over a terrifyingly profound view of the world and the most acute sensitivity to suffering. But how rarely is that complete enthrallment in the beauty of semblance which we call naïve actually achieved" (Nietzsche 1999, §3, p.24). It seems straightforward to Nietzsche that to a people who were strong and confident enough to look directly at the truth of existence, the Apolline aesthetic experience would not only become extremely fragile, but also artificial, even repulsive. Nietzsche is not interested, as the early parts of *The Birth of*

---

[7] See Nietzsche (2001), §78. This claim constitutes Nietzsche's therapeutic strategy against the pathology of thought: the capacity to see ourselves, unburdened by shame and guilt, from the outside perspective, as spectators. This view will be therapeutic only if it is ironic, if it engenders laughter: "No, you should first learn the art of comfort in this world, you should learn to laugh, my young friends, if you are really determined to remain pessimists. Perhaps, then, as men who laugh, you will some day send all attempts at metaphysical comfort to Hell—with metaphysics the first to go!" *An Attempt at Self-Criticism* §7 (Nietzsche 1999). Laughter occurs with the realization that our lives are not measured by any transcendent ideal.

[8] Nietzsche 1999, §3, p. 25. Nature's goal is self-preservation. Thus, the human condition is torn between two contrary tendencies: the rational desire to be rid of aimless suffering and the natural impulse or drive to continue to exist and thus to create or fabricate the conditions under which continued existence becomes possible. Spinoza provides the classic definition of this drive: "*conatus in suo esse perseverandi*" [striving to persevere in one's being], in *Ethics* III, P7. This becomes one of the sources for Nietzsche's will to power, which is important for understanding his notion of the ascetic ideal.

Tragedy make abundantly clear, in describing an aesthetic experience of wonder and amazement at the artifact's enticing semblance of reality—enticing us to reach for mere appearance, delighting us with its deception.[9] The semblance and deception, which interest Nietzsche, take place not at the aesthetic, but at a much deeper psychological and metaphysical level.

What led Nietzsche to suspect a deeper dimension to Greek tragic art? The role of the Chorus in tragedy convinced him that at some level, the spectator was himself transformed by a vision that was not just a semblance of the mundane world, but also the appearance of a deeper, truer reality (Nietzsche 1999, §7). Nietzsche begins to personify the Dionysiac drive of nature as itself an artist, a creator of transfiguring appearances. "Man is no longer an artist, he has become a work of art; all nature's artistic power reveals itself here, amidst shivers of intoxication, to the highest, most blissful satisfaction of the primordial unity [das Ur-Eine]" (Nietzsche 1999, §1). The Dionysiac intoxicating semblance in contrast to the Apolline dream state is not referential, it does not point or gesture to a higher realm of the gods beyond the work of art. It is, itself, transformative:

> The more I become aware of those all-powerful artistic drives in nature, and of a fervent longing in them for semblance, for their redemption and release in semblance, the more I feel myself driven to the metaphysical assumption that that which truly exists, the eternally suffering and contradictory, primordial unity, simultaneously needs, for its constant release and redemption, the ecstatic vision, intensely pleasurable semblance (Nietzsche 1999, §4).

In an unpublished essay, *The Dionysiac World View,* written two years before *The Birth of Tragedy,* Nietzsche postulates that what reconciled the Greeks to reality could not have been the aesthetic semblance of an ideal world, but a metaphysical cognition of being a part of an eternally self-manifesting and self-destructive primordial chaos. "For there are two states in which human beings attain to the feeling of delight in existence, namely, in dream and in intoxication. Every human being is fully an artist when creating the worlds of dream, and the lovely semblance of dream is the father of all the arts of image-making ... We dream with pleasure as we understand the figure directly; all forms speak to us . . ."[10] But, as in any dream state, we awaken and see through the illusion as enticing, but also transitory and fanciful. What happens when we awaken from the dream, from the fantasy? Nietzsche would agree with Kant's remark that we have rational insight only into that which we create after our own plans. To repress this aspect of our dream-making activity from reaching consciousness is to embark on a pathological course:

> Yet even while this dream-reality is most alive, we nevertheless retain a pervasive sense that it is semblance; only when this ceases to be the case do the pathological effects set in whereby dream no longer enlivens and the healing natural energy of its states ceases . . . Things which are grave, sad, gloomy, and dark are contemplated with just as much

[9] Titian once remarked that his aesthetic aim was to have birds fly into his workshop to pluck the newly painted grapes off the canvass. Nietzsche would call this art a "semblance of a semblance," for even the real grapes on the real vine do not represent the deepest layer of reality—that which interests Nietzsche.

[10] *The Dionysiac World View* (1870); see Nietzsche (1999), p. 119.

> pleasure, always provided that here too the veil of semblance is in fluttering movement and does not completely cover up the basic forms of the real (Nietzsche 1999, p. 119).

In this first mention of pathology in his writings, Nietzsche conceives of it as a failure to distinguish our own life-enhancing illusions from reality.[11] The healing natural energy of dreaming ceases and is replaced by the noxious effects associated with the forgetfulness of the true nature of reality. The "fluttering movement" of the veil of illusion, the fluttering of consciousness itself, indicates the intentional, subjective aspect of semblance—the subtle reminder that the image is a mere appearance covering up a deeper dimension.[12] This nice distinction, however, is more difficult to maintain in the intoxicating and ecstatic condition symbolized by the experience of Dionysiac art. The festivals "forge a bond between human beings" and reconcile human beings with nature:

> Yet it is more than this: they feel themselves to have been transformed by magic, and they really have become something different. [The participant] feels himself to be a god; that which had previously lived only in his imagination he now feels in his own person. What does he now care for images and statues? *Man is no longer an artist, he has become a work of art*; man himself now moves with the same ecstasy and sublimity with which, in dream, he once saw the gods walk. *The artistic force of nature, not that of the individual artist*, reveals itself here; a nobler clay, a more precious marble is kneaded and chiseled here: the human being (Nietzsche 1999, p. 121; my emphases).

This is an extraordinary statement of the anti-aesthetic experience of participating in the "force of nature," which "transforms" the individual into a "work of art." The transfigured human being replaces ideal art objects as the actual appearing of the power of "nature." Yet, a fateful line has been crossed, and the fluttering movement marking the art object as semblance has disappeared. Nietzsche obviously perceives a psychological threat in its disappearance, that is, the vanishing from consciousness of difference, so he constructs an ambivalent safeguard into the Dionysiac experience, which he describes as "rather like dreaming and at the same time being aware that the dream is a dream. Thus the attendant of Dionysos must be in a state of intoxication and at the same time he must lie in ambush, observing himself from behind. Dionysiac art manifests itself, not in the alternation of clear-mindedness and intoxication, but in their co-existence" (Nietzsche 1999, p. 121).

But now, we might ask, who's kidding whom—a clear-minded intoxication? Nietzsche is advocating an impossible unity of self-consciousness in the midst of a profound division, a consciousness fully caught up in the intoxicating illusion, yet observing itself precisely in this ecstatic dream of oneness. Nietzsche compares it to a dream state in which one becomes aware of dreaming. But how does this slight awareness of dreaming function to control the

---

[11] In *The Future of an Illusion*, Freud writes, "Thus we call a belief an illusion when a wish-fulfillment is a prominent factor in its motivation, and in doing so we disregard its relation to reality, just as the illusion itself sets no store by verification" (Freud 1995, p.704).

[12] Later in *The Dionysiac World View*, Nietzsche writes, "But the image of Apollo must also include that delicate line which the dream image must not overstep if its effect is not to become pathological, in which case the semblance does not simply deceive but also cheats" (Nietzsche 1999, p. 120). The line here is the psychological line separating self-knowledge from delusion or fantasy. When one passes over the line, the semblance will necessarily "cheat" by not delivering the promised goods, by not fulfilling the wish embodied in the "outstretched hand" of the spectator. The "ironic spectator" sees it for what it's worth. See above footnote 7.

illusion? One might ask, what motivated Nietzsche to construct this self-conscious perspective on illusion, this "observing himself from behind"? It is obviously an attempt to control rationally an uncontrollable will to illusion. Nietzsche will later call this attempt to get a grip on illusion, the will to truth, a desire for truthfulness, cleanliness of spirit and psychological honesty, profoundly at odds with psychic consolations. The rational desire not to abandon truth, especially self-knowledge, and to be honest with oneself, Nietzsche contends, are necessary aspects of human freedom. Nietzsche's unargued idea is that truth is as important for human beings as illusion, but how can a single consciousness sustain both simultaneously? This is what he has to say later in *The Birth of Tragedy* about the inevitable return to lucid consciousness of self-knowledge: "In the consciousness that follows his awakening from intoxication, he sees the terrible and absurd aspects of human existence wherever he looks; it disgusts him. Now he understands the wisdom of the wood-god... What mattered above all was to transform those repulsive thoughts about the terrible and absurd aspects of existence into representations with which it was possible to live." Nietzsche is too honest a thinker to accept an obvious dodge for long, for he realizes that all aesthetic representations do not just transfigure but also cover up the real: "[The sublime and comical representations] cast a veil over truth, which, although it is more transparent than beauty, nevertheless remains a veil" (Nietzsche 1999, p. 130). Yet, it will take the young Nietzsche some time to comprehend the error and romantic deception into which he had fallen. I want to interpret this early text, however, as Nietzsche's honest attempt to stake out uncharted territory, as explorations for a future psychological reinterpretation of the human condition that the young philologist is not yet capable of instituting.

The clue the psychologist will follow to reinterpret the split consciousness of Dionysiac intoxication has already been placed in *The Birth of Tragedy*: "The metaphysical consolation, which, I wish to suggest, we derive from every true tragedy, the consolation that in the ground of things, and despite all changing appearances, life is indestructibly mighty and pleasurable, this consolation appears with palpable clarity in the chorus of the satyrs, a chorus of natural beings whose life goes on ineradicably behind and beyond all civilization, as it were, and who remain eternally the same despite all the changes of generations and in the history of nations."[13] At bottom, this metaphysical consolation remains nothing but the intoxicating effect of a trivial illusion embodied by the chorus of satyrs that exhorts us—appearances to the contrary: "you remain part of a deeper flow of life cycles of rejoicing and delight at unending destruction of your own appearance." Already in the Foreword to *The Birth of Tragedy*, Nietzsche had enthusiastically proclaimed that the discovery of art's consoling power was the supreme achievement of Richard Wagner: "... my conviction that art is the highest task and the true metaphysical activity of life is based on an understanding which I share with the man and fighter whose sublime lead I follow and to whom I now wish to dedicate this work" (Nietzsche 1999, p. 14). The metaphysical task of art is to console the human being, to mitigate the stark vision of Silenus, by revealing the eternal depths of appearance and destruction, in which he participates as an appearance, as nature's "work of art."

> At this point we need to take a bold run-up and vault into a metaphysics of art, as I repeat my earlier sentence that only as an aesthetic phenomenon do existence and the world

[13] Nietzsche (1999), §7 (translation slightly altered).

appear justified; which means that tragic myth in particular must convince us that even the ugly and disharmonious is an artistic game which the Will, in the eternal fullness of delight, plays with itself (Nietzsche 1999, §24).

Even if, by means of this metaphysical vault, we imagine the world as a play of some demonic or benign force of nature, how should this help us live? In his mature evaluation of *The Birth of Tragedy*, after his break with Wagner, Nietzsche began to think of metaphysical consolation as nothing other than a symptom of weakness and decadence: "Knowledge, saying Yes to reality, is just as necessary for the strong as cowardice and the flight from reality—as the "ideal" is for the weak, who are inspired by weakness." The weak shun a knowledge that, on the contrary, enables the strong to affirm existence. In this 1888 reflection on *The Birth of Tragedy* that he composed for *Ecce Homo*, Nietzsche hits the decisive point that changed his entire view of illusion and the value of artistic semblance: "[The weak] are *not free to know*: the decadents *need* the lie—it is one of the conditions of their preservation" (Nietzsche 1989, p. 272; my emphasis). Nietzsche's earlier view in *The Birth of Tragedy* that the Dionysian enthusiast could maintain a healthy "split" consciousness, balancing two distinct wills, being both spectator and transformed "art object" of the self-destructive world of appearance, has been replaced by what is clearly a psychological diagnosis of a pathology. The drive of self-preservation (conatus) simply blocks out the thought, "this is all a dream, an illusion of intoxication," because such a thought would not be enough to "console" and persuade the weak to endure their meaningless suffering. "The weak are not free to know," Nietzsche now asserts—misunderstood or repressed "needs" disable human freedom; the will to survive is stronger than the will to truth. When one gives up any knowledge of the objective situation of appearances, one loses grip on the possibility of healthy affirmation of life exactly as it is, not as we wish it could be.[14] But is it, in fact, healthier to see existence exactly as it is?

The two autobiographical commentaries that Nietzsche wrote about his misdirected failure, first in the Preface for the new edition of *The Birth of Tragedy* in 1886, which he entitled *An Attempt at Self-Criticism,* and then in *Ecce Homo* two years later, I would suggest are the two essential texts for understanding both his diagnosis and prognosis of the pathology of thought. In the 1886 Preface, Nietzsche calls *The Birth of Tragedy* a "questionable book," one that he finds "an impossible book today ... badly written, clumsy, embarrassing with a rage for imagery and confused in its imagery, emotional ..."[15] Yet, he did not hesitate to republish it. It would be too easy to conclude that the value of the earlier effort was simply to mark how far he had advanced, or to highlight by sharp contrast his mature views on art and metaphysics. The book failed not just because it represented the mistaken metaphysical and romantic views of Schopenhauer and Wagner, but more significantly, it failed to express adequately in a language of his own what Nietzsche had for himself correctly grasped about the Greeks' strength of will and capacity to affirm existence.[16] In his 1886 reevaluation, Nietzsche realized that the earlier book had disclosed

---

[14] In the classic *Formulations on the Two Principles of Mental Functioning,* Freud writes, "We have long observed that every neurosis has as its result, and probably therefore as its purpose, a forcing of the patient out of real life, an alienating of him from reality ...Neurotics turn away from reality because they find it unbearable—either the whole or parts of it" (Freud 1995, p. 301).

[15] *An Attempt at Self-Criticism*, §3 (Nietzsche 1999).

[16] "I now regret very much that I did not yet have the courage at the time to permit myself a *language of my own* for such personal views and acts of daring ..." *An Attempt at Self-Criticism*, §6 (Nietzsche 1999).

some highly original insight about the Greek character that would prove invaluable to his analysis of the pathology of contemporary Western culture.

Nietzsche continued to value the book because it presented, for the first time in Western thought, a question that would open up a new path of critical inquiry, a path that would eventually lead to the unmasking and undermining of the entire European metaphysical, moral, and religious tradition. The question underlying the book was "a most stimulating and supremely important question" as well as "a profoundly personal one":

> The finest, most beautiful, most envied race of men ever known, the people who made life seem most seductive, the Greeks—what, they of all people needed tragedy? Or even—art? What purpose was served by Greek art? You will guess here the big question mark concerning the value of existence had thus been raised. Is pessimism necessarily a sign of decline, decay, failed existence, of tired and debilitated instincts …?

Nietzsche here presents the motivating question of his entire philosophical development: how can existence be justified, what is the value of existence? All other problems, from metaphysics to science, from religion to morality, stem from this vital, life-defining problem and struggle for existence. His fundamental insight into the roots of the dichotomy of a radically devalued existence (pessimism) and a radically idealized existence (optimism), he characterized as essentially "psychological" insights into the root motivations and pathologies of *all* human evaluation: our moral, religious, and philosophical judgments about good and evil coalesce around the problem of justifying human existence to ourselves. Nietzsche continues his reflection upon the above paragraph:

> Is there pessimism of strength? An intellectual preference for the hard, gruesome, evil, and problematic aspects of existence which comes from a feeling of well-being, from overflowing health, from an abundance of existence? Is there perhaps a suffering from superabundance itself? Is there a tempting bravery in the sharpest eye, which demands the terrifying as its foe against which it can test its strength and from which it intends to learn the meaning of fear?[17]

This original insight became the great question mark that Nietzsche would place next to existence: if life is a chaos of aimless and pointless suffering culminating in the routine destruction of individual life, how did the Greeks—who knew the truth better than any people—affirm existence and affirm it unblinkingly and joyfully? Consequently, it is the solution offered by his youthful and emotional text—metaphysical consolation of art—not its underlying question that Nietzsche comes to reject. If tragedy and its apparent pessimism are, in fact, symptoms of strength and the affirmation of life in the face of the worst aspects of existence, then it follows that the optimistic aspects of subsequent Greek culture, especially the rationalistic morality of Socrates as well as its progressive views of science, are to be reinterpreted as symptoms of weakness and decay. The young Nietzsche's psychological examination of the Dionysiac cult had led him to the doorstep of a critique of Western culture.

[17] *An Attempt at Self-Criticism*, §1 (Nietzsche 1999); translation slightly altered.

> Conversely, those things which gave rise to the death of tragedy—Socratism in ethics, the dialectics, smugness and cheerfulness of theoretical man—might not this very Socratism be a sign of decline, of exhaustion, of sickness, of the anarchic dissolution of the instincts? ... And science itself, our science—what indeed is the meaning of all science, viewed as a symptom of life? What is the purpose, and, worse still, what is the origin of all science? What? Is scientific method perhaps no more than fear of and flight from pessimism? A subtle defense against—truth? (Nietzsche 1999, §1).

Knowledge in philosophy and science, sublime beauty in art, progress in culture—are these all opposed to truth, repressions of truth? The mature Nietzsche thought that this question was the fundamental insight of his entire philosophical endeavor. Thus, in the 1886 *Self-Criticism*, he writes: "What I had got hold of at the time was something fearsome and dangerous, a problem with horns, not necessarily a bull, but at any rate a new problem; today I would say that it was the problem of science itself, science grasped for the first time as something problematic and questionable" (Nietzsche 1999, §2). Who had ever before questioned the value of knowledge for human well-being? Yet Nietzsche's seminal discovery that motivated his future inquiry was that knowledge itself is the great problem: the human claim of knowledge of the world of appearances is, in fact, a truth-suppressing drive, a metaphysical illusion that has provided a pragmatic foothold for sustaining life and defending it against unsettling truth. Once Nietzsche had removed the hypothesis of the metaphysical consolation from the Dionysiac affirmation and embrace of life in all its tragic aspects, then the question became urgent of how the will to truth might possibly coincide with a new affirmation of life; in view of his psychological insights, are they not mutually exclusive? To hope and to forget is the goal of life, not truth. Nietzsche concluded *The Birth of Tragedy* with a thought that subsequently he will struggle to refute: the power of art and illusion "to hold fast within life the animated world of individuation."

> If you could imagine dissonance assuming human form—and what else is man?—this dissonance would need, to be able to live, a magnificent illusion which would spread a veil over its own nature ... all those countless illusions of beautiful semblance which, at every moment, make existence at all worth living at every moment and thereby urge us on to experience the next (Nietzsche 1999, §25).

Why are we of all living beings a dissonant species? Our dissonance springs from a particular drive in our will, a drive to truth, to know the truth of ourselves, that introduces the dissonant cord in our being and that we must suppress in order to continue living—for us, truth is dissonance. For the natural consonance of the will is to act, to impose itself, to overcome obstacles, to strengthen itself in deed, not in thought, without regard for the way things really are. On the contrary, knowledge and self-consciousness impede action. And Nietzsche's own goal—truth and willing—about which he wrote in *Ecce Homo*, springs directly from this insight: "... the will to power as no man ever possessed it, the ruthless courage in matters of spirit, the unlimited power *to learn without damage to the will to act*."[18]

[18] Nietzsche (1999), §4; my emphasis. In *Beyond Good and Evil* (1886), Nietzsche had previously written: "Learning transforms us, it acts like all other forms of nourishment that do not just "preserve" —But at our foundation, "at the every bottom," there is clearly something that will not learn, a brick wall of spiritual *fatum*, of predetermined decisions and answers to selected, predetermined questions. In any cardinal problem, an

This is the crucial therapeutic remedy to the pathology of thought built on illusion, but it is a remedy, like Silenus' counsel, that we cannot immediately put into practice. Unlike the Greeks, Nietzsche thought that in modern European culture, the more we learned and discovered about ourselves, the weaker, more decadent the will became and the more we needed the psychic mechanism of illusion and semblance. What would be, Nietzsche questioned, the value of living without psychic defenses? In *Beyond Good and Evil*, written at the same time as *An Attempt at Self-Criticism*, Nietzsche characterized his goal of freeing human beings from the "lures of the metaphysical bird catchers" as an attempt "to translate humanity back into nature … to make sure that, from now on, the human being will stand before the human being." But this is the fruit of a self-effacing, cold-sighted knowledge that humans might not ultimately desire:

> Why do we choose it, this insane task? Or to ask it differently: "Why knowledge at all?"—Everyone will be asking us this. And we who have been prodded so much, we who have asked ourselves the same question a hundred times already, we have not found and are not finding any better answers…(Nietzsche 2002, §230).

An extraordinary admission that he has no better answer than the one given above: to stand before the terrible text of human nature without the bright gloss of fantasy and human vanity. But is this a reason; could this provide a therapy for the self-deceiving will, an alternate value to illusion? Nietzsche remains perplexed by the question, but to his credit, he makes no attempt to improvise an answer. "Above all, the problem that a problem exists here—and that, for as long as we have no answer to the question, 'What is Dionysiac?' the Greeks will remain as utterly unknown and unimaginable as they have always been …" (Nietzsche 1999, §3). How to understand the Dionysiac answer? *The Birth of Tragedy* offered a deeply felt analysis and solution, but one that was misconceived and shared in the dissembled pessimism and will to illusion of the entire rationalistic Apolline culture. Nietzsche saw clearly, however, that without an answer to how the Greeks affirmed life precisely by means of tragedy, a culture sustained by illusion and semblance, turning aside from truth, will inevitably lead to nihilism. Nihilism is a kind of knowledge, a species of truth: the acute recognition of the pathology of our thought, namely, that what we produce are lies—without hope either of a better way to live or a deeper truth to counteract it. Nihilism is a kind of dead-end truth, a truth that negates the future of truth.

THE PATHOLOGY OF THOUGHT II: THE ASCETIC IDEAL

What is the meaning of a life whose every thought is a prophylactic illusion of health and well-being, a life, however, that, in fact, accomplishes what it sets out to achieve—a certain rational control of the self as a means of continued existence and mitigated flourishing? Like Freud, Nietzsche defines thought physiologically; and like all else, there are strong and weak, healthy and sick, physiologies.

immutable "that is me" speaks up (Nietzsche 2002, §231). But this hitting the wall, "that is me," can be the beginning of psychic health.

> But the awakened, the knowing one says: body am I through and through, and nothing besides; and soul is just a world for something on the body.
>
> The body is a great reason, a multiplicity with one sense ... Your small reason, what you call "spirit" is also a tool of your body, a small work—and plaything of your great reason...
>
> Behind your thoughts and feelings stands a powerful commander, an unknown wise man—he is called self. He lives in your body; he is your body.
>
> The self says to the ego: "Feel pain here!" And then it suffers and reflects on how it might suffer no more—and just for that purpose it is supposed to think.
>
> The self says to the ego: "Feel pleasure here!" Then it is pleased and reflects on how it might feel pleasure more often—and for that purpose it is supposed to think![19]

This is one of the fundamental insights that guide the development of Nietzsche's mature analysis of the thought processes, by which illusion is created and sustained. Similar to Freud's argument in *Formulations on Two Principles of Mental Functioning,* Nietzsche located the physiological origin of thought in the body's search for satisfaction and its need to release frustration by means of the bodily "action" of thinking (Freud defined thinking as "essentially an experimental kind of acting") (Freud 1995, p. 303). Nietzsche's point (as his writings from the late notebooks prove) is not so much that the two principles of pleasure and pain determine our actions, but that the bodily will uses mental life to achieve its own satisfaction, namely, the exercise and expression of strength. The body commands thought—thought is an instrument of a bodily drive of dominance over obstacles. Pleasure and pain are the guideposts to an end, not the end itself. In a notebook entry from the winter of 1888, Nietzsche qualifies the 1883 remark in *Zarathustra*: "the satisfaction of the will is not the cause of pleasure: I particularly want to combat this most superficial of theories . . . instead, that the will wants to move forward, and again and again becomes master of what stands in its way: the feeling of pleasure lies precisely in the dissatisfaction of the will, in the way it is not yet satiated unless it has boundaries and resistances . . ." (Nietzsche 2003, 11 [75]). Thus, the body's encounter with obstacles and resistance, though a cause of frustration and dissatisfaction, is a spur to its fundamental drive and a chance to will further expansion. Our dissatisfied drives, Nietzsche continues, are not necessarily dispiriting, rather,

> the greater the resistances a force seeks out in order to master them, the greater is the magnitude of the failure and misfortune thus provoked: and as every force can only expend itself on what resists, every action necessarily contains an ingredient of unpleasure. But the effect of that unpleasure is to stimulate life—and to strengthen the will to power! (Nietzsche 2003, 11 [77]).

At first glance, this claim seems absurdly counterintuitive. Nietzsche, however, is aware that on certain psychological natures failure, misfortune, and dissatisfaction can produce the opposite effect, not to stimulate the affirmation of life, but in fact to weaken—without destroying—the will to power. Instead of increasing action in the direction of life and the worldly action, some natures react against resistance by turning inwardly, by becoming spiritual and ascetic. Nietzsche's association of weak and hypersensitive natures with religion is a constant in his publications of the 1880s:

---

[19] Nietzsche 2006, First Part: *On the despisers of the body.*

> With humans as with every other type of animal, there is a surplus of failures and degenerates, of the diseased and the infirm, of those who necessarily suffer. Even with humans, successful cases are always the exception and, since humans are still the undetermined animals, the infrequent exception. But it gets worse: people who represent more nobly bred types are less likely to turn out well. Chance … is most terribly apparent in its destructive effect on the higher men. So how is this surplus of failures treated by the two great religions [Christianity and Buddhism]? They try to preserve, to keep everything living that can be kept in any way alive. In fact, they take sides with the failures as a matter of principle, as religions of the suffering (Nietzsche 2002, § 62).

I take Nietzsche's comment that we are still "undetermined animals" to mean that our psycho-physiological tendencies have not achieved a stable organization of action and reaction to external stimuli. There is still a degree of openness and variability about how the organism acts and responds to obstacles in its environment. The strong and the successful must be seen as exceptional cases of an ideal potentiality that most humans, even those of superior natures, fail to achieve. At the nexus of striving and failure, the will makes use of thought to construct new possibilities of affective discharge, even if it implies a diminishment of overall satisfaction and a weakening of life.

Beginning with the publication of *Human All Too Human* in 1878, Nietzsche began to associate decadence of the will with Socratic rationalism and metaphysics. Nietzsche has learned well the lessons of the *Birth of Tragedy*: the cognitive representation of metaphysical reality serves some deep psychological need arising from the physiological affect that Nietzsche calls will to power. It is important to keep in mind that even though the physiological drives and needs are individual, as are the feelings of failure, when these drives are frustrated, the cognitive response of weak natures is necessarily mediated by language and symbolic representations of a culture's self-understanding, whether by means of myth, tragedy, religious morality or metaphysics. The virtue of Nietzsche's cultural semiotics is that it offers a rational explanation of the universal appeal of the ascetic ideals of the ascetic priesthood.[20] These ascetic groups Nietzsche derisively refers to as "the herd": "The formation of a herd is a significant victory and advance in the struggle against depression. With the growth of the community, a new interest grows for the individual, to, and often lifts him above the most personal element in his discontent, his aversion to himself. All the sick and sickly instinctively strive after a herd organization as a means of shaking off their dull displeasure and feeling of weakness" (Nietzsche 1967, III, 18). The physiological root of the religious or ascetical reinterpretation of existence from the perspective of the weak and sick Nietzsche calls "depression" [Depressions-Zustände]. He defines depression as an unpleasurable affect, "a feeling of physiological inhibition" (Nietzsche 1967, III, 17). It stems from the physiological failure to direct drives outwardly towards their fulfillment or satisfaction in the world. One is thrown back upon oneself, and the natural response is to seek a reason for one's suffering, a reason, which is not truth-directed, but serves the needs of the "body-self" to relieve, or at least, to dull pain and to regain some degree of satisfaction from willing. And, of course, the ascetic priest, whom Nietzsche views as a medicating physician, responds to the depressed person's assertion, "I suffer: someone must be to blame for it," with

[20] Nietzsche (1967), III, 11. In this text, Nietzsche characterizes ascetic valuations as "the most widespread and enduring phenomena," which would lead an objective observer to conclude that "the earth was [a] distinctively ascetic planet."

exactly what the suffering person wishes to hear: "But you yourself are this someone, you alone are to blame for it—You alone are to blame for yourself!" (Nietzsche 1967, III, 15).

It is not farfetched to argue that Nietzsche's entire published work after the *Birth of Tragedy*, beginning with *Human, All Too Human* (1878) and culminating in *Genealogy of Morals* (1887), *Twilight of the Idols* (1888), and *The Antichrist* (1888), are attempts to offer a sustained argument—based on physiology and psychology—against the metaphysical and religious responses to cultural depression and decadence of the will. The key methodological insight of a cultural genealogy, he articulates in *Twilight of the Idols*, but it was an idea present from the start of his inquiry:

> Morality is just an interpretation of certain phenomena, or speaking more precisely, a misinterpretation . . . Thus, moral judgments can never be taken literally: literally, they always contain nothing but nonsense. But they are semiotically invaluable all the same; they reveal, at least to those who are in the know, the most valuable realities of cultures and inner states that did not know enough to "understand" themselves. Morality is just a sign language, just a symptomatology: you already have to know what it's all about in order to get any use out of it.[21]

The whole system of cultural signs, the rational achievement of Western culture initiated by the Greeks, is, on the surface, sheer nonsense because the claim to represent "reality" as it is in itself is nonsense. Cultural signs are, however, valuable as symptoms of disease below the surface appearance of health and vitality. Thus, we read Nietzsche's earliest application of this method in the opening section of *Human, All Too Human* directed at the semiotics of metaphysics: " ... but all that has hitherto made metaphysical assumptions valuable, terrible, delightful [to people], all that has begotten these assumptions, is passion, error and self-deception; the worst of all methods for acquiring knowledge . . . When one has disclosed these methods as the foundation of all extant religions and metaphysical systems, one has refuted them!" (Nietzsche 1986, § 9).

THE PARADOX OF THE ASCETIC IDEAL IN *GENEALOGY OF MORALS*

> And what if Euripides was correct when he said: "Who can know if living is not dying and dying is not living?" Perhaps our life is in reality a death. Moreover, I have heard it said, even by wise men, that we are now dead and that the body is a tomb for us.
>
> Plato, *Gorgias*, 492e—493a

Genealogy of Morals analyzes the ascetic ideal in the context of its revaluation of values, especially, the value of moral judgments of good and evil. "Under what conditions did man devise these value judgments good and evil? And what value do they themselves possess?" Nietzsche asks and then provides criteria, based on his dichotomy of healthy and weak natures, to evaluate moral judgments: "Have they hitherto hindered or furthered human prosperity? Are they signs of distress, of impoverishment, of the degeneration of life? Or is

[21] Nietzsche 1997, §1. And in the 1886 Preface to *Human, All Too Human*, Nietzsche defines the psychologist as a "reader of signs" (Nietzsche 1986).

there revealed in them, on the contrary, the plentitude, force, and will of life, its courage, certainty, future?" (Nietzsche 1989, Preface §3). Nietzsche asks his reader to interpret moral judgments as signs of underlying psychological states of healthy or sickly reactions to external stimuli. To ask, as Nietzsche does, what is the value of our moral values, is it to redirect our attention from surface interpretations to ascertain the kind of willing that such judgments promote? Nietzsche's extraordinary insight is that weak, decadent, and reactive natures have gained the upper hand over healthier ones. The three essays of *Genealogy of Morals* constitute Nietzsche's best attempt to answer this question. "Let us articulate this new demand: we need a critique of moral values, the value of these values themselves must first be called in question—and for that is needed a knowledge of the conditions and circumstances in which they grew, under which they evolved and changed ..." (Nietzsche 1989, Preface §6).

The first two essays articulate the central question of the book that, when properly understood, complete his demand for a critique of moral values based on an analysis of origins: "What is the meaning of ascetic ideals?" Nietzsche assumes the textbook definition of "ascetic" as the practice of self-abnegation and self-discipline, but attaches an "ideal" to it. The ideal aspect of asceticism is that which penetrates and fills suffering with meaning and purpose insofar as the person wills to suffer in a certain way. Suffering as chosen and willed has meaning only because it serves a purpose beyond the isolating and individualizing sensations of pain. The third essay clarifies the ideal further:

> Apart from the ascetic ideal, man, the human animal, had no meaning so far. His existence on earth contained no goal; "why man at all?"—was a question without an answer; the will for man and earth was lacking; behind every great human destiny there sounded as a refrain a yet greater "in vain!" This is precisely what the ascetic ideal means; that something was lacking, that man was surrounded by a fearful void—he did not know how to justify, to account for, to affirm himself; he suffered from the problem of his meaning. He also suffered otherwise, he was in the main a sickly animal: but his problem was not suffering itself, but that there was no answer to the crying question, "why do I suffer?"
>
> In it suffering was interpreted; the tremendous void seemed to have been filled; the door was closed to any kind of suicidal nihilism. This interpretation—there is no doubt of it—brought fresh suffering with it, deeper, more inward, more poisonous, more life-destructive suffering: it placed all suffering under the perspective of guilt.
>
> But all this notwithstanding—man was saved thereby, he possessed a meaning, he was henceforth no longer like a leaf in the wind, a plaything of nonsense—he could now will something; no matter at first to what end, why, with what he willed; the will itself was saved (Nietzsche 1989, III, 28).

Nietzsche means that the fundamental striving of the will not only to remain in being but also to assert and affirm its being has no final sense or purpose beyond itself. Nietzsche draws out the consequences of this position for human consciousness: if bodily willing is both an end and means to the end, then implicit in all our acts of willing is the thought "in vain," that is, our lives exhaust themselves in their striving; they die out and of them nothing remains. Here, Nietzsche has returned with extraordinary verve and clarity to the central nerve of *The Birth of Tragedy*: Consciousness—our cognitive self-awareness—seeks consolation in some metaphysical purpose outside of itself, but in order to be effectively consoled, consciousness cannot see behind the veil of its self-created meaning and purpose. As we have already seen, if existence is to have value, human willing must be thought as aiming at some goal, some ideal. But now in his mature understanding of the psychology of this self-deception, Nietzsche realizes that the remedy proposed by the ascetic ideal could in fact be worse, "more poisonous, more life-destructive," than the depressive illness of the "in vain." Nevertheless, willing seeks to continue its life of willing at all costs: "That the ascetic ideal has meant so many things to man, however, is an expression of the basic fact of the human will, its *horror vacui*: it needs a goal—and it will rather will nothingness than not will" (Nietzsche 1989, III, 1).

This last thought requires additional attention for it unites two psychological aspects of the ascetic will that tend to become separated in analysis. In the opening paragraph of the third essay, Nietzsche suggests that the ascetic ideal had its origin in the desire of the suffering and sick to be free of pain: "What does it mean when a philosopher pays homage to the ascetic ideal?—he wants to gain release from a torture" (III, 6). But this, obviously, doesn't explain why the ascetic intensifies other negative, life-defeating and deadening affects to escape his torture. Here, Nietzsche puts his finger on the paradoxical nature of ascetic ideals and all psychological conditions that exhibit acts of willing that turn back destructively against the agent: "It will immediately be obvious that such a self-contradiction as the ascetic appears to represent, 'life against life,' is, physiologically considered and not merely psychologically, a simple absurdity. It can only be apparent; it must be a kind of provisional formulation, an interpretation and psychological misunderstanding of something whose real nature could not for a long time be understood or described as it really was." (III, 14)[22] Nietzsche is obviously correct: physiologically, the body strives to persevere in existence and to expand its power. A life force that seeks to destroy its own conditions of willing is paradoxical, but its contradictoriness is merely apparent. Nietzsche provides an explanation based in two disguised aims of the ascetic ideal: power and self-affirmation.

> In that ideal, the ascetic priest preserves, not merely his faith, but also his will, his power, his interest. His right to existence stands and falls with that ideal. No wonder that here we run into a fearful opponent—an opponent of the sort who fights for his existence against those who deny the ideal ... (Nietzsche 1989, III, 11).

The very existence of the ascetic (his will to live on) is tied to the ideal. Nietzsche underlines in his genetic account the ideal element of the negation, namely, the rationalized other worldly existence that legitimizes both the philosophical and the priestly life. The power and self-affirmation of the ascetic is possible only on the condition of some ideal confirmation of such an existence. Consequently, he understands his life "as a bridge to that other existence." The ascetic ideal thus preserves in modern guise both elements of Greek art, the Apolline and the Dionysiac: the affirmation of the ideal through the destruction and negation of the real. This transcendence, or passing over into another world by means of negation, is in fact a "passing over" to a different interpretation of life, a different valuation of

[22] At III, 3, Nietzsche had already noted the paradox in his formulation, "die Widernatur des asketischen Ideals" (the anti-nature of the ascetic ideal).

good and bad, a turning of the tables on the noble, powerful, and successful elites of this world.

> We should consider how regularly, how commonly, how in almost all ages, the ascetic priest makes an appearance. He does not belong to one single race. He flourishes everywhere . . . There must be a high-order necessity which makes this species hostile to life always grow again and flourish — *it must be in the interest of life itself not to have such a type of self-contradiction die out*. For an ascetic life is a self-contradiction. Here, a ressentiment without equal is in control, something with an insatiable instinct and will to power, which wants to become master, not over something in life but over life itself, over its deepest, strongest, most basic conditions; here, an attempt is being made to use one's power to block up the sources of that power; here, one directs one's green and malicious gaze against one's inherent physiological health, particularly against its means of expression—beauty, joy—while *one experiences and seeks for a feeling of pleasure in mistrust, atrophy, pain, accident, ugliness, voluntary loss, self-denial, self-flagellation, self-sacrifice*. All this is paradoxical to the highest degree. Here, we stand in front of a dichotomy which essentially wants a dichotomy, which enjoys itself in this suffering and always gets even more self-aware and more triumphant in proportion to the decrease in its own prerequisite, the physiological capacity for life. "Triumph precisely in the ultimate agony"—under this supreme sign the ascetic ideal has fought from time immemorial. Inside this riddle of seduction, in this picture of delight and torment, it sees its highest light, its salvation, its final victory (Nietzsche 1989, III, 11; my emphases).

The ascetic ideal, consequently, is a function of life itself, a strategy of life—its unconscious calculation to maintain this, as yet, unstable and indeterminate animal in existence until it can develop some other, less contradictory and self-destructive, means of thriving. Certainly, the ascetic ideal brings about an intensification of self-consciousness to the "body-self," whose will denies the value of the body by asserting the deepest ontological distinction between what the self ideally is in contrast to what the material, changing body actually is. It is, as Nietzsche writes, a dichotomy that wants to be and remain a dichotomy; that is, a consciousness that is split in itself and wants to remain split, torn between its natural self (body) and an idealized, spiritual self as the condition of power and self-assertion. And, as Nietzsche was the first to admit, this self-diremption at the core of ascetic will works and succeeds brilliantly. But, since it has been built on mendacity, its veil will "flutter," and the lie will undermine itself: the moral values of truthfulness and honesty will force it into the light of day. At that point, the human being, the de-deified and naturalized human being, will stand once again naked before Silenus without an answer (Nietzsche 2001, §109).

CONCLUSION

Nietzsche's analysis of cultural pathologies revolves around his awareness that human ideals (metaphysical, religious, or moral) provide an indispensable incentive for life. Existence is willed, and suffering is interpreted as the means to the actualization of an ideal. Yet Nietzsche also realized that ideals are value judgments of a peculiar kind. For the world they display is a world of our own making, a world of illusions in constant tension with our will to truth and our desire to know how things really are. The problem with deception, Nietzsche judged, was not its falsification of how things are, but the implication that every deception is a species of self-deception. Yet, even when Nietzsche acknowledged this, he never completely refuted the thought that semblance and illusion have greater value for life than truth and honesty. As far as I can judge, this haunting possibility remains an open question in his late works. [23]

In his critique of romantic delusion in *The Birth of Tragedy*, Nietzsche clearly acknowledged that without the veil of semblance and illusion of metaphysical consolation, there would be an irresistible movement of existence towards nihilism, in fact so irresistible that even he succumbed to it. Yet, when consciousness sees the truth of this kind of self-deception, it turns to an act of revenge against the (self)-deception that its former ideals and values have practiced upon it. Consequently, when the "ideal" is removed from the ascetic, all that is left is his bare nihilistic will, a pure revenge against the world, the body, and the natural conditions of existence; depression in the face of the relentless "in vain" of all life. A will stripped of all illusion and metaphysical consolation rejoices in its own destructive power in the absence of any other creative goal. Recall Nietzsche's conclusion to *Genealogy of Morals* quoted above:

> In [the ascetic ideal] suffering was interpreted; the tremendous void seemed to have been filled; the door was closed to any kind of suicidal nihilism—man was saved thereby, he possessed a meaning, he was henceforth no longer like a leaf in the wind, a plaything of nonsense.

And in *Zarathustra*, the suicidal nihilism is seen as a consequence of the will's inability to will creatively:

> Even in your folly and contempt, you despisers of the body, you serve your self. I say to you: your self itself wants to die and turns away from life.
>
> No longer is it capable of that which it wants most: to create beyond itself. This it wants most of all, this is its entire fervor.
>
> But now it is too late for that, and so your self wants to go under, you despisers of the body … .
>
> And that is why you are angry now at life and earth. There is an unknown envy in the looking askance of your contempt.[24]

Nietzsche apprehended the modern crisis of meaning as "suicidal nihilism"—once value, aim, and purpose had been unmasked as metaphysical deceptions, the human being—at least a certain kind of human being with an acute sense of self-consciousness—feels himself to be "a leaf in the wind," blown about aimlessly by natural forces like a "plaything of nonsense," unable to create beyond himself. The perception of oneself as the plaything of nonsense is not just an instance of existential anxiety, but a contradiction in the very heart of willing. In order

[23] Nietzsche (2001), §344. Nietzsche again considers the claim that the will to truth might not be as valuable to life as "error, deception, simulation, blinding, self-blinding…" etc.

to will something, ideals must feel like purposes to be grasped and realized by means of action. But the truth that springs from the drive of self-disclosure and honesty reveals that the will itself is the sole origin of all its ends and ideals. If this is true, why not illusion, why not deception? What is the value of truth and self-knowledge, if it brings us to the doorstep of despair and suicide? In an illuminating passage from the *Gay Science*, Nietzsche contrasts "knowledge" with truth: the value of knowledge in human culture has never been its alleged correspondence to objective reality, but simply its usefulness for existence. "Knowledge" has always been rife with errors and deceit. Truth, on the other hand, is the result of a will to honesty, but not necessarily useful for life.. Can one lead a life directed by honest self-appraisal and transparency that would not culminate in suicidal nihilism? Can we will a self-contradictory truth that places in question the very nature of willing? What would such a life look or feel like? How would it be nourished, or would it not necessarily will to starve itself, to negate its own negations? Nietzsche comments on this "battle" being enacted [in himself] between the drive to truth and life-preserving errors:

> In relation to the significance of this battle, everything else is a matter of indifference; the ultimate question about the condition of life is posed here, and the first attempt is made here to answer the question through experiment. To what extent can truth stand to be incorporated into life?—that is the question; that is the experiment.[25]

As we know, Nietzsche's personal experiment in answering this question came to an unhappy end; yet it seems clear that in a culture that has to an astonishing degree institutionalized the denial of its own nihilistic drives, perhaps we should view anorexics as the first appearance of decent and honest human beings—whom Nietzsche called "free spirits"—free from the need of semblance and illusion only because they have reached an end with nothing left to lose—women who have pushed the experiment and the battle between error and truth to the limits of their own bodies, to the limits of their wills.[26]

REFERENCES

Brumberg, Joan Jacobs (1988), *Fasting Girls*. New York: Vintage Books.

Freud, Sigmund (1995), *The Freud Reader*, edited by P. Gay. New York: Norton.

Kant, Immanuel (1997), *Foundations of the Metaphysics of Morals*, trans. by L.W. Beck. New Jersey: Prentice-Hall.

[24] Nietzsche (2006). Envy arises when one sees his imagined "ideal" self realized in another, but continues to desire it as his own birthright. It is an acute observation that beholding one's ideal self in another provokes contempt for the actual self.

[25] Nietzsche (2001), §110. For "incorporation," the German text has "Einverleibung," which literally means assimilating something into the body. Whether it is possible to bring "truth" into the actual self, that is, into the body, Nietzsche does not think can be answered a-priori. For this reason, he intends to "experiment" on himself by attempting to live a life-affirming existence without the intoxications of ideals and deceptions—a new, experimental "birth of tragedy" as life affirming in his own body.

[26] Nietzsche's first and clearest definition of "free spirit" is found in the 1886 *Preface* to *Human, All Too Human*: "Indeed, the free spirit henceforth has to do only with things—and how many things!—with which he is no longer concerned…" (Nietzsche 1986, §4). No longer being concerned about becoming someone you are not creates freedom to become who you are.

Malson, Helen (1998), *The Thin Woman: Feminism, post-structuralism and the psychology of anorexia nervosa.* London: Routledge.

Nietzsche, F. (1967), *Genealogy of Morals*, edited by W. Kaufmann. New York: Vintage Books.

Nietzsche, F. (1967), *Genealogy of Morals*, edited by W. Kaufmann. NY: Vintage Books.

Nietzsche, F. (1972), *Nietzsche Werke, Kritische Gesamtausgabe*, edited by Giorgio Colli and Mazzino Montinari. Berlin: Walter de Gruyter.

Nietzsche, F. (1986), *Human, All Too Human*, translated by R.J. Hollingdale. Cambridge: Cambridge University Press.

Nietzsche, F. (1989), *On The Genealogy of Morals and Ecce Homo*, edited and translated by W. Kaufmann. New York: Vintage Books.

Nietzsche, F. (1997), *Twilight of the Idols*, trans. R. Polt. Indianapolis: Hackett Publishing Co..

Nietzsche, F. (1999), *The Birth of Tragedy and Other Writings*, edited by R. Geuss and R. Speirs. Cambridge: Cambridge University Press.

Nietzsche, F. (2001), *Gay Science*, edited by B. Williams. Cambridge: Cambridge University Press.

Nietzsche, F. (2002), *Beyond Good and Evil*, edited by R.P. Horstmann and J. Norman. Cambridge: Cambridge University Press.

Nietzsche, F. (2003), *Writings from the Late Notebooks*, edited by R. Bittner. Cambridge: Cambridge University Press.

Nietzsche, F. (2006), *Thus Spoke Zarathustra*, edited by A. del Caro and R. Pippin. Cambridge: Cambridge University Press.

Pippin, R. (2009), "How to overcome oneself: Nietzsche on Freedom," in *Nietzsche on Freedom and Autonomy*, ed. K. Gemes and S. May. Oxford: Oxford University Press.

Porter, James (2000), *The Invention of Dionysus: An Essay on The Birth of Tragedy*. Stanford, California: Stanford University Press.

CONCLUSION

The three sections of the book have underlined different approaches to the complex picture of AN. Biological aspects concern the regulation of appetite, based on a network of neural circuits and the balance between orexigenic and anorexigenic substances; many peptides and neurotransmitters are altered in AN, but no single and univocal alteration explains the whole status. Similarly, only single-case genetic alterations, evaluated by molecular methods, have been identified. Many endocrine alterations have been described in Chapter 1, including the resistance to action of GH, typical of malnutrition; the activation of the stress system (particularly the axis hypothalamus-pituitary-adrenal gland); the altered metabolism of thyroid hormones (with the so called "low T3 syndrome" or "non-thryoidal illness," suggesting, therefore, that it represent an adaptive mechanism to negative energetic balance); and the reduced secretion of leptin due to reduced amount of adipose tissue and low secretion of insulin, perhaps with an enhanced sensitivity to the hormone itself. Most of these endocrine disturbances are secondary to malnutrition, but the picture is not entirely overlapping to that of a normal woman undergoing a forced or experimentally prolonged period of fasting. In Chapter 2, the focus centered on cytokines, molecules produced by immunocompetent system, showing the strict interaction between endocrine and immune systems. More recently investigated molecules are the adypocytokines, synthesized in adipose tissue; in particular adiponectin, which is increased in AN, can induce some particular negative phenomena, such as a depression of hematic cell formation and worsen the weight loss. In Chapter 3, we have described, with more attention, the pituitary-gonadal axis, which shows a return to a prepubertal stage, causing amenorrhea, which is a diagnostic criteria of AN according to DSM.IV.

Clinical consequences that can be fatal are described in Chapter 4; the dietetic approach, which sometimes needs forced alimentation, is described in Chapter 5. Therefore, still remaining in the biological point of view, dangerous vicious circles can induce more aggravating processes. However, every physic status has a co-respective psychological correspondence, and a further vicious cycle confounds the psychic and organic causes (Fig.1), criticizing the classical concept of causality, to which we are confident in philosophical debates.

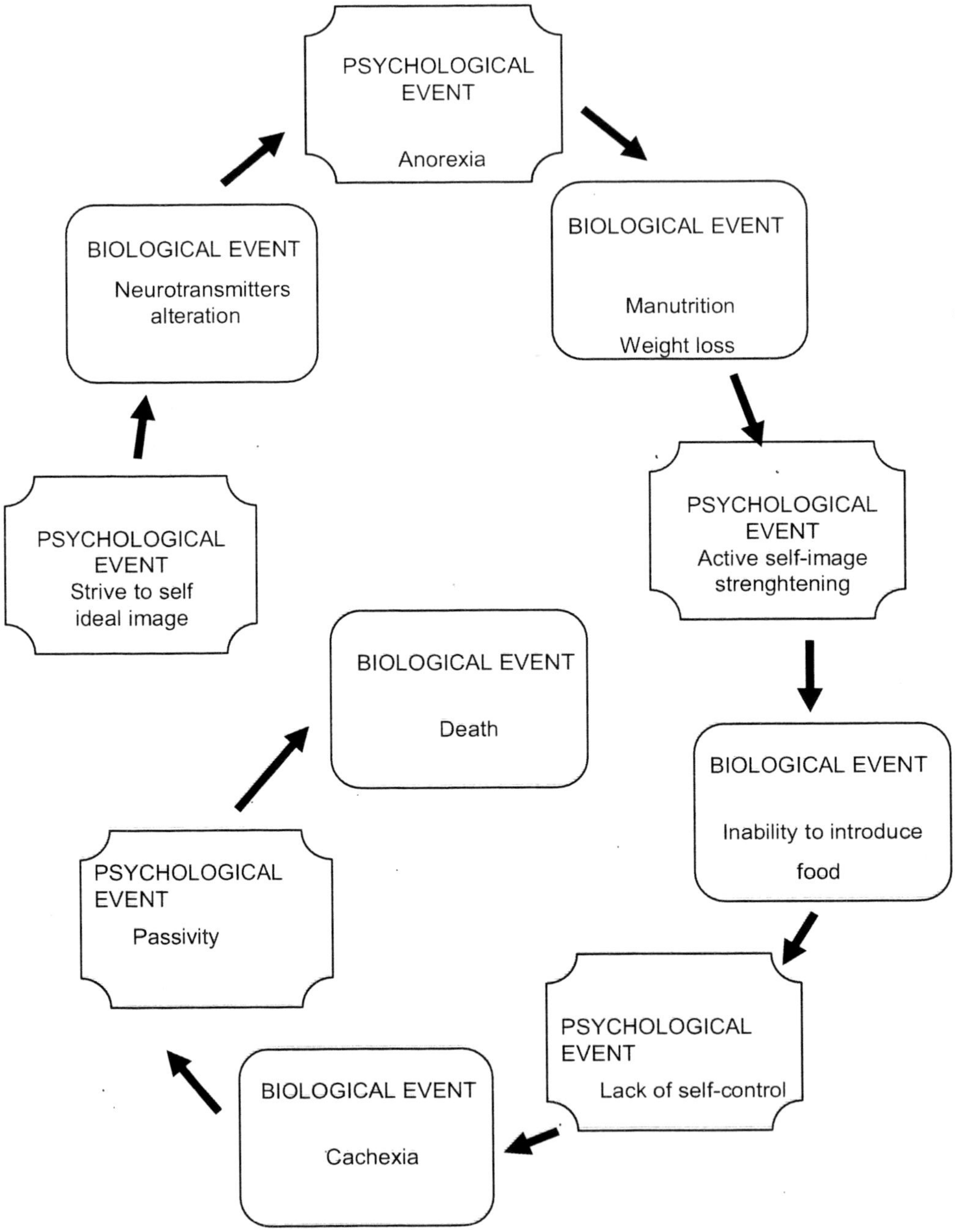

Figure 1.

Different psychiatric schools have approached the eating disorders; we particularly underlined the problems occurring in childhood, often overlooked by parents but possible precursors of later disorders. The relation with nurturant mother constitutes the first learning environment to express one's own personality through feeding behavior, and family relations are the mediating factors of social and cultural influences throughout the development period. In lack of this mediation, the heightened need for affective relations, external to family ones, that starts in adolescence, could be related to fears and psychological closure, to which anorexic starvation not only follows, but what it also symbolically represents. The interpersonal bereers, often hidden behind an apparent social compliance, are a fundamental obstacle for therapeutic interventions: so, the lowering of psychological defenses in the critical periods can be the occasion for starting a therapeutic relationship, otherwise impossible. The emergency psychological intervention is, therefore, another key step in the treatment. At the same time, cognitive and emotional support to the parents, particularly in these critical periods, can allow a psychological separation and individuation of the anorexic patients, overcoming abandonment fears and promoting more mature family relations.

The school of logotherapy, based on the existential analysis by V.E. Frankl, realizes a bridge from the psychological to philosophical plane, since it involves the search of meaning in life and opens a hope for a man, not entirely conditioned by his past life or cognitive schemes.

The third and final part of the volume was dedicated to philosophical issues. With regard to ethics, two main conclusions were drawn: first, that careful understanding of the cultural and ethical meaning of eating, of body construction and of relationships is indispensable for ethical reasoning about anorexia; secondly, that it is necessary to integrate, on the one hand, the principle of respect for the anorexic's autonomy and, on the other hand, the duty of responsibility of both the patient and the physician towards the objective good of life. The next chapter highlighted the crucial importance of a deeper understanding of introspection and interpretation. The conclusion here was that, when dealing with expressions involving bodily states, one should avoid the simplistic model of internal-perception. Moreover, to interpret responsibly what the anorexic says, the best procedure seems to be to consider the anorexic's utterances lying somewhere between two worlds of meaning, lying on the boundary between the accepted meaning and the anorexic's own private space of meaning. This philosophical study was followed by another one that focused on the link between anorexia and self-deception. The conclusion here was expressed in the form of a warning. When diagnosing anorexia and treating those who suffer from it, we tend to consider them self-deceived and, at the same time, often forget how self-deception can be pervasive in the society within which we, ourselves, are situated. The suggestion, therefore, was to acknowledge more openly that the phenomenon of anorexia could, in fact, be expressing a widespread cultural bias or self-deception on the large-scale. The final chapter introduced some insights deriving from Friedrich Nietzsche's theory of the ascetic ideal. The main focus was on how humans, in various destructive ways, seek release from the anguish and pointlessness of existence. It was concluded that, in line with this view, new insights may become available for empirical and cultural researchers if anorexics are seen as ascetics deprived of an otherworldly ideal as their goal.

An obvious conclusion is that an integrated approach is needed to manage this difficult condition, with the collaborations of endocrinologists, expertise in internal medicine, psychiatrists and psychologists, dieticians, and so on. The cooperation of different professional profiles must go beyond the treatment of specific aspects, which can remain based on separate competences organized in watertight compartments.

The method that inspired this book and that analyzes different aspects, is, on one side, necessary due to the enormous literature in the field, but it is enriched, on the other side, by a global vision; biological and psychological aspects are separated in heuristic way, but what emerges is the reciprocal influence of the different plans. This is the provoking message for training students and matter of debating for those who are involved in the clinical management of this kind of patient.

Our aim is also to open a debate to reach a new interpretation that involves notions from biological and human sciences interpreted in a unique model, which could allow a new method to treat the disease. Self-deception is not only a psychological entrapment, but sinks its roots in existential choices. The real way of prevention, in a familiar context, characterized by true communication, can bring adolescents to correctly use their capacities, their faculties of auto-determination, and to answer to challenges of life in a meaningful frame. This vision of human beings, which studies specific molecules and biochemical language without lowering itself to a reductionistic and mechanicistic view, is directed to a global vision of spiritual man and is our proposal to reach a better knowledge of this still mysterious disease.

About Editors and Contributors

Editors

Antonio Mancini, MD, Researcher and Aggregate Professor, Dept. of Internal Medicine, Division of Endocrinology, Catholic University of Sacred Heart, Rome, Italy; M. Phil., PhD, Pontificial Gregorian University, Rome, Italy.

Silvia Daini, MD, Researcher and Aggregate Professor, Institute of Psychiatry, Catholic University of Sacred Heart, Rome, Italy.

Louis Caruana, S.J., PhD, Senior Lecturer, Department of Philosophy, Heythrop College University of London, UK.

Contributors

Bernardini, Lucia, MD, Institute of Psychiatry, Catholic University of Sacred Heart, Rome, Italy.

Bianchi, Antonio, MD, Endocrinologist, Assistant Professor, Division of Endocrinology, Catholic University of Sacred Heart, Rome, Italy.

De Marinis, Laura, MD, Endocrinologist, Associate Professor, Division of Endocrinology, Catholic University of Sacred Heart, Rome, Italy.

Di Donna, Vincenzo, MD, Division of Endocrinology, Catholic University of Sacred Heart, Rome, Italy.

Di Pietro, Maria Luisa, MD, Associate Professor, Institute of Bioethics, Catholic University of Sacred Heart, Rome, Italy.

Festa, Roberto, MD, Institute of Clinical Pathology, University "Politecnica delle Marche," Ancona, Italy.

Giacchi, Elena, MD, Gynecologist, Center for Study and Research on Natural Fertility Regulation, Catholic University of the Sacred Heart, Rome, Italy.

Giraldi, Alessandra, RD, Dietician, Dietetics Service; Dept of Laboratory Medicine; Policlinico Universitario "A. Gemelli," Rome Italy.

Leone, Erika, MD, Division of Endocrinology, Catholic University of Sacred Heart, Rome, Italy.

Magini, Marinella, RD, Dietician, Dietetics Service; Dept of Laboratory Medicine; Policlinico Universitario "A. Gemelli," Rome, Italy.

Martorana, Giuseppe Ettore, MD, Associate Professor of Cellular Biochemistry; Institute of Biochemistry and Clinical Biochemistry School of Medicine, Catholic University; Dietetics Service; Dept of Laboratory Medicine; Policlinico Universitario "A. Gemelli," Rome, Italy.

Meniconi, Paola, RD, Dietician, Dietetics Service; Dept of Laboratory Medicine; Policlinico Universitario "A. Gemelli," Rome Italy.

Meucci, Elisabetta, BD, Biochemist, Associate Professor of Applied Biochemistry, Institute of Biochemistry and Clinical Biochemistry School of Medicine, Catholic University, Rome, Italy.

Moltisanti, Dino, M. Phil., Ph.D., Institute of Bioethics, Catholic University of Sacred Heart, Rome, Italy.

Panetta, Carla, MD, Institute of Psychiatry, Catholic University of Sacred Heart, Rome, Italy.

Petrongolo, Luana, MD, Institute of Psychiatry, Catholic University of Sacred Heart, Rome, Italy.

Sultana, Mark, PhD, Lecturer, Department of Fundamental & Dogmatic Theology, University of Malta.

Tartaglione, Linda, MD, Division of Endocrinology, Catholic University of Sacred Heart, Rome, Italy.

Tilaro, Laura, MD, Division of Endocrinology, Catholic University of Sacred Heart, Rome, Italy.

Veltri, Flora, MD, Division of Endocrinology, Catholic University of Sacred Heart, Rome, Italy.

Virdis, Andrea, M. Phil., Ph.D., Institute of Bioethics, Catholic University of Sacred Heart, Rome, Italy.

Walsh, Terrance, S.J., PhD, Lecturer, Department of Philosophy, Heythrop College University of London, UK.

INDEX

A

absorption, 9, 79
abstinence, 17
acanthocytosis, 82
accounting, 36
accuracy, 192
achievement, 19, 66, 126, 128, 210, 217
acid, 12, 21, 36, 37, 39, 46, 48, 63, 72, 82, 93
acrocyanosis, 76
acromegaly, 26, 28
ACTH, 15, 17, 18, 28, 33, 34, 60, 63
activation, 8, 15, 16, 21, 37, 39, 63, 65, 80, 102, 227
activators, 49
acute, 10, 15, 16, 20, 25, 26, 27, 29, 32, 46, 79, 80, 82, 85, 92, 102, 106, 115, 118, 125, 137, 140, 207, 214, 221, 222
acute stress, 15, 16
acylation, 35
adaptation, 3, 4, 101, 104, 109, 110, 119, 125
addiction, 154, 188
ADH, 19, 20, 79
adhesion, 45, 47, 163
adipocyte, 16, 35, 37, 40, 45, 46, 47, 48
adipocytes, 3, 7, 30, 35, 37, 40, 41, 45, 48, 83
adipocytokines, 3, 21, 30, 31, 34, 35, 39
adipogenic, 37, 46
adiponectin, 22, 29, 30, 31, 35, 42, 44, 45, 46, 47, 48, 49, 227
adipose tissue, viii, 5, 7, 11, 19, 21, 23, 30, 31, 33, 35, 36, 37, 38, 39, 40, 41, 42, 44, 45, 46, 48, 227
adiposity, 6, 7, 9, 36, 38
administration, 12, 14, 17, 19, 22, 25, 40, 42, 47, 53, 57, 58, 59, 60, 61, 79, 130
adolescence, vii, 3, 66, 67, 73, 81, 118, 120, 127, 134, 150, 163, 175, 228
adolescent female, 54, 66, 67
adolescent patients, 19, 119, 120, 135
adolescents, 23, 52, 53, 54, 56, 66, 67, 69, 73, 77, 78, 84, 91, 93, 94, 95, 102, 111, 121, 131, 132, 134, 166, 170, 177, 230
adrenal cortex, 15, 16, 63, 64
adrenal gland, 4, 16, 227
adrenal glands, 4
adrenocorticotropic hormone, 15, 20, 63
adult, vii, 53, 62, 73, 103, 107, 111, 121
adulthood, 177
adults, 12, 27, 68, 91, 93, 102, 131
advertising, 163
aetiopathogenesis, 99
affective disorder, 14, 18, 65, 116, 132
affective states, 177
afferent nerve, 179
age, vii, x, 13, 19, 38, 52, 53, 54, 55, 66, 67, 81, 118, 120, 130, 150, 198
agent, 189, 191, 194, 195, 196, 219
agents, 103, 131
aggregation, 116, 117
aggressive behavior, 113, 139
aggressiveness, 101
aging, 123
aging process, 123
agonist, 33, 37, 46
air, 189
Akrasia, 200
alcohol, 8, 24, 106, 137, 154
alcohol abuse, 106
alcohol consumption, 8
alcoholism, 62, 65
aldosterone, 79
alimentation, 227
allele, 6, 8
alpha, 20, 43, 44
ALS, 12
alternative, 13

alternatives, 138
alters, 44, 69
ambiguity, 168
ambivalence, 146
ambivalent, 109, 209
amenorrhea, ix, x, 17, 25, 51, 52, 53, 54, 55, 56, 57, 61, 62, 63, 67, 69, 71, 153, 227
American Psychiatric Association, vii, x, 51, 93, 199
amino, 21, 36, 63, 93
amino acid, 21, 36, 63, 93
amino acids, 93
amorphous, 54, 83
amphetamine, 6, 9
amplitude, 11, 15, 52, 61
ampulla, 77
amygdala, 15
amylase, 80
anabolic, viii, 5, 6, 9, 79
anabolism, 89
androgen, 54, 59
androgens, 21
anemia, 33, 41, 75, 76, 82, 83
anger, 102, 103, 104, 105, 141
angiogenesis, 39, 48
angiotensin II, 15
Anglo-Saxon, 141, 166
animal models, 37, 39
animals, 10, 32, 36, 37, 58, 70, 216
anisocytosis, 82
antagonism, 152
antagonist, 6, 11, 33, 43, 64
antagonistic, 16
antagonists, 8
anterior pituitary, viii, 15, 65, 72
anthropological, viii, ix, 150, 151, 152, 153, 154, 161, 162, 163
anthropology, 150, 152, 155
anti-atherogenic, 31, 36, 38, 39
antidepressant, 14, 27, 80
antidepressant medication, 27, 80
antidepressants, 20, 80
antidiabetic, 39, 46
antidiuretic, 19, 20
antidiuretic hormone, 19, 20
antioxidant, 80
anxiety, 32, 56, 62, 91, 100, 101, 106, 107, 109, 119, 121, 136, 139, 142, 221
anxiety disorder, 56, 121
apathy, 155
aplastic anemia, 83
apoptosis, 58, 70
appendix, 102
appetite, 3, 4, 5, 7, 8, 9, 10, 16, 20, 21, 24, 32, 33, 35, 42, 71, 101, 109, 195, 227
ARC, 6, 7, 16
arginine, 15, 17, 20, 63
argument, 167, 174, 193, 196, 206, 215, 217
Aristotelian, 200
Aristotle, vii, 190
arousal, 18, 63
arrest, 19, 53, 66, 93
arrhythmia, 78
arrhythmias, 75, 77, 92
arteries, 36
artery, 36, 38
articulation, 164
artistic, 208, 209, 211
ascetic, ix, 198, 203, 205, 206, 207, 215, 216, 217, 218, 219, 220, 221, 229
aseptic, 66
aspirate, 83
aspiration, 153
assessment, 22, 44, 47, 70, 88, 106, 112, 142, 144, 170
assumptions, 180, 217
asthma, 64
asthma attacks, 64
atherosclerosis, 36, 37, 39
athletes, 55, 69
athleticism, 65
atmosphere, 127, 131
atoms, 13
ATPase, 79
atresia, 57
atrioventricular block, 84
atrophy, viii, 13, 14, 20, 26, 75, 76, 83, 91, 94, 220
attachment, 102, 104, 106, 108, 109, 112, 113
attachment theory, 106, 108
attacks, 64, 165
attitudes, 6, 51, 56, 67, 119, 121, 128, 131, 151, 178, 180
attractiveness, 166
authority, 142
autoantibodies, 20
autocrine, 57
autoimmune, 62, 65
autoimmune disorders, 65
autonomic nervous system, 63, 78
autonomy, viii, 100, 106, 109, 117, 118, 119, 124, 142, 143, 152, 161, 166, 168, 169, 229
availability, vii, 55, 61, 69, 108, 127
aversion, 216
avoidance, 122, 198
awareness, 127, 139, 142, 144, 145, 146, 162, 163, 178, 181, 209, 218, 220

B

babies, 101
back, 76, 99, 101, 149, 155, 156, 176, 183, 214, 216, 219
bacterial, 37
bacterial cells, 37
baroreflex sensitivity, 84
barrier, 9, 12, 59
basal metabolic rate, 38, 41, 79, 89
behavior modification, 148, 157
behavior therapy, 189
behavioral aspects, 143
behavioral change, 4
behavioral effects, 16
behavioral manifestations, 181
behavioral theory, 122
behaviorism, 155
behaviours, vii, ix, 8
beliefs, ix, 87, 167, 173, 177, 180, 182, 183, 187, 189, 190, 191, 192, 193, 194, 195
benchmark, vii
beneficial effect, 57
benefits, 126, 148, 166, 176, 184
benevolence, 166
benign, 211
bias, 199, 229
binding, 8, 11, 12, 13, 17, 21, 24, 36, 45, 54, 65
binding globulin, 17, 54
binge eating disorder, 134, 148
bioassay, 33
bioavailability, 41
bioethics, 166
biological activity, 33
biological markers, 68
biomarker, 39
biomedical model, 175
biopsy, 83
biosynthesis, 65, 72
birds, 208
birth, 52, 99, 100, 106, 118, 133, 222
blame, 216
blastocyst, 58, 62
blocks, 41, 211
blood, viii, 9, 10, 31, 36, 38, 39, 44, 75, 78, 79, 82, 83, 84, 90, 91
blood flow, 39, 91
blood glucose, 36, 78, 79
blood plasma, 10
blood pressure, 38, 39, 84, 90
blood urea, 79
blood vessels, 83
bloodstream, 9
body composition, 3, 10, 27, 30, 66, 88
body dissatisfaction, 166
body fat, 9, 11, 21, 34, 36, 39, 41, 42, 51, 54, 55, 60, 61, 67, 69, 83
body image, vii, 10, 41, 56, 66, 137, 142, 155, 162, 166, 170, 177, 180, 187, 188, 197, 198
body mass index (BMI), 11, 12, 18, 21, 34, 36, 38, 40, 42, 44, 53, 54, 55, 61, 68, 82, 87, 88, 91, 92, 141
body shape, 143, 166, 178, 192
body temperature, 12, 38
body weight, x, 6, 8, 13, 17, 18, 19, 26, 40, 42, 49, 53, 54, 55, 60, 67, 68, 69, 71, 88, 89, 90, 91, 92, 136, 140, 141, 142, 147, 187, 188, 192, 198
bonding, 101, 131
bonds, 124
bone density, 30, 55, 73, 75, 81
bone growth, 66, 73, 81
bone loss, 81, 85
bone marrow, 32, 48, 82, 83
bone marrow biopsy, 83
bone mass, 55, 66, 67, 75, 81, 82
bone resorption, 81
borderline personality disorder, 137, 140
bovine, 57, 59, 70
bowel, 80
boys, 3, 52, 70
bradycardia, 75, 76, 77
brain, 6, 8, 9, 15, 20, 21, 29, 32, 33, 35, 49, 60, 61, 67, 72, 73, 91, 94, 102, 179
brain stem, 8, 15
brain structure, 67
brainstem, 7, 63
breakdown, 204
breakfast, 142
bronchial asthma, 64
bubble, 205
Buddhism, 216
bulimia, vii, x, 20, 24, 27, 28, 29, 30, 41, 43, 44, 49, 69, 80, 84, 85, 116, 118, 119, 121, 132, 134, 135, 137, 138, 141, 147, 189
bulimia nervosa, vii, x, 20, 24, 28, 29, 30, 41, 43, 44, 49, 69, 80, 84, 85, 116, 118, 121, 132, 147, 189 199, 200, 201
burn, 126
buttocks, 191

C

cachexia, viii, 23, 32, 43
calcium, 81, 88, 90
caloric intake, 12, 18, 34, 55
caloric restriction, 12, 55, 120

calorimetry, 22
cAMP, 26, 58, 59
cancer, 43
capsule, 58
carbohydrate, 9, 27, 34, 79, 88, 93
carbohydrate metabolism, 79
carbohydrates, 14, 16, 35, 90
cardiac arrhythmia, 92
cardiac muscle, 77
cardiac output, 12, 77, 90
cardiomyopathy, 77, 84
caregiver, 100, 104, 106, 107, 108, 109, 110
caregivers, 100, 104, 108
case-studies, 177
cast, 210
catabolic, 5, 9, 10, 12, 15, 18, 32
catabolism, 32, 40, 81, 89
cataract, 154
catecholamine, 37
catecholamines, 32, 40, 65
Catholic, 3, 31, 51, 75, 87, 99, 115, 135, 149, 161, 225, 226
cattle, 59
Caucasians, 40
causal relationship, 18
causality, 227
causation, 176
cell, viii, 5, 34, 38, 43, 48, 57, 80, 82, 83, 91, 227
central nervous system, viii, 5, 6, 9, 32, 52, 56, 65
cerebral damage, 121
cerebrospinal fluid, 10, 17, 20, 67, 94
cerebrovascular, 30
cerebrovascular disease, 30
CFI, 120
c-fos, 64
changing environment, 38
chaos, 208, 212
chemokines, 32
chemoreceptors, 6
chemotaxis, 32
chemotherapy, 134
chest, 77
chickens, 58
childhood, vii, ix, 67, 70, 73, 99, 107, 132, 150, 163, 178, 181, 228
children, 44, 49, 52, 60, 67, 99, 100, 102, 106, 108, 109, 110, 113, 118, 123, 124, 162, 163, 166, 170, 177, 181, 206
cholesterol, 12, 38, 40, 47, 48, 79, 90, 92, 93
cholinergic, 11, 56
Christianity, 216
chronic disease, 26
chronic illness, 13, 87
chronic stress, 15, 16, 63
circadian, 15, 21, 60
circadian rhythm, 15, 60
circulation, 15, 54, 59, 80
cirrhosis, 10
c-jun, 64
classes, 6, 118, 175
classical, 143, 227
classification, 103, 104, 132
clay, 209
cleavage, 48, 58, 122
clinical presentation, viii
clinical psychology, 157
clinical symptoms, 52
clinics, 140
clonidine, 11, 25
cloning, 45
closure, 228
CNS, 4, 6, 9, 24, 25, 32, 33, 34, 85
Co, 223
coding, 8, 22
coercion, 92, 102
co-existence, 209
cofactors, 79
cognition, ix, 67, 68, 167, 173, 174, 175, 176, 177, 178, 184, 208
cognitive behavior therapy, 189
cognitive deficit, 67, 91
cognitive deficits, 67, 91
cognitive function, 66, 67, 68, 73, 91
cognitive impairment, 91
cognitive performance, 73
cognitive psychology, 168
cognitive system, 189
cohesion, 147
cohort, 56
colic, 99
collaboration, 124, 127, 136
collagen, 36, 45
collateral, 119
collusion, 122
colony stimulating factors, 33
colony-stimulating factor, 32, 41
colors, 154
coma, 75, 77, 79
communication, viii, 60, 65, 99, 103, 106, 122, 123, 125, 126, 130, 134, 145, 153, 184, 230
community, 73, 134, 140, 143, 163, 166, 175, 182, 196, 197, 216
comorbidity, 69, 137
compensation, 137
competence, 70, 108, 129, 138, 161, 167, 168, 169, 170, 193, 197

competency, 167, 168
competition, 177
complement, 36, 48
complexity, 4, 16, 78, 144, 149, 180
compliance, 136, 139, 229
complications, vii, ix, 3, 4, 27, 31, 33, 36, 39, 41, 48, 66, 73, 75, 76, 77, 78, 79, 80, 84, 87, 88, 89, 90, 92, 99, 137, 140, 169
components, 12, 15, 16, 32, 62, 66, 121
composition, 3, 10, 21, 27, 30, 66, 88, 152
compounds, 79
comprehension, 128, 164
computed tomography, 91, 94
concentration, 12, 13, 19, 20, 22, 36, 47, 168
conception, 123, 150, 151, 152, 167
concrete, 146, 150, 204
concreteness, 128
conditioning, 151, 154, 166
confidence, 108, 191
conflict, viii, 105, 106, 109, 110, 119, 122, 123, 124, 127, 142, 161, 165, 166, 171, 204
confrontation, 125
confusion, 75, 79, 146, 174, 178, 181, 185
consciousness, 130, 152, 154, 169, 190, 192, 208, 209, 210, 211, 213, 218, 220, 221
consensus, 91
consent, 166, 167, 169
conservation, 41, 56
consolidation, 183
constipation, 80, 101
construction, ix, 131, 161, 163, 164, 229
consumption, 8, 9, 13, 16, 35, 79, 165
contingency, 105, 106
continuity, 198
contracts, 93
control, viii, 3, 4, 5, 6, 7, 8, 9, 10, 11, 13, 15, 16, 20, 23, 24, 25, 29, 33, 35, 37, 41, 48, 54, 64, 69, 70, 71, 92, 93, 104, 105, 106, 110, 116, 120, 122, 130, 135, 137, 138, 139, 142, 163, 164, 165, 177, 178, 184, 188, 199, 206, 209, 214, 220
control group, 13, 41, 116, 120, 130
controlled studies, 118, 130
convergence, 5
conversion, 12, 59
conviction, 188, 191, 210
cooking, 137
coping strategies, 126
coronary artery disease, 36, 38
correlation, vii, 11, 22, 34, 36, 53, 121, 183
correlations, 20, 22, 40, 82, 175
corruption, 198
cortex, 15, 16, 63, 64
corticotropin, 28, 63, 66, 71, 72
cortisol, 15, 16, 17, 18, 23, 28, 34, 38, 52, 54, 56, 60, 62, 63, 64, 65, 67, 69
costs, 126, 219
counsel, 214
counseling, 87, 88, 90, 125
couples, 122, 124, 127
covering, 209
cows, 59
creatinine, 79
credibility, x, 203
credit, 214
CRH, 6, 9, 15, 16, 17, 18, 20, 24, 28, 29, 34, 52, 56, 62, 63, 64, 65, 66, 72
critical period, 146, 229
critical thinking, 141
critically ill, 92
criticism, 120, 152, 153, 206
cross-sectional, 20, 47, 67
cross-talk, 39, 48
crying, 181, 218
CSF, 17, 20, 21, 29, 32, 33, 67
cultural factors, 175
cultural influence, 228
cultural values, 162
culture, x, 37, 152, 164, 174, 175, 177, 182, 197, 198, 199, 203, 204, 206, 207, 212, 213, 214, 217, 222
curing, 154
curiosity, 101, 145
Cushing's syndrome, 52, 62
cyanosis, 76
cycles, x, 51, 53, 58, 60, 62, 65, 69, 100, 210
cycling, 26
cysteine, 35
cysteine-rich protein, 35
cystic fibrosis, 120, 133
cysts, 19
cytokine, 21, 32, 33, 34, 35, 36, 41, 43, 44
cytokine receptor, 33, 34
cytokines, viii, 14, 15, 21, 22, 31, 32, 33, 34, 35, 36, 42, 43, 80, 227
cytopenias, 83
cytoplasm, 65
cytotoxicity, 35

D

dairy, 88
dairy products, 88
danger, 101, 108, 150, 168, 182, 205
DCA, 140
de novo, 59

death, 23, 75, 76, 77, 78, 79, 84, 107, 118, 137, 138, 146, 147, 168, 169, 196, 197, 205, 213, 217
debates, ix, 170, 173, 227
decay, 212
decision-making process, 168
decisions, 139, 168, 169, 170, 171, 178, 186, 195, 213
deconvolution, 11
defects, 20, 39, 40, 60
defence, 169
defense, 16, 36, 45, 122, 128, 139, 177, 198, 213
defenses, 128, 136, 145, 146, 214, 229
deficiency, 12, 33, 35, 37, 44, 54, 58, 59, 61, 70, 82, 92, 122, 155
deficit, 57
deficits, 67, 73, 76, 81, 91, 94
definition, vii, 42, 91, 123, 138, 183, 207, 218, 222
dehydration, 75, 79
delayed gastric emptying, 80
delirium, 93
delivery, 62, 101
delusion, 187, 196, 197, 198, 199, 209, 221
delusions, 207
dementia, 121
demographic characteristics, 117, 118
denial, x, 127, 139, 146, 164, 168, 169, 173, 187, 188, 193, 197, 204, 220, 222
density, 23, 30, 39, 40, 47, 55, 67, 73, 75, 81, 82, 85, 87, 88, 92, 94, 95
deposition, 83
depressed, 91, 103, 133, 136, 216
depression, ix, 18, 20, 28, 56, 62, 65, 77, 106, 109, 121, 124, 132, 136, 137, 139, 146, 154, 216, 217, 221, 227
depressive disorder, 18, 20, 116, 132
depressive symptomatology, 14
depressive symptoms, 14, 18, 121, 136
deprivation, viii, 20, 22, 35, 61, 178
deregulation, 33, 34
destruction, 165, 176, 207, 210, 212, 219
detachment, 139
detection, ix, 134
determinism, 152
developed countries, 175
developmental disabilities, 99, 100
developmental disorder, 112
developmental process, 103
deviation, 106
dexamethasone, 11, 17, 18, 25, 28, 46
dexamethasone suppression test, 17, 28
diabetes, 10, 19, 29, 36, 37, 38, 39, 40, 44, 45, 46, 47, 48, 121, 140
diabetes mellitus, 10, 37, 46, 140
diabetic patients, 39, 47
diacylglycerol, 35
Diagnostic and Statistical Manual of Mental Disorders, 199
diagnostic criteria, vii, ix, 51, 102, 132, 227
diastolic blood pressure, 38, 90
dichotomy, 212, 217, 220
diet, 9, 13, 21, 27, 35, 37, 38, 79, 88, 90, 92, 95, 122, 136, 169, 192, 198
dietary, ix, 10, 38, 87, 88, 89
dietary intake, 88
dieting, ix, 13, 192, 198
diets, 47, 87, 92, 137
differential diagnosis, 19, 137
differentiation, 38, 56, 59, 163
diffusion, vii
digestion, 9, 16
dignity, 152
dilation, 80
dimensionality, 152
dimorphism, 72
direct observation, 99
disability, 138
disappointment, 165, 205
discipline, 32, 193, 199, 218
disclosure, 222
discomfort, 105, 108, 122, 123, 125, 144
discourse, 165
disease model, 61
diseases, 34, 83
disordered systems, 165
dispersion, 84
disposition, 192
dissatisfaction, 121, 144, 155, 166, 215
distortions, 20, 164, 178
distraction, 105
distress, 102, 107, 217
distribution, vii, 21, 46, 47
diuretic, 78, 137
diuretics, 90, 122
division, 124, 209
dizygotic, 117
dizygotic twins, 117
DNA, 64
doctors, vii, 120, 136, 141, 142, 146, 147, 182
dominance, 215
dopamine, 5, 10, 32
dosage, 58
down-regulation, 17, 22, 32
dream, 207, 208, 209, 211
dreaming, 209
drug-induced, 51
DSM-IV, x, 102, 187, 188, 192, 199

duality, 164
duration, 11, 15, 20, 53, 55, 58, 62, 81, 83, 103, 118, 121, 127, 130, 137, 140, 141, 142, 143
dysregulation, 9, 10

E

ears, 19
earth, 216, 218, 221
eating behavior, 32, 55, 87, 89, 90, 107, 163, 165
economic development, 163
ecstasy, 209
edema, 75, 76, 78, 79, 92
educators, 129, 144, 162
egg, 58
ego, 151, 164, 215
elaboration, 123, 152, 179
electrocardiogram, 84
electrolyte, 75, 77, 78, 79, 90
electrolyte depletion, 75, 79
electrolytes, 79, 92
ELISA, 33
emotion, 120, 133, 134
emotional, 103, 106, 108, 111, 115, 119, 122, 123, 125, 128, 131, 137, 143, 145, 146, 150, 184, 192, 199, 211, 212, 229
emotional conflict, 184
emotional experience, 130
emotional reactions, 146
emotional state, 103, 108
emotions, 108, 119, 123, 126, 137, 143, 150, 179, 180
empathy, 119, 125
employees, 129
encephalopathy, 102
encouragement, 119, 125
endocrine, viii, 3, 4, 9, 13, 18, 20, 23, 25, 26, 27, 28, 31, 32, 34, 35, 39, 57, 59, 69, 170, 227
endocrine disorders, 13, 27
endocrine system, 31, 34
endocrinological, viii
endocrinology, 144
endometrium, 54, 62, 66, 72
endothelial cell, 36, 39, 48
endothelial cells, 36, 39, 48
end-stage renal disease, 48
endurance, 177
energy, 7, 8, 9, 10, 11, 12, 13, 14, 16, 21, 22, 27, 34, 35, 41, 54, 55, 56, 60, 61, 69, 80, 81, 87, 88, 89, 91, 92, 93, 95, 164, 187, 208, 209
energy density, 87, 92, 95
engagement, 145, 182
enlargement, 76, 91, 94
enterprise, 184
entertainment, 198
entrapment, 230
environment, 51, 107, 108, 110, 115, 124, 130, 131, 137, 138, 139, 145, 146, 147, 150, 162, 165, 216, 228
environmental conditions, 38
environmental factors, 117, 166
enzymatic, 54
enzymes, 8, 13, 58, 59, 75, 79, 81
epidemic, 198
epistemological, 150
equilibrium, ix, 16, 123
erythropoietin, 41
essential fatty acids, 9, 88
estradiol, 34, 38, 51, 52, 53, 55, 61, 62, 64, 65, 66, 71, 72
estrogen, 18, 19, 21, 52, 54, 62, 64, 66, 67, 68, 73, 81, 94
estrogens, 81
ethical questions, ix
ethicists, 162
ethics, 170, 213, 229
etiologic factor, 90, 149
etiology, ix, 4, 18, 22, 51, 67, 116, 162, 166, 198, 203, 205
etiopathogenesis, 42, 115, 117
eukaryotic cell, 37
Europe, 198
euthanasia, 169
euthyroid sick syndrome, 13
evil, 212, 217
evolution, 119, 123, 124, 125, 127
evolutionary process, 102
excitability, 4
exclusion, 51
excretion, 17, 40
execution, 64
exercise, 30, 51, 55, 61, 62, 67, 69, 90, 142, 163, 169, 170, 187, 188, 194, 215
exercisers, 55
expertise, 229
exploitation, 198
exposure, 15, 46
expressivity, 144
external environment, 107
external influences, 168
extracellular matrix, 36
extrusion, 57
eye, 154, 179, 212
eyes, 100, 207

F

fabricate, 207
facilitators, 129
failure, 66, 67, 73, 75, 76, 77, 79, 81, 84, 100, 109, 111, 112, 121, 137, 165, 183, 209, 211, 215, 216
failure to thrive, 100, 109, 111, 112
faith, 219
false belief, 191
familial, ix, 117, 118, 119, 120, 123, 125, 127, 128, 130, 165
familial aggregation, 117
family environment, 137, 145
family functioning, 119
family history, 116, 127, 132
family life, 123
family members, 115, 116, 117, 119, 120, 121, 123, 124, 125, 126, 128, 129, 130, 131
family relationships, 122, 124
family structure, 127
family studies, 122
family support, 122, 124, 125
family system, 103, 123, 175
family therapy, 120, 123, 124, 126, 131, 134
family units, 128
fashion industry, 199
fasting, vii, 8, 17, 38, 46, 71, 76, 155, 174, 227
Fasting, 10, 61, 185, 222
fat, x, 3, 4, 7, 9, 11, 14, 16, 19, 21, 22, 30, 31, 34, 36, 38, 39, 40, 41, 42, 44, 46, 47, 48, 51, 54, 55, 56, 60, 61, 67, 69, 79, 81, 82, 83, 88, 90, 93, 162, 170, 173, 176, 178, 182, 187, 190, 191, 192, 197
fatigue, 65
fats, 92
fatty acids, 9, 38, 81, 88
fear, vii, x, 41, 107, 135, 173, 176, 190, 212, 213
fears, 56, 110, 136, 144, 168, 192, 228
feedback, 3, 4, 5, 7, 9, 10, 11, 15, 16, 17, 25, 37, 40, 41, 52, 56, 64, 153
feedback inhibition, 37
feeding problems, 110, 113
feelings, ix, 101, 108, 125, 126, 127, 131, 137, 145, 173, 183, 192, 195, 215, 216
feet, 76
females, x, 51, 53, 54, 55, 59, 61, 66, 67, 71, 73
femininity, 164
femur, 81
ferritin, 82
fertility, 57, 58, 60
fertilization, 58
fetus, 52
FHA, 55, 63
fiber, 93
fibrinolysis, 39
fibromyalgia, 65
fibrosis, 79, 120, 133
fidelity, 190, 191, 194, 195, 196
flexibility, 91
flight, 203, 211, 213
float, 180
flow, 39, 91, 210
fluctuations, 62, 65
fluid, 10, 17, 20, 59, 65, 67, 75, 78, 79, 94, 191
fluid balance, 79
focusing, 91, 107, 115, 125, 126, 176, 180
folic acid, 82
follicle, 54, 57, 65, 70
follicles, 57, 58, 59, 62
follicle-stimulating hormone, 65
follicular, 19, 52, 53, 57, 59, 62, 65, 70
follicular fluid, 59, 65
food intake, 6, 7, 8, 9, 10, 12, 16, 21, 23, 24, 28, 32, 33, 41, 42, 80, 188
foreigner, 31
forgetfulness, 209
forgetting, 149
fracture, 91
fractures, 67, 75, 81
fragility, 83, 184
fragmentation, 122
free will, 146
freedom, 141, 150, 151, 152, 153, 154, 155, 156, 168, 210, 211, 222
freedom of choice, 152, 156
freedom of will, 150, 151
Freud, Sigmund, viii, 101, 102, 107, 111, 113, 149, 151, 152, 156, 204, 209, 211, 214, 215, 222
frontal cortex, 15
frustration, 197, 215
FSH, 19, 51, 52, 53, 55, 57, 59
fuel, viii, 10, 36, 62
fulfillment, 151, 152, 153, 156, 204, 209, 216
functional changes, 67

G

G protein, 24
GABA, 9
games, 194
gametes, 57
gametogenesis, 56
gastric, vii, 75, 80, 170
gastrointestinal, vii, 7, 8, 11, 20, 22, 75, 80, 81
gastrointestinal involvement, 75
gastrointestinal tract, vii, 7, 80
gelatin, 36, 45

gender, 39, 164, 165, 198
gender ideology, 165
gene, 6, 8, 22, 23, 24, 30, 36, 37, 45, 46, 48, 59, 61, 62, 64, 70, 71, 72
gene expression, 22, 30, 36, 37, 46, 48, 72
gene promoter, 24, 62
genealogy, 217
General Health Questionnaire, 130
generation, 12, 13, 65, 131
genes, 8, 37, 46, 170
genetic alteration, 8, 227
genetic factors, 116
genotype, 8
geriatric, 13
germ cells, 59
gestation, 52
GHQ, 130
Ghrelin, 7, 11
Gibbs, 29
gift, 207
girls, vii, 3, 25, 28, 30, 52, 53, 66, 67, 68, 69, 72, 73, 93, 94, 95, 135, 177, 198
gland, 3, 4, 5, 13, 15, 16, 19, 20, 21, 26, 29, 80, 227
glaucoma, 154
globulin, 17, 54
GLP-1, 7, 9
glucagon, 12, 78
glucocorticoid receptor, 17, 52, 64, 65, 72
glucocorticoids, 4, 12, 15, 16, 21, 36, 61, 62, 64, 72
gluconeogenesis, 38
glucose, 6, 7, 10, 11, 12, 22, 23, 29, 30, 32, 35, 36, 37, 38, 39, 40, 42, 44, 49, 56, 78, 79, 81
glucose metabolism, 12, 22, 29, 30, 36, 37, 42, 49
glucose tolerance, 22, 23, 35
glucose tolerance test, 22
glycogen, 22, 79
GM-CSF, 33
goals, 129
gold standard, 83
gonad, 59
gonadotropin, 19, 52, 53, 57, 58, 59, 62, 64, 65, 66, 68, 71, 72
gonadotropin secretion, 52
gonadotropin-releasing hormone (GnRH), 52, 53, 65
gonads, 4, 5, 19, 21, 59
grades, 177
grandparents, 123
granulocyte, 33, 41
granulopoiesis, 33, 41
granulosa cells, 57, 59
grapes, 208
gravity, 169
gray matter, 67, 73, 91, 94
grief, 182
groups, 8, 36, 41, 42, 54, 55, 109, 120, 128, 129, 130, 144, 163, 165, 216
growth, viii, 3, 4, 5, 9, 10, 13, 23, 25, 26, 27, 32, 39, 41, 43, 45, 53, 54, 56, 57, 63, 64, 65, 66, 67, 70, 71, 72, 73, 81, 82, 100, 109, 123, 155, 216
growth factor, 10, 25, 26, 32, 43, 64, 70, 71, 82
growth factors, 32, 64
growth hormone, viii, 3, 4, 5, 23, 25, 26, 27, 70
guardian, 122, 170
guidelines, 108, 140
guilt, 127, 137, 166, 207, 218
guilty, 153, 164, 165

H

half-life, 11, 17
handling, 101, 173
hands, 76, 101, 206, 207
harm, 140, 168
harmonization, 101
HDL, 12, 39
healing, 185, 208, 209
health, vii, ix, 30, 34, 53, 68, 121, 122, 127, 135, 138, 139, 141, 142, 143, 146, 163, 167, 169, 187, 196, 198, 212, 214, 217, 220
health problems, vii
healthcare, 127, 129, 130, 164
heart, 3, 13, 31, 51, 75, 76, 77, 79, 84, 87, 90, 92, 99, 102, 115, 135, 140, 149, 161, 170, 193, 221, 225, 226
heart block, 77
heart failure, 77, 79
heart rate, 13, 79, 92
Hebrew, vii
height, x, 54, 69
hematologic, 73, 75, 79
hematological, 31, 41, 79, 82, 83
hematology, 85
hematopoiesis, 35, 41
hematopoietic, 12, 83
hematopoietic cells, 83
hematopoietic system, 12
hemodialysis, 41
hemoglobin, 82
heritability, 117
heterogeneity, 11
heterogeneous, 33, 58, 92, 99, 142
heuristic, x, 229
high fat, 47
high risk, 78, 81, 127, 137, 168
high-density lipoprotein, 47
high-fat, 38

high-level, 69
high-risk, 146
hip, 55, 82
hippocampus, 15, 65
holism, 178, 179, 180, 182, 183
holistic, viii, 180
holistic approach, viii
homeostasis, 9, 15, 21, 22, 36, 37, 44, 47, 60, 71, 104, 106, 118
homolog, 37
homology, 36
honesty, 210, 220, 221, 222
hormone, viii, 3, 4, 5, 6, 7, 8, 10, 12, 13, 15, 17, 19, 20, 21, 22, 23, 24, 25, 26, 27, 28, 30, 35, 38, 39, 44, 46, 52, 53, 54, 55, 56, 59, 60, 61, 62, 63, 64, 65, 66, 68, 70, 71, 72, 82, 85, 227
hormones, 3, 4, 5, 7, 8, 9, 13, 14, 15, 16, 22, 23, 24, 27, 35, 36, 38, 52, 55, 57, 58, 59, 61, 62, 66, 67, 71, 227
hospital, 88, 115, 125, 135, 138, 139, 140, 141, 142, 145, 147
hospitalization, 89, 90, 119, 127, 135, 136, 138, 139, 140, 141, 142, 143, 145
hospitalizations, 126
hospitalized, 13, 87, 92, 138, 139, 141, 144, 196
hospitals, 140
host, 43
hostility, 103, 104, 120
household, 134
HPA, 14, 15, 16, 17, 18, 20, 32, 34
HPA axis, 15, 16, 17, 18, 20, 34
human animal, 218
human behavior, 174, 180
human condition, 207, 210
human dimensions, 151
human nature, 214
human sciences, viii, x, 230
human subjects, 60, 72
human will, 219
humanism, 152
humanity, 214
humans, ix, 3, 6, 10, 11, 15, 16, 24, 26, 27, 36, 37, 38, 39, 40, 41, 45, 47, 60, 206, 214, 216, 229
husband, 190, 196
hyperactivity, 18, 20, 28, 29, 34, 162
hyperalimentation, 76
hyperinsulinaemia, 38
hyperinsulinemia, 39, 48
hypersensitive, 100, 215
hypersensitivity, 10, 139
hypoglycemia, 64, 84
hypogonadism, 3, 4, 19, 23, 52, 60, 62
hypokalemia, 78, 80, 90
hypomagnesemia, 79
hyponatremia, 90
hypophosphatemia, 79, 82
hypotension, 75, 76, 77, 92
hypothalamic, 4, 7, 8, 9, 10, 11, 12, 13, 14, 15, 16, 17, 19, 20, 21, 22, 23, 25, 26, 27, 28, 29, 32, 51, 52, 53, 55, 56, 59, 60, 61, 62, 63, 64, 65, 68, 69, 71, 72, 90
hypothalamic-pituitary axis, 4
hypothalamic-pituitary-adrenal axis, 27, 28, 29, 62, 63, 64, 65, 71, 72
hypothalamus, 3, 4, 5, 6, 7, 8, 9, 15, 16, 17, 19, 21, 23, 32, 52, 63, 64, 65, 66, 227
hypothalamus-pituitary-adrenal, 227
hypothermia, 77
hypothesis, 6, 7, 8, 18, 19, 20, 22, 54, 59, 60, 61, 62, 69, 101, 141, 191, 213
hypothyroidism, 13
hypovolemia, 79
hysteria, viii

I

ICD, 102, 187, 188, 192, 200
id, 61
ideal body weight, 54, 55, 91, 92
identification, 68, 109, 124, 125, 126, 146
identity, ix, 117, 122, 124, 146, 147, 150, 161, 163, 164, 166, 182, 188, 206
ideology, 165
idiopathic, 82, 83
IFN, 34
IFNγ, 31, 32, 33
IGF, 5, 10, 11, 12, 13, 14, 26, 55, 56, 57, 58, 59, 62, 63, 66, 70, 82
IGF-1, 5, 10, 11, 12, 13, 14, 62, 63
IGF-I, 10, 12, 26, 55, 56, 57, 58, 59, 62, 66, 70, 82
IgG, 20
IL-1, 31, 32, 33, 34, 35, 80
IL-2, 32, 33, 43
IL-4, 33, 43
IL-6, 31, 32, 33, 34, 35, 80
illusion, 192, 207, 208, 209, 210, 211, 213, 214, 215, 221, 222
illusions, 207, 209, 213, 220
imagery, 211
images, 129, 146, 147, 166, 209
imagination, 142, 209
imaging, 20, 29, 73, 91, 94
imbalances, 136
immune function, 33, 34
immune system, 31, 33, 34, 227
immunity, 36, 41

immunoassays, 33
immunocompetent cells, 41
immunodeficiency, 34
immunosuppression, 35
immunosuppressive, 15
impaired glucose tolerance, 22
implementation, 143
impotence, 144
impulsive, 140
in situ, 116, 196
in vitro, 13, 22, 27, 37, 40, 41, 44, 48, 59, 70
in vivo, 23, 27, 38, 39, 40, 41, 48, 57, 59
inactivation, 8
inactive, 13
incentive, 207, 220
incidence, vii, 3, 55, 58, 65, 75, 82, 83, 87, 173, 198
incomes, 79
incubation, 39, 58
independence, 92, 118, 152
Indians, 40
indication, 87, 101, 176, 197
indicators, 12, 95, 143
indices, 6, 82
indirect effect, 32, 60
individual character, 103
individual characteristics, 103
individual differences, 100, 112
individuality, 118, 162, 164
induction, 37, 46, 57, 58, 59, 60
industry, 199
ineffectiveness, ix, 177
infancy, 104
infants, 100, 102, 107, 110, 111, 113
infection, 34, 88
infections, 41, 102
infectious, 41, 48
infertile, 58, 70
infertility, 4, 58
inflammation, 15, 32, 43
inflammatory, 31, 32, 33, 34, 36, 37, 39, 48, 62, 65, 66, 72, 81
inflammatory disease, 62
inflammatory response, 33
infrastructure, 140
ingestion, 6, 7
inherited, 24, 194
inhibition, 8, 33, 37, 56, 64, 65, 72, 216
inhibitor, 35
inhibitory, 5, 7, 8, 15, 34, 37, 41, 59, 62, 64
inhibitory effect, 38, 62, 64
initiation, 15, 26, 60, 195
innovation, 103
insane, 214
insecurity, 112, 144, 145
insight, 43, 204, 208, 212, 213, 217, 218
insomnia, 136
inspiration, 128, 207
instability, 94, 118
instinct, 155, 163, 220
institutions, 164
instruments, 104
insulin, 6, 7, 8, 9, 10, 21, 22, 23, 25, 26, 27, 29, 30, 31, 35, 36, 37, 38, 39, 40, 41, 42, 43, 44, 45, 46, 47, 48, 51, 62, 63, 64, 71, 78, 81, 82, 227
insulin resistance, 22, 29, 30, 35, 36, 37, 38, 39, 40, 43, 44, 45, 47, 48, 62
insulin sensitivity, 22, 30, 31, 35, 36, 37, 38, 39, 40, 41, 42, 46, 47, 62
insulin-like growth factor, 10, 25, 26, 71, 82
insulin-like growth factor I, 25, 26, 82
integration, viii, ix, 3, 124, 144, 146, 147, 161
integrity, 118, 123, 164, 166
intelligence, 142
intentionality, 150, 164
intentions, 103, 191, 195
interaction, 15, 32, 64, 71, 103, 104, 106, 107, 108, 109, 110, 112, 118, 153, 174, 175, 181, 227
interactions, 8, 15, 16, 103, 106, 147, 165
interdependence, 180
interdisciplinary, viii, ix, 130
interface, 51
interference, 35, 168
interferon, 43
interleukin-1, 43, 44, 66, 71, 72
interleukin-2, 43
interleukin-6, 43, 44
interleukine, 43
interleukins, 21, 32
internal organization, 147
internalization, ix
International Classification of Diseases, 188, 200
internist, 138
internists, 144
interpersonal relations, 131, 152, 165
interpersonal relationships, 152
interrelations, 31, 146
interstitial, 59, 79
interval, 53, 76, 78
intervention, 27, 87, 88, 91, 122, 123, 125, 126, 128, 129, 130, 131, 138, 139, 140, 142, 143, 144, 145, 146, 147, 229
interview, 116, 120, 143
interviews, 119, 143, 144
intimacy, 122
intoxication, 208, 209, 210, 211
intravenous, 22, 64, 92

intrinsic, 18, 20, 40, 191
introspection, ix, 173, 179, 180, 182, 184, 229
invasive, 107
inversion, 194
investment, 145
iodine, 13
iron, 88, 122
irrationality, 184
irritability, 104, 136
ischemic, 30
isoforms, 11, 37
isolation, 126, 130, 136, 145, 146, 153
Italy, 3, 31, 51, 75, 87, 99, 115, 118, 127, 135, 141, 142, 143, 149, 161, 225, 226

J

JAMA, 71
Japan, 175
Japanese, 47
judge, 191, 194, 195, 221
judges, 141, 196
judgment, 153, 191, 194, 196
justice, 189
justification, 167, 170, 192

K

Kant, 204, 222
kidneys, 79
kinase, 30, 37, 39, 48
kinetics, 57

L

L1, 30, 48
labor, 62
lactation, 61
language, viii, ix, 67, 103, 173, 174, 176, 178, 180, 182, 183, 184, 190, 211, 216, 217, 230
late-onset, 19
laughter, 206, 207
law, 135, 141, 142, 166
laws, 182
laxatives, 122
LDL, 12, 38, 40
lean body mass, 53, 81, 82
learning, 70, 143, 152, 178, 181, 228
learning environment, 228
learning process, 152
left ventricular, 75, 76, 77, 90
legumes, 102
leptin, 4, 5, 6, 7, 8, 9, 10, 14, 16, 21, 22, 23, 24, 27, 29, 30, 35, 36, 38, 41, 42, 44, 46, 48, 49, 51, 54, 55, 60, 61, 63, 65, 67, 70, 71, 82, 227
leukaemia, 82
leukemia, 34
leukopenia, 33, 82
liberty, 166
libido, 113, 153
LIF, 34
life cycle, 123, 210
lifestyle, 88, 130, 166
lifestyles, 125
life-threatening, 40, 75, 82
lifetime, 61, 198
ligand, 64
ligands, 37, 46
light cycle, 15
likelihood, 55
limbic system, 9
limitation, 153
limitations, 121
linear, 10, 66, 68, 73
linguistic, 174, 175, 176, 180, 181, 182, 183, 196, 197
links, 34, 44, 146, 175
lipase, 35, 40
lipid, 9, 14, 15, 37, 38, 39, 40, 47
lipid metabolism, 9, 14, 37, 39, 40
lipid oxidation, 38
lipids, 9, 10, 38, 40
lipodystrophy, 39, 40
lipolysis, 30
lipoprotein, 40, 93
liquids, 101, 110
listening, 126, 130
liver, 5, 10, 11, 22, 37, 75, 79, 80
liver cirrhosis, 10
liver enzymes, 75, 79
LMW, 38
locus, 3, 8, 15, 16, 63, 65, 198
locus coeruleus, 8, 15, 16
logical reasoning, 177
logistics, 129
long distance, 66
longitudinal studies, 40
losses, 109
love, 152, 196
lumbar, 81
lumbar spine, 81
lutein, 65, 72
luteinizing hormone, 52, 61, 62, 64, 65, 68, 71, 72
lying, 189, 190, 229
lymphocyte, 34, 35, 43

lymphocytes, 31, 32

M

machinery, 88
macrophage, 33, 41
macrophages, 31, 32, 45, 46, 49
magnesium, 77, 79, 88
magnetic resonance imaging, 20, 29, 73, 91, 94
maintenance, 4, 8, 34, 35, 54, 55, 60, 69, 120, 122, 134, 141, 150, 153, 162, 166
major depression, 132, 137
malabsorption, 10, 75
males, vii, 59, 173
malicious, 220
malnutrition, vii, 4, 10, 11, 13, 17, 18, 23, 26, 31, 34, 35, 41, 42, 44, 49, 55, 56, 62, 66, 80, 82, 85, 89, 109, 137, 227
mammalian cells, 37
mammals, 63
management, ix, x, 76, 84, 87, 88, 89, 93, 99, 115, 126, 129, 134, 143, 161, 162, 167, 169, 230
manifold, 203, 205
manipulation, 11, 56
manners, 195
marriage, 124
married couples, 124
marrow, 32, 48, 75, 76, 82, 83
maternal, 101, 105, 106, 108, 109, 110, 111, 120
matrix, 36, 111, 139, 147
maturation, 52, 56, 57, 60, 70, 100, 155
maturation process, 100
meals, 8, 88, 89, 102, 104, 105, 106, 110
mean corpuscular volume (MCV), 82
meanings, 153, 163, 180, 183
measurement, 28, 33, 120, 152
measures, 18, 87, 91
meat, 88
media, 162, 166
media messages, 162, 166
mediation, 146, 228
mediators, 15, 38
medication, 27, 80, 115
medulla, 15
meiosis, 57
melancholic, 62, 65
melanin, 6
melatonin, 8, 14
memory, 67, 91
men, 3, 21, 39, 61, 73, 82, 180, 207, 212, 216, 217
menarche, x, 19, 52, 54, 55, 66, 68, 69
menopause, 65
menstrual cycle, x, 51, 52, 53, 54, 55, 58, 60, 62, 64, 65, 69, 71, 82
menstruation, 53, 62, 64, 65, 68
mental disorder, x, 147, 168
mental illness, 129, 141
mental life, 215
mental model, 104, 108
mental representation, 108
mental state, 104
messages, 108, 139, 162, 165, 166, 205
messenger ribonucleic acid, 72
meta-analysis, 24, 147
metabolic, viii, 10, 12, 17, 27, 29, 38, 39, 40, 42, 46, 48, 55, 60, 66, 77, 78, 81, 87, 88, 89, 90, 91, 92, 93, 94, 95, 137
metabolic disturbances, 78
metabolic rate, 27, 38, 41, 77, 79, 89, 95
metabolic syndrome, 27, 29, 39, 46
metabolism, viii, 4, 6, 9, 10, 12, 13, 17, 19, 22, 28, 29, 30, 32, 35, 36, 37, 39, 40, 42, 43, 44, 49, 54, 64, 79, 81, 90, 93, 227
metabolite, 10
metabolites, 13, 17
meta-message, 139
MHC, 82
mice, 22, 36, 37, 40, 42, 44, 45, 48, 57, 58, 60, 61, 70
Middle Ages, 176
milk, 100
mimicking, 82
mind-body, 142
minerals, 79
mirror, 40, 182, 190, 192, 197, 207
misinterpretation, 139, 217
misunderstanding, 122, 173, 219
mitochondria, 38, 46
mitral, 75, 77, 78, 84
mitral valve, 75, 77, 78, 84
mitral valve prolapse, 75, 77, 78, 84
modality, 163, 196
models, vii, 35, 37, 39, 58, 104, 106, 107, 108, 109, 122, 126, 129, 131, 151, 153, 163, 166, 175, 176, 195, 198
modulation, 4, 11, 24, 40, 102
molecular mechanisms, 43, 64, 92
molecular weight, 38
molecules, viii, 4, 31, 35, 37, 45, 47, 227, 230
momentum, 108
monkeys, 37, 40, 46, 64
monocytes, 32, 35
monozygotic twins, 117
mood, 24, 62, 64, 65, 69, 71, 91, 136, 170
mood disorder, 65, 69, 136

moral judgment, 217
morality, 198, 203, 204, 212, 216
morals, 170
morbidity, 68, 75, 79, 116, 134, 142
morning, 15
morphogenetic processes, 123
morphological, 82, 83
morphology, 20, 29
mortality, 3, 4, 75, 79, 140, 141, 142, 148
mortality rate, 141, 142
mothers, 101, 107, 109, 110, 119, 121
motion, 77
motivation, 88, 92, 137, 140, 209
motives, 117, 128
mountains, 179
mouse, 46, 60
mouse model, 60
mouth, 101
movement, 12, 32, 79, 155, 209, 221
MRI, 20, 67, 73
mRNA, 21, 36, 37, 39, 40
multidimensional, 149, 174, 177, 185
multidisciplinary, 110, 141, 142
multiple factors, 144
multiplicity, 122, 215
multivariate, 40
murine model, 35
murine models, 35
muscle, 22, 38, 48, 77, 81, 179
muscles, 37
muscular contraction, 77
mutation, 6, 24, 71
mutations, 23, 24, 39, 45, 60, 61

N

naloxone, 11, 25
narcissism, 199
narcissistic, 110, 145, 146, 165
nasogastric tube, 87, 93
National Health Service, 138
natural, 35, 110, 204, 207, 208, 209, 210, 213, 216, 220, 221
necrosis, 21, 30, 43, 44, 46, 80
negative influences, 119
neglect, 169
negligence, 103, 109
negotiation, 88, 100
nerve, 218
nerves, 179
nervous system, viii, 5, 6, 9, 23, 24, 32, 52, 56, 63, 65, 77, 78
network, 3, 7, 8, 33, 34, 110, 131, 183, 227
neuroanatomy, 23
neurobiological, 16, 85
neuroendocrine, 4, 6, 9, 20, 21, 25, 27, 28, 60, 61, 62, 66, 69, 71, 162
neuroendocrine system, 6
neuromodulation, 25
neuronal circuits, 6
neurons, 4, 6, 7, 8, 14, 15, 16, 20, 24, 32, 63, 64, 71
neuropeptide, 6, 7, 8, 10, 15, 20, 21, 23, 24, 27, 65, 72
neuropeptide Y, 6, 9
neuropeptides, 4, 8, 10, 16, 21, 24, 29
neuroscience, 179
neuroses, 150, 154
neurotic, 133
neuroticism, 117
neurotransmission, 4, 43
neurotransmitter, 3, 5, 8, 16
neurotransmitters, viii, 4, 6, 8, 227
New Jersey, 222
Newton, 156
Nietzsche, 203, 204, 205, 206, 207, 208, 209, 210, 211, 212, 213, 214, 215, 216, 217, 218, 219, 220, 221, 222, 223
nitric oxide, 48
nitrogen, 13
NO synthase, 39
norepinephrine, 15, 16, 32, 64, 65
normal, vii, x, 10, 11, 12, 13, 14, 17, 18, 19, 21, 22, 25, 26, 28, 35, 37, 38, 39, 42, 46, 52, 53, 54, 55, 57, 58, 60, 62, 63, 66, 70, 72, 75, 78, 81, 82, 83, 88, 89, 90, 91, 155, 178, 181, 182, 183, 188, 198, 227
normal children, 60
normalization, 12, 17, 18, 21, 61
norms, 54, 181
Norway, 117
NOS, 39
NS, 30, 43
NTS, 7
nuclear, 37, 46, 57, 142
nuclear receptors, 46
nuclei, 6, 8, 15, 151
nucleus, 6, 7, 8, 16, 63, 154
nurse, 101
nurses, 182
nursing, 141
nurturance, 104
nutrient, 88
nutrients, 16, 35, 88
nutrition, 6, 10, 13, 17, 30, 34, 55, 60, 78, 80, 87, 88, 89, 90, 91, 92, 95, 110, 122, 169, 196

O

obese, 8, 11, 24, 28, 34, 36, 38, 39, 40, 47, 70
obese patients, 34, 40
obesity, vii, 10, 24, 25, 27, 28, 29, 30, 35, 36, 37, 38, 39, 40, 41, 43, 44, 45, 46, 47, 48, 60, 71, 116, 168
objectification, 147
objective reality, 174, 222
obligation, 169, 175
observations, 12, 37, 61, 104, 108, 116, 118, 122, 125, 131, 198
observed behavior, 103
obsessive-compulsive, 24, 116, 136, 137, 140
obsessive-compulsive disorder, 24, 136, 137, 140
omentum, 38
one dimension, 176
oocyte, 57, 58
oocytes, 57, 70
openness, 136, 216
opioid, 10, 16
opioids, 16
opposition, vii, 102, 109
optimism, 188, 212
oral, 22, 67, 89, 92, 100, 101, 107
orexin A, 8
organ, vii, ix, 15, 23, 110
organic, vii, viii, 55, 100, 102, 109, 112, 144, 153, 154, 227
organism, 15, 216
originality, viii, 162
orthostatic hypotension, 77
oscillation, 61
osmosis, 79
osteocalcin, 81
osteopenia, 81, 85, 94
osteoporosis, 4, 33, 55, 69, 73, 81, 85
outpatient, 89, 92, 121, 137, 140, 141, 142, 145
outpatients, 89, 92, 138
ovarian failure, 73
ovarian follicular, 70
ovariectomized, 72
ovaries, 21, 54, 58, 59, 65, 72
ovary, 52, 59, 62, 66, 70, 72
overweight, 10, 91, 132, 166, 176, 187, 188, 198
oviduct, 60
ovulation, 52, 56, 57, 58, 61, 62, 64, 65, 66, 69
ovum, 65
oxidation, 10, 22, 29, 36, 37, 38, 44, 48
oxidation rate, 29
oxidative, 22
oxygen, 9, 13, 79
oxygen consumption, 9, 13
oxytocin, 6, 19, 29

P

Pacific, 201
PAI-1, 35
pain, 16, 77, 80, 181, 192, 195, 215, 216, 218, 219, 220
palpitations, 77
pancreas, 7, 8, 80
pancreatic, 22
pancreatic islet, 22
pancreatitis, 75, 80, 85
paracrine, viii, 31, 35, 57, 70
paradox, x, 193, 203, 206, 219
paradoxical, 11, 40, 56, 169, 189, 219, 220
parallelism, 152
parameter, 42
parasympathetic, 16, 78
paraventricular, 6, 8, 15, 63
paraventricular nucleus, 6, 8, 15, 63
parent-child, 103, 163
parenteral, 87, 89, 90, 92, 95
parents, ix, 99, 100, 102, 104, 110, 111, 115, 118, 119, 120, 121, 123, 124, 127, 128, 129, 130, 131, 133, 135, 142, 143, 144, 162, 163, 228
parotid, 80
parotid gland, 80
particles, 40
parvicellular, 63
passive, 169
paternal, 111
pathogenesis, 31, 33, 35, 36, 37, 40, 43, 116, 162
pathogenic, 101, 128
pathogens, 31
pathologist, viii
pathology, 18, 20, 68, 109, 117, 120, 121, 128, 129, 135, 137, 138, 140, 141, 143, 146, 162, 205, 207, 209, 211, 214
pathophysiological mechanisms, 18
pathophysiology, 29
pathways, ix, 4, 6, 7, 9, 39, 64, 155
pedagogical, 154
pediatrician, 111
pelvic, 54
pelvic ultrasound, 54
peptide, 7, 9, 10, 11, 26, 33, 37, 39, 43, 63, 70
peptides, 6, 7, 8, 10, 20, 31, 33, 34, 62, 227
percentile, 54
perception, ix, 119, 121, 130, 166, 168, 173, 174, 175, 176, 177, 178, 179, 181, 182, 184, 221, 229
perceptions, 164, 178, 181, 196
perfectionism, ix
perforation, 80
pericardial, 77

pericardial effusion, 77
peripheral, 76, 78, 79
peripheral blood, 82, 83
peripheral nervous system, 63, 77
permit, 211
peroxisome, 37
personal identity, 150
personality, 11, 26, 99, 103, 106, 107, 137, 138, 140, 144, 146, 150, 162, 182, 195, 228
personality disorder, 106, 137, 140
personality test, 144
personality traits, 11
persuasion, 142, 193
perturbations, 39
pessimism, 212, 213, 214
pessimists, 207
pharmacological, 8, 16, 37, 57, 126, 129, 131, 142, 146
pharmacological treatment, 129, 131
pharmacology, 115
phenomenology, 63, 152
phenotype, 36
philosophers, 153, 179, 183
philosophical, viii, ix, 153, 164, 174, 177, 178, 179, 180, 183, 184, 187, 188, 203, 206, 212, 213, 219, 227, 229
philosophy, 173, 174, 175, 176, 178, 179, 184, 185, 204, 213
phobia, 136
phosphate, 78, 92
phosphorous, 79
phosphorus, 77, 78, 90
phosphorylation, 26, 39
physical activity, 143
physical diagnosis, 176
physical exercise, 169
physical health, 53
physical properties, 179
physicians, 162, 169
physiological, 4, 8, 11, 16, 32, 35, 36, 52, 53, 57, 82, 101, 102, 110, 142, 215, 216, 220
physiological regulation, 4, 102
physiology, ix, 7, 21, 36, 52, 61, 62, 68, 71, 217
physiopathology, 14, 42, 149
pig, 59
pigs, 58, 59
pilot study, 133
pioglitazone, 39
pituitary, viii, ix, 3, 4, 5, 11, 12, 14, 15, 16, 17, 18, 19, 20, 21, 22, 26, 28, 29, 32, 51, 52, 53, 56, 57, 59, 60, 61, 62, 63, 64, 65, 68, 69, 71, 90, 227
pituitary gland, 3, 4, 5, 15, 19, 20, 29
pituitary gonadotroph, 64
placenta, 21
placental, 52, 57, 59, 62, 66, 70
placental hormones, 52
planning, 123, 142, 144, 150, 152
plasma, 10, 11, 12, 16, 17, 18, 21, 26, 27, 28, 30, 32, 34, 35, 36, 37, 38, 39, 40, 45, 46, 47, 48, 49, 62, 64, 72, 79
plasma levels, 10, 11, 30, 32, 34, 36, 39, 48, 49, 62
plasminogen, 35, 58
plasticity, 122
platelet, 24, 83
plausibility, 180
play, 6, 8, 14, 20, 23, 31, 34, 37, 39, 62, 78, 81, 82, 99, 101, 107, 162, 165, 166, 174, 189, 211
pleasure, 101, 106, 153, 208, 209, 215, 220
PMA, 133
poisonous, 218, 219
polar body, 57
politics, 204
polycystic ovary syndrome, 58
polymorphism, 6, 8, 24
polymorphisms, 8
poor, 10, 18, 70, 80, 103, 119, 179, 190, 195
population, 40, 47, 53, 66, 68, 82, 118, 132
positive correlation, 36
positive reinforcement, 110
positivist, 156
postmenopausal, 67
postmenopausal women, 67
postpartum, 62
postpartum period, 62
postsynaptic, 4
potassium, 79
poverty, 109
power, 123, 153, 164, 165, 166, 177, 195, 198, 199, 206, 207, 208, 209, 210, 213, 215, 216, 219, 220, 221
PPAR ligands, 37
PPARγ, 37, 39
praxis, 150, 151, 153
prediction, 53, 134
predictors, 30, 95, 132, 133
pre-existing, 169
preference, 212
pregnancy, 52, 60, 61, 62, 71, 112
premature death, 75
premature ovarian failure, 67, 73
premenopausal, 47
pressure, 38, 39, 84, 90, 146, 176, 179, 198
presynaptic, 4
prevention, 68, 84, 92, 126, 162, 166, 230
preventive, 127
primates, 40, 60, 65, 72

prisoners, 64
probability, 175
probands, 8, 132
problem solving, 126
procreation, 61
production, 4, 5, 6, 9, 13, 14, 16, 17, 19, 22, 28, 32, 33, 34, 35, 37, 39, 40, 41, 43, 44, 48, 57, 58, 59, 64, 82
profit, viii, 178
progenitors, 41, 45
progesterone, 21, 59, 62, 64, 65, 66
prognosis, 14, 68, 117, 119, 133, 136, 145, 211
prognostic value, 28
program, 87, 89, 90, 91, 110, 125, 126, 127, 130, 131, 138, 140, 142, 144
proinflammatory, 66, 80
pro-inflammatory, 31, 32, 33, 34
prolactin, 5, 19, 25, 27, 28, 58, 70
prolapse, 75, 76, 77, 78, 84
proliferation, 32, 36, 57, 59
promoter, 8, 22, 24, 37, 62, 64
promoter region, 8, 22
propagation, 15
prophylactic, 214
prosperity, 217
prostaglandins, 48
proteases, 81
protection, 106, 108, 109, 155
protective role, 37, 39
proteic, 21, 57
protein, 11, 12, 14, 17, 21, 22, 30, 34, 35, 36, 37, 38, 39, 44, 45, 46, 47, 48, 54, 59, 64, 79, 80, 81, 88, 90, 93
protein synthesis, 22, 59
proteins, 5, 10, 11, 12, 13, 34, 36
proteolysis, 12
protocol, 142
protocols, 139, 140, 145
prototype, 101, 107
pseudo, 18
psyche, 135, 146, 147, 149, 153
psychiatric disorder, 75, 106, 132, 137
psychiatric disorders, 106, 132
psychiatric hospitals, 140
psychiatric illness, 131, 133, 134
psychiatric morbidity, 134
psychiatric patients, 130, 141
psychiatrist, 127, 129, 138, 146
psychiatrists, 144, 229
psychoanalysis, 106, 111, 150, 151, 153, 155, 156, 175
psychoanalytic theories, 151
psychoeducational intervention, 126, 128, 130, 131
psychoeducational program, 126, 130, 131
psychological problems, 122
psychological processes, 125
psychological states, 218
psychological stress, 28, 51, 67
psychological stressors, 51, 67
psychologist, 127, 129, 141, 204, 210, 217
psychology, 125, 129, 146, 151, 152, 153, 157, 162, 168, 175, 179, 186, 204, 217, 219, 223
psychopathology, x, 100, 102, 107, 109, 116, 128, 129, 137, 185
psychopharmacological, 154
psychosocial factors, 106
psychosocial stress, 66, 106, 109
psychosomatic, vii, viii, 41, 122, 133, 156, 147, 149, 150
psychotherapeutic, 111, 126, 128, 130, 131, 136, 144, 145, 147, 150, 151
psychotherapy, 76, 92, 112, 124, 136, 139, 142, 145, 146, 147, 150, 153
psychotic, 126
psychotic symptoms, 126
pubertal development, 52, 58, 66, 68
puberty, 19, 52, 53, 60, 65, 66, 68, 70, 72, 88
public, 138
public health, 138
pulse, 11, 52, 55, 56, 61, 62, 64, 72, 76, 90
pulses, 15, 52
pupil, 154
putative cause, 33
PVN, 6

Q

QT interval, 76, 78
QT prolongation, 78
quality of life, 88, 125, 130
query, 189, 194, 196
question mark, 212
questioning, 146, 193
questionnaire, 134, 144
questionnaires, 130

R

race, 206, 212, 220
range, 8, 11, 53, 54, 67, 75, 137
rat, 43, 59, 65, 70, 72
rating scale, 121, 134
ratings, 66
rationality, 125, 167, 176
rats, 6, 11, 32, 59, 61

RDA, 90
reactivity, 20
reading, 67, 161, 163, 165
reality, 123, 139, 146, 151, 153, 161, 163, 164, 165, 167, 174, 176, 183, 189, 193, 195, 196, 197, 203, 204, 207, 208, 209, 211, 216, 217, 222
reasoning, 91, 177, 178, 181, 184, 191, 197, 229
recall, 67, 175, 179
receptors, 4, 6, 8, 9, 11, 17, 21, 23, 29, 32, 33, 34, 37, 43, 46, 52, 59, 62, 65
reciprocity, 105, 106, 108
recognition, 84, 124, 214
reconcile, 209
reconstruction, 131, 145
recovery, ix, 3, 4, 11, 12, 13, 17, 18, 26, 28, 29, 35, 52, 53, 54, 56, 58, 67, 69, 73, 75, 76, 82, 84, 89, 90, 93, 95, 119, 120, 124, 128, 131, 132, 136, 138, 140, 146, 151, 152
recurrence, 4
red blood cell, 75, 82
red blood cells, 75, 82
red meat, 88
REE, 13, 14
refining, 191
reflection, 124, 129, 130, 155, 162, 180, 192, 211, 212
regional, 77, 91, 94
regression, 19, 53, 115, 122, 125, 139
regressions, 107, 124
regular, 37, 52, 53, 55, 88, 89, 92, 106, 110
regulation, 4, 6, 8, 9, 10, 15, 17, 19, 21, 22, 25, 26, 27, 28, 30, 32, 35, 37, 42, 46, 48, 57, 59, 71, 72, 102, 106, 109, 110, 144, 227
regulators, 62, 63
rehabilitation, 35, 75, 76, 87, 89, 90, 91, 93, 129, 138, 140, 141, 142, 143
reinforcement, 110, 128, 136
relapse, 87, 92, 95, 132, 134, 147, 195
relapses, 128, 131
relationships, ix, 31, 40, 104, 107, 113, 119, 122, 123, 124, 135, 147, 152, 161, 163, 165, 196, 229
relatives, 14, 125, 129, 132, 139
relevance, 19, 166
reliability, 104, 132
religion, 203, 207, 212, 215
religions, 216, 217
religious beliefs, 87
remission, 119, 137
renal, 20, 48, 75, 79, 121
renal disease, 48
renal failure, 121
renin, 79
repair, 88, 164
repolarization, 77
reproduction, 29, 57, 60, 63, 67, 70
resentment, 107
reserves, 60, 61
residential, 143
resistance, 3, 4, 10, 11, 12, 22, 23, 24, 29, 30, 35, 36, 37, 38, 39, 40, 43, 44, 45, 47, 48, 51, 56, 57, 62, 63, 77, 126, 152, 215, 227
resistin, 30, 35, 36, 41, 42, 44
resolution, 142, 150, 182
resources, 60, 123, 124, 125, 126, 129, 143, 144
respiratory, 79
responsibilities, 136
responsiveness, 19, 53, 56, 58, 78, 108
restaurant, 191
resting energy, 27, 89
restructuring, 143
retardation, 111
retention, 12, 20
retinoic acid, 46
returns, 13, 21, 53, 142
revaluation, 217
rhythm, 15, 19, 60, 100
rhythmicity, 61
ribonucleic acid, 72
rigidity, 118, 123
rings, 126
risk, vii, 18, 48, 67, 72, 75, 78, 81, 91, 92, 116, 117, 119, 124, 127, 128, 132, 133, 137, 138, 139, 140, 142, 143, 146, 147, 168, 169
risk factors, 48, 132, 133, 143
risks, 79, 92, 119, 136
rodents, 37
rosiglitazone, 39
routines, 137
rumination, 99, 111

S

safeguard, 209
safety, 95
salivary glands, 76
sample, 33, 118, 119, 120, 130, 132
SASS, 130
satisfaction, 100, 101, 107, 142, 166, 170, 208, 215, 216
scandalous, 163
scarcity, 119, 120, 122, 127
schizophrenia, 119, 120, 121, 126, 134
schizophrenic patients, 120, 121
school, viii, 149, 151, 153, 154, 156, 177, 228, 229
scientific community, 140
scientific method, 213

sclerosis, 79
scores, 92, 106, 130
search, ix, 108, 124, 149, 150, 152, 163, 206, 215, 229
searching, 165
seasonal affective disorder, 65
secondary sexual characteristics, 19
secrete, 34, 64
secretion, viii, 4, 5, 6, 8, 10, 11, 13, 14, 15, 16, 18, 19, 20, 21, 23, 24, 25, 26, 27, 29, 33, 34, 37, 40, 51, 52, 53, 55, 56, 58, 59, 60, 61, 62, 63, 64, 65, 66, 68, 72, 78, 79, 81, 227
sedentary, 55
selenium, 77
self-actualization, 156
self-awareness, 218
self-concept, 166
self-confirmation, 155
self-consciousness, 130, 190, 192, 209, 213, 220, 221
self-control, 177, 178
self-discipline, 218
self-esteem, 120
self-expression, 156
self-help, 195
self-identity, 161, 164
self-image, ix, 185, 187, 199
self-knowledge, 149, 190, 192, 193, 209, 210, 222
self-organization, 104
self-understanding, 204, 216
self-worth, 178
semantic, 107, 174, 175, 176, 177, 180, 182, 183, 184
semiotics, 216, 217
sensation, vii, 10, 16
sensations, 177, 181, 188, 192, 218
sensitivity, 13, 18, 20, 22, 29, 30, 31, 34, 35, 36, 37, 38, 39, 40, 41, 42, 46, 47, 58, 62, 72, 84, 107, 198, 207, 227
sensitization, 37
sentences, 129, 180
separation, 100, 104, 106, 109, 112, 115, 117, 118, 125, 142, 144, 145, 229
sequelae, 79
series, 78, 137
serine, 58
serotonin, 8, 9, 10, 14, 24, 32
Sertoli cells, 59
serum, 7, 11, 12, 13, 14, 20, 21, 30, 33, 36, 37, 38, 41, 42, 45, 47, 49, 52, 53, 55, 60, 61, 79, 80, 82, 92, 95
serum ferritin, 82
services, 122
severity, 4, 18, 34, 77, 83, 118, 121, 127, 168
sex, vii, 13, 52, 54, 58
sex hormones, 52
sexual abuse, 104
sexual dimorphism, 72
sexuality, 198
shame, 207
shape, x, 91, 122, 143, 165, 166, 177, 178, 182, 187, 191, 192, 204
shares, 18
sharing, 128
sheep, 57, 58
shock, 79
shortness of breath, 77
short-term, 14, 17, 21, 29, 92, 119, 142, 148, 167
sign, 94, 107, 194, 204, 212, 213, 217, 220
signal transduction, 26, 64
signaling, 39, 48
signaling pathway, 39
signaling pathways, 39
signals, 3, 4, 6, 7, 16, 32, 34, 42, 54, 61, 123
signs, 10, 83, 92, 100, 103, 105, 106, 107, 108, 110, 139, 144, 165, 174, 205, 217
similarity, 179
simple vocabulary, 183
simulation, 221
singular, 151, 180, 182
sinus, 77
sites, 59, 66
skeletal muscle, 37
skills, 99, 101, 104, 109, 126, 134, 141
skills training, 126, 134
skin, 76, 197
sleep, 19, 52, 53, 68
smiles, 105
smooth muscle, 36
smooth muscle cells, 36
social behavior, 131
social class, 118, 119, 175
social consequences, 75
social context, 166
social desirability, 198
social environment, 131, 139, 150
social exchange, 106
social factors, 118, 133, 141
social group, 198
social influence, 188
social influences, 188
social isolation, 136
social network, 131
social perception, 175
social phobia, 136
social psychology, 175

social relations, 130
social responsibility, 177
social skills, 126, 134
social skills training, 126, 134
sociocultural, 166
socioeconomic, 118
socio-emotional, 129, 130
sociological, viii, 151, 165
Socrates, 180, 212
sodium, 79
somatization, 121
somatosensory, 179
somatostatin, 5, 11, 56, 59
somatostatin, 10, 70
sounds, 183
spatial, 91
species, 57, 58, 59, 63, 213, 214, 220, 221
specificity, 144, 150, 151, 154
spectrum, 142
speech, 195
spheres, 197
spinal cord, 179
spine, 55, 81, 82
spiritual, 150, 151, 152, 153, 154, 155, 164, 203, 204, 206, 213, 215, 220, 230
spouse, 124
springs, 213, 222
stability, 3, 94, 118, 167
stabilization, 18, 89
stages, 20, 34, 52, 107, 155
standard deviation, 66
standards, 54, 170
starvation, 3, 4, 17, 18, 22, 23, 34, 35, 40, 61, 65, 77, 89, 91, 93, 133, 164, 175, 198, 229
statistical analysis, 130
stenosis, 45
steroid, 13, 19, 34, 36, 59, 60, 65, 72
steroidogenesis, 56, 59
steroids, 19, 52
stigma, 166
stimulus, 181
stomach, 7, 8, 21, 37, 55, 178, 205
storage, 8, 11, 16, 22
strains, 79
strategies, 101, 108, 109, 126, 127, 131
strength, 152, 166, 168, 169, 205, 211, 212, 215
stress, viii, 14, 15, 16, 18, 20, 27, 28, 29, 32, 43, 51, 56, 62, 63, 64, 65, 66, 69, 71, 72, 106, 109, 126, 131, 150, 227
stress factors, 131
stressors, 51, 67
strikes, 130
stroma, 65
structuralism, 165, 223
structuring, 102, 103
students, viii, x, 230
subgroups, 116
subjective, 103, 104, 121, 123, 126, 144, 149, 152, 156, 164, 209
subjective experience, 103, 104
substance abuse, 116
substances, 4, 6, 8, 9, 99, 137, 140, 227
substitution, 14
substrates, 10, 12
success rate, 138
suffering, ix, 17, 82, 126, 131, 155, 161, 165, 168, 174, 197, 203, 205, 207, 208, 211, 212, 216, 218, 219, 220, 221
suicidal, 140, 218, 221
suicide, vii, 64, 137, 222
suicide attempts, 64, 137
summaries, x
superiority, 153
superstitious, 178, 191
supervision, 87, 91
supplemental, 79
supplements, 27, 89, 92
supply, 115, 126, 127, 129, 131, 137, 176
suppression, 11, 16, 17, 18, 28, 32, 33, 37, 46, 55, 56, 62, 90
surplus, 216
survival, 16, 95, 163, 166
susceptibility, 4, 24
swallowing, 99, 100
Sweden, 117
symbolic value, 164
sympathetic nervous system, 77
symptom, vii, ix, 51, 123, 138, 141, 150, 162, 187, 211, 213
symptoms, ix, 14, 18, 31, 52, 55, 73, 90, 99, 103, 117, 119, 121, 123, 126, 127, 135, 136, 137, 139, 140, 141, 144, 150, 153, 165, 166, 174, 175, 176, 187, 198, 203, 205, 212, 217
synapses, 4
synaptic transmission, 4
synchronization, 15
syndrome, viii, x, 3, 4, 12, 13, 14, 18, 23, 24, 26, 27, 29, 39, 46, 52, 58, 62, 63, 65, 67, 73, 75, 76, 78, 82, 84, 85, 87, 90, 93, 100, 109, 117, 162, 165, 198, 227
synergistic, 15, 16
synthesis, 10, 14, 22, 35, 37, 48, 58, 59, 79, 108, 161, 164
systemic circulation, 15, 59
systolic blood pressure, 90

T

T cells, 43
targets, 4, 87, 95
taste, 100
TBG, 12
teaching, 196
teenage girls, 68
teenagers, 162
temperament, 113
temperature, 12, 38, 54, 76, 100
temporal, 4, 67, 128
tendon, 179
tension, 65, 100, 103, 126, 179, 206, 220
territorial, 122
territory, 210
testes, 59
testis, 59, 70
testosterone, 38, 68
testosterone levels, 38
test-retest reliability, 104
Texas, 200
TGFβ, 33
therapeutic interventions, 229
therapeutic process, 152
therapeutic relationship, 135, 139, 141, 169, 229
therapists, 118, 121, 124, 127, 130, 131
therapy, ix, 39, 58, 70, 78, 82, 85, 90, 92, 95, 111, 119, 120, 123, 124, 126, 128, 129, 131, 133, 134, 136, 137, 138, 142, 143, 144, 145, 146, 150, 151, 169, 170, 174, 189, 201, 214
thiazolidinediones, 38, 40
thinking, 141, 147, 152, 164, 165, 168, 171, 178, 188, 191, 195, 197, 204, 206, 215
third party, 167
threat, 101, 102, 209
threatening, 15
threshold, 40, 54, 61, 116
threshold level, 116
thrombocytopenia, 82, 83
thrombosis, 35
thyroid, viii, 4, 5, 11, 12, 13, 14, 26, 27, 36, 38, 61, 227
thyroid gland, 4, 13, 26
thyrotropin, 27, 56
time series, 78
timing, 58, 62
tissue, viii, 5, 7, 10, 11, 12, 13, 15, 19, 21, 22, 23, 30, 31, 33, 34, 35, 36, 38, 39, 40, 41, 42, 44, 45, 47, 48, 58, 66, 72, 78, 83, 88, 227
tissue plasminogen activator, 58
title, 111, 112, 113, 156, 157, 177
TNF-α, 22, 35, 37, 80
toddlers, 110, 113
tolerance, 22, 23, 35
tonic, 11
torture, 219
total cholesterol, 40
total parenteral nutrition, 89, 92
total plasma, 36
trabecular bone, 55
trace elements, 90
tradition, 212
training, x, 14, 110, 113, 126, 134, 164, 230
traits, 11, 29, 144
trajectory, 54
transcendence, 149, 150, 151, 152, 154, 155, 156, 219
transcript, 6, 9, 45
transcription, 21, 64
transcription factor, 64
transcriptional, 37, 39
transducer, 21
transduction, 26, 34, 64
transfer, 4, 107, 124
transference, 146
transformation, 35, 76, 83
transformations, 123
transforming growth factor, 43
transgenic, 70
transgenic mice, 70
translation, 185, 210, 212
transmission, 4, 115
transparency, 131, 222
transparent, 126, 210
transport, 21, 37
transportation, 31
trauma, 182
trees, 179
trial, 134
tricyclic antidepressants, 80
triggers, 108
triglyceride, 35, 40
triglycerides, 36, 38, 39
triiodothyronine, 12, 26
trimolecular complex, 12
true belief, 190, 191
trust, 136, 193
trusts, 193
trypsin, 80
tryptophan, 8
TSH, 12, 13, 14, 27
tumor, 21, 30, 43, 44, 46
tumor necrosis factor (TNF) , 21, 22, 30, 33, 34, 35, 3743, 44, 46, 80
tumour, 102

turnover, 81
twins, 117, 132
type 1 diabetes, 36, 47
type 2 diabetes, 36, 38, 40, 45, 46, 48
type 2 diabetes mellitus, 36
tyrosine, 26

U

ultrasonography, 69
ultrasound, 54
ultra-thin, 198
undergraduates, viii
undernutrition, 69
United Kingdom, 200
United States, 66, 198
universality, 151
unmasking, 212
urbanization, 118
urbanized, 118
urea, 79
uric acid, 39
urinary, 17, 20, 81
uterus, 54, 60

V

valence, 123
validation, 134
validity, 132
values, vii, 19, 67, 89, 106, 123, 151, 152, 153, 155, 157, 162, 167, 168, 169, 171, 186, 204, 217, 218, 220, 221
variability, 84, 89, 117, 216
variables, 42, 100, 107, 117, 119, 120, 121, 175
variance, 6, 12, 117
variation, 17, 21, 25, 52
variety of domains, 67
vascular disease, 39
vasodilator, 39
vasopressin, 15, 17, 19, 20, 29, 63
vasopressin level, 29
vegetables, 76
vegetarians, 88
ventilation, 79
ventricle, 6, 77
ventricles, 67
ventricular arrhythmia, 78
verbal abuse, 104
vero, 163
very low density lipoprotein, 40
vessels, 83
victims, 165, 198
violence, 109
violent, 153
visible, 197
vision, x, 104, 151, 153, 155, 206, 207, 208, 210, 229, 230
vitamin A, 76
vitamin B1, 82
vitamin B12, 82
vitamin D, 81, 88, 90
vitamin supplementation, 88
vitamins, 88, 90, 92
VLDL, 40
vocabulary, 183, 205
voice, 167
vomiting, 44, 76, 79, 80, 90, 99, 122, 137, 140
vulnerability, 62, 65, 117, 118, 125, 135

W

water, 6, 20, 90, 110
watershed, 204
weakness, 211, 212, 216
web, 166
websites, 166, 196
weight changes, 88
weight gain, 11, 12, 14, 17, 18, 26, 33, 34, 51, 53, 55, 69, 71, 89, 91, 92, 93, 95, 167
weight loss, vii, viii, ix, 9, 17, 18, 21, 26, 28, 31, 32, 34, 40, 48, 51, 55, 56, 61, 68, 81, 89, 92, 117, 136, 137, 167, 168, 173, 188, 190, 227
weight reduction, 40
weight status, 14
wellbeing, 130, 203, 204, 206, 212, 213, 214
Western culture, 164, 198, 204, 212, 217
western models, vii
Western philosophy, 164
Western societies, 198
white matter, 73, 91, 94
wind, 218, 221
winter, 215
wisdom, 207, 210
withdrawal, 52, 62, 131
women, 3, 18, 21, 25, 26, 28, 39, 42, 47, 49, 51, 52, 53, 54, 55, 56, 58, 59, 61, 63, 64, 66, 67, 69, 70, 71, 73, 77, 81, 82, 84, 94, 130, 132, 137, 138, 156, 166, 174, 175, 176, 198, 199, 205, 206, 222
wood, 210
workers, 127, 129, 130
working memory, 67
workload, 79
World Health Organisation, 200
worldview, 182

worry, 100, 117, 139, 143
writing, 176, 191, 197

Y

yield, 175, 189
young adults, 91, 93
young women, 3, 55, 56, 63, 77, 84, 166, 175, 205
younger children, 162

Z

zinc, 88
zygote, 57